D1507679

SCHOOL-AGE PREGNANCY AND PARENTHOOD

Biosocial Dimensions

SCHOOL-AGE PREGNANCY AND PARENTHOOD

Biosocial Dimensions

Edited by

Jane B. Lancaster

Beatrix A. Hamburg

Sponsored by the
Social Science Research Council

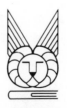

ALDINE
DE GRUYTER
New York

ABOUT THE EDITORS

Jane B. Lancaster is presently Professor of Anthropology, University of
New Mexico and was formerly Professor of Anthropology, University of Oklahoma. Dr. Lancaster chairs the Social Science Research Council's Committee on Biosocial Science Perspectives on
Parenthood and Offspring Development. She has been a major
contributor to various books and journals and is the co-author of
Eve and Adam: The Origins of Sex and the Family.

Beatrix A. Hamburg is Clinical Professor of Psychiatry and Pediatrics,
Mt. Sinai School of Medicine. Dr. Hamburg is a member of the
Institute of Medicine, National Academy of Sciences and the Na-
tional Research Council Commission on Behavioral and Social
Sciences and Education. She is the recipient of the Gallagher
Award for Outstanding Achievement in Adolescent Medicine, the
Distinguished Service Award from the Alcohol, Drug Abuse and
Mental Health Administration, and is editor of *Behavioral and Psy-
chosocial Issues in Diabetes*.

ALDINE DE GRUYTER
Division of Walter de Gruyter, Inc.
200 Saw Mill River Road
Hawthorne, New York 10532

Library of Congress Cataloging in Publication Data

School-age pregnancy and parenthood.

   Includes bibliographies and index.
   1. Pregnancy, Adolescent.   2. Pregnancy, Adolescent
—Social aspects.   I. Lancaster, Jane Beckman, 1935–
II. Hamburg, Beatrix A.   III. Social Science Research
Council (U.S.)
RG556.5.S36   1985   306.8'5   86–1054
ISBN 0-202-30321-7 (lib. bdg.)

Printed in the United States of America
10 9 8 7 6 5 4 3 2

CONTENTS

v

FOREWORD

David A. Hamburg*

The social context in which ancient human biology is embedded is rapidly changing because of the profound transformation that our species has brought about since the industrial revolution. In a moment of evolutionary time, we have drastically changed the world of our ancestors. We have changed our technology, our diet, our activity patterns, the substances of daily use and exposure, patterns of reproductive activity, tension-relief, and human relationships. These changes are laden with new benefits and new risks, and the long-term consequences are little understood. Extreme population growth in much of the world, drastic urbanization with its crowding of strangers beyond any prior experience, environmental damage, resource depletion, the risks of weapons technology, new patterns of disease, and the prolongation of adolescence to a decade or more—all are largely products of changes which have occurred only in the most recent phase of human evolution.

We are all so much a part of the present that it takes a great mental effort to comprehend the time scale of human life on earth. Human ancestors have been separate from the apes for about 5 million years. For nearly all of that five-million year period there were fewer than a million people on earth, all of whom subsisted by hunting and gathering in small, nomadic groups. Agriculture and large, settled populations have existed for less than .005% of those five million years, and our technical world has been present for only .00005% of that time—a tiny interval on the time scale of human evolution. This means that the way we live today is, in many important respects, a novelty for our species.

Insights from the past few decades of careful, systematic, interdisciplinary research help to illuminate the long path by which the human species has arrived in its present predicament. Our endless curiosity about the roots of human nature has been stimulated by unprecedented

*President, Carnegie Corporation of New York.

scientific advances, involving not only a revitalization of traditional lines of inquiry (such as stones and bones), but the contributions of physical, biological, and behavioral sciences over a wide front. There have recently been major discoveries pertinent to human origins in molecular biology, geology, and methods of measuring time. Despite centuries of fascination with monkeys and apes, little was firmly established about the behavior of non-human primates in their natural habitats until the past quarter century. In that period, the study of non-human primates has rapidly developed into a productive area of research that links biological and social sciences. Basic human relationships and primary social groups have deep roots in our evolutionary past. These roots now grow in a soil largely different from that of the past. The old biology is in a new social and technological setting. There are formidable advantages and also profound dislocations in this circumstance.

For reasons of this kind, the editors have devoted a substantial portion of this volume to an evolutionary-historical perspective on adolescent pregnancy: examining adolescence in non-human primates and preindustrial societies, using animal models for precocious pregnancy and parenthood, studying comparative anatomy and biology, and illuminating special circumstances in modern society that affect adolescence.

Adolescence is a time in non-human primates and humans when extensive changes in behavior occur along with drastic changes in physiological and biochemical systems. The timing of puberty is controlled in the brain. Signals from the brain in turn stimulate the secretion of sex hormones. These sex hormones have biochemical influences throughout the organism, including effects on cells and circuits in the brain. Much evidence has accumulated on the coordinated functioning of nervous and endocrine systems in the adaptation of the whole organism to environmental conditions. In this respect, the neuroendocrine coordination of reproduction, especially in females, emerges as one of the most complex regulatory systems of the human organism. It has evolved gradually over millions of years.

A crucial focal point for research in this field has been the structural and functional connection between the hypothalamus and the pituitary. Several decades ago, it was known that there were no connecting nerves between the brain and the anterior pituitary; they were therefore believed to be functionally unrelated. An important advance came with discovery of a distinctively rich network of blood vessels that link the hypothalamus at the base of the brain with the pituitary gland located immediately beneath it. These blood vessels carry chemical signals from brain to pituitary and to the gonads in both sexes (as well as the adrenals and thyroid). Over years of difficult inquiry, the controlling substances in the brain were isolated, purified, and characterized.

These hypothalmic hormones play a central role in coordination of the body. They provide a way in which the molecular and cellular components of the body can function as a whole in adapting to changes in the life cycle and in environmental conditions. Thus, the brain and endocrine system are a functional unit in adaptation.

The cells and circuits of the brain involved in the secretion of the hypothalamic hormone that regulates the reproductive system (GnRH) are mediated chemically in various ways. Biogenic amines, opiate-like peptides, and sex steroids all have roles to play. Their interaction is complex and is not yet fully elucidated. The cells in the pituitary that respond to this hypothalamic hormone secrete two hormones (LH and FSH) in pulses and which, in turn, bring about the far-reaching effects of the sex steroids when these are secreted by the ovary and testis (and to some extent by the adrenal as well).

The basic machinery of these neuroendocrine coordinations of puberty is not only found widely among the primates but is in essence common to mammalian species. This is not to say that the machinery is identical across these millions of years of evolution. There are enough differences between rhesus monkeys, chimpanzees, and humans to be of practical significance in research on contraception; but the core of the machinery is shared by a great variety of species over a very long time in evolution. The research that has clarified this ancient biological system has made puberty one of the frontiers of the neurosciences. It is now, as evidenced by this volume, becoming a frontier of the behavioral and social sciences as well.

Clearly, the operation of this machinery is linked to environmental influence and social context. A major thrust of the present volume is the drastic change in social context of puberty onset and, indeed, of adolescence altogether. These social changes not only affect the timing of puberty but the whole nature of the adolescent experience—not least the incidence and consequences of adolescent pregnancy.

In pre-modern times, preparation for adult roles typically extended over much of childhood. Children had abundant opportunity for directly observing their parents and other adults performing the same adult roles that they would also adopt when the changes of puberty endowed them with adult physique and capabilities. In today's highly technological and rapidly changing world, such learning opportunities are greatly diminished. What is the adult world anyway? Is television the main window on adult roles?

The lengthy period of human adolescence is an evolutionary novelty. We now have two largely non-overlapping, critical periods in the transition from childhood to adulthood. At the beginning of adolescence there is a change in biological status and at the end of adolescence a change in psychosocial status. Not only does adolescence start earlier than it used to, but it ends later. Individuals with biological maturity are being required to remain in childlike roles, or in any case, non-adult status for a decade or more. Indeed the end of adolescence tends to be ambiguous. When is a person fully adult in modern circumstances? How does the modern adolescent adapt to the lengthy transition?

This volume does much to clarify the special and distinctive problems of *early* adolescence in modern societies. By and large, it is not until about the end of the teen years that the various systems of the brain reach a fully adult state of development in biological terms—let alone social maturity. So, in the 10–15 age range, psychosocial risk is intensified by relative immaturity in knowledge, social experience, and cognitive development. Yet this is a time of heavy exposure not only to sexuality but to alcohol and other drugs, smoking, and temptation to a variety of health-damaging behaviors. The biological, cognitive, psychological, and social differences between the 13 year old and the 19 year old are so great that it is barely meaningful to subsume both under the label "teenage pregnancy."

A great deal of research converges on the negative outcomes of *early* adolescent pregnancy, some of it occurring even before the teen years. Such pregnancies are at high risk for maternal toxemia, low birth weight infants, and a variety of adverse outcomes for mother and child. In the United States, the women at highest risk are very young, black, have a low gynecologic age, are marginally nourished, are from a low socioeconomic status, and do not seek prenatal care. This does not mean that all outcomes are necessarily undesirable. The present volume makes many useful distinctions, including some conditions under which adolescent pregnancy may turn out favorably. But these differentiations also highlight high-risk groups, where preventive intervention deserves utmost consideration.

Viewing the situation of contemporary adolescents in an evolutionary-historical perspective illuminates an important set of recent changes that intensify the problems of adolescent pregnancy.

Through most of human history, adolescent childbearing was common—within 4 years of menarche while the mother was in her late teens. But in those societies the community provided relatively predictable networks of social support and cultural guidance for the young parents. For such adolescents in preindustrial societies to set up a household apart from either family was rare. Even more rare was the single-parent family and still more rare was a socially isolated very young mother largely lacking any effective network of social support.

A perplexing human novelty is the current large number of school-age parents without support of cultural institutions, so there is little experience by which adaptive strategies can be assessed. Social isolation and other socioeconomic stresses put both early adolescent mothers and fathers at very high risk in our society. Studies show that the adolescent father appears to be just as much at risk as the school-age mother in modern society. He experiences negative trajectory for his life course similar to that shown in studies of adolescent mothers—low educational and employment opportunities, poverty, early divorce, and frequent changes of marital partner.

Altogether, this is an exceptionally informative volume. The Social Science Research Council has performed a valuable service by bringing together excellent scholars over a wide range of disciplines. Taken together, they bring to bear converging biological, psychological, and social perspectives that illuminate the world-wide epidemic of adolescent pregnancy and its distinctively modern associated problems. The old biology of the mammalian–primate–human organism is set in a very new social context. We have not yet learned how to adapt. The insights provided here, and the specific challenges to thoughtful people of good will, give us new light on paths to adaptation.

ACKNOWLEDGMENTS

All aspects of the program of the Committee on Biosocial Perspectives on Parent Behavior and Offspring Development which have focused on school-age pregnancy and parenthood have been funded by the William T. Grant Foundation (New York). The committee and the Council are very appreciative of the support provided by the Foundation, and wish particularly to thank Dr. Robert Haggerty, President of the Foundation, for his deep interest and intellectual support. A previous grant to the Council from the National Institute of Child Health and Human Development provided funding for a series of planning workshops that led to the formation of the committee. The editors of the volume wish also to thank the Social Science Research Council for its support of the committee.

Among the early activities relating to the topic, School-Age Pregnancy and Parenthood, the committee held a conference at the Belmont Conference Center, Elkridge, Maryland in May of 1982. The committee wishes also to express its appreciation to the staff of the Belmont Center.

During the several years of planning and preparation following this conference, that have resulted in the present volume, the editors were assisted by the members of the committee and the staff of the Social Science Research Council. A particular expression of appreciation is due Terry Ciatto at the SSRC who has handled all of the daily aspects of typing, mailing, distributing proofs, telephoning authors, and generally keeping the volume progressing. The management and staff at Aldine de Gruyter were of invaluable assistance throughout all phases of production of the volume.

LIST OF CONTRIBUTORS

Jeanne Altmann
Allee Lab of Animal Behavior
University of Chicago
Department of Biology
Chicago, Illinois 60637

Victoria K. Burbank
Department of Anthropology
Harvard University
Cambridge, Massachusetts 02139

Catherine S. Chilman
School of Social Welfare
University of Wisconsin
Milwaukee, Wisconsin 53201

Lisa Crockett
Individual and Family Studies
College of Human Development
Pennsylvania State University
University Park, Pennsylvania 16802

Mercedes de Cubas
Mailman Center for Child
Development
University of Florida Medical Center
Miami, Florida 33101

Arthur B. Elster
Department of Pediatrics
University of Utah Medical Center
Salt Lake City, Utah 84132

Phyllis B. Eveleth
Epidemiology and Disease Control
Study Section I
Division of Research Grants
National Institute of Health
Bethesda, Maryland 20205

Tiffany Field
Mailman Center for Child
Development
University of Florida Medical School
Miami, Florida 33101

Frank F. Furstenberg, Jr.
Department of Sociology
University of Pennsylvania
Philadelphia, Pennsylvania 19104

Stanley M. Garn
Center for Human Growth and
Development
University of Michigan
Ann Arbor, Michigan 48109

Richard J. Gelles
Department of Sociology and
Anthropology
University of Rhode Island
Kingston, Rhode Island 02881

Beatrix A. Hamburg
Mt. Sinai School of Medicine
Child and Adolescent Psychiatry
New York, New York 10029

David Hamburg
Carnegie Corporation of New York
New York, New York 10022

Roberta Herceg-Baron
Department of Sociology
University of Pennsylvania
Philadelphia, Pennsylvania 19104

Lorraine V. Klerman
Division of Health Services
Department of Epidemiology and
Public Health
Yale University
New Haven, Connecticut 06510

Melvin Konner
Departments of Anthropology and
Psychiatry
Yerkes Regional Primate Center
Emory University
Atlanta, Georgia 30322

Jane B. Lancaster
Department of Anthropology
University of New Mexico
Albuquerque, New Mexico 87131

Michael E. Lamb
Department of Psychology
University of Utah
Salt Late City, Utah 84132

Shelly D. Pesick
Center for Human Growth and
Development
University of Michigan
Ann Arbor, Michigan 48109

Anne C. Petersen
Individual and Family Studies
College of Human Development
Pennsylvania State University
University Park, Pennsylvania 16802

Audrey S. Petzold
Center for Human Growth and
Development
University of Michigan
Ann Arbor, Michigan 48109

Mitchell S. Ratner
Department of Anthropology
Harvard University
Cambridge, Massachusetts 02138

Edward O. Reiter
Bay State Medical Center
Department of Pediatrics
Springfield, Massachusetts 01107

Judy Shea
Department of Sociology
University of Pennsylvania
Philadelphia, Pennsylvania 19104

Marjorie Shostak
Departments of Anthropology and
Psychiatry
Emory University
Atlanta, Georgia 30322

Sherilyn Stoller
Mailman Center for Child
Development
University of Florida Medical Center
Miami, Florida 33101

Charles M. Super
Department of Nutrition
Harvard School of Public Health
Boston, Massachusetts 02115

Maris A. Vinovskis
Department of History
University of Michigan
Ann Arbor, Michigan 48104

David Webb
Department of Sociology
University of Pennsylvania
Philadelphia, Pennsylvania 19104

John W. M. Whiting
Department of Anthropology
Harvard University
Cambridge, Massachusetts 02138

Susan Widmayer
Mailman Center for Child
Development
University of Florida Medical Center
Miami, Florida 33101

Carol M. Worthman
Laboratory of Human Reproduction
and Reproductive Biology
Harvard Medical School
Boston, Massachusetts 02115

FOUNDATIONS OF HUMAN BEHAVIOR

An Aldine de Gruyter Series of Texts and Monographs

Edited by
Sarah Blaffer Hrdy, *University of California, Davis*
Melvin Konner, *Emory University*
Richard W. Wrangham, *University of Michigan*

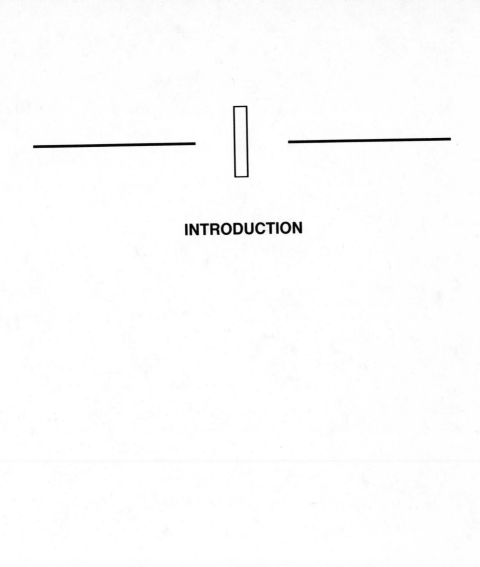

INTRODUCTION

1

THE BIOSOCIAL DIMENSIONS OF SCHOOL-AGE PREGNANCY AND PARENTHOOD: AN INTRODUCTION

Jane B. Lancaster
Beatrix A. Hamburg

THE BIOSOCIAL PERSPECTIVE

This volume is the first of a series of volumes sponsored by the Social Science Research Council Committee on Biosocial Perspectives on Parent Behavior and Offspring Development. The Committee is a multidisciplinary group of biological, behavioral, and social scientists who seek to promote exchange of concepts, methods, and data across disciplines. The goals of the Committee's program are: to develop conceptualizations of social phenomena relying on biosocial science; to explore the interface between biological and social phenomena; and to advance our understanding of human social behavior.

Biosocial science is particularly relevant to research on human family systems and parenting behavior because the family is the universal social institution within which the care of children has been based and where cultural traditions, beliefs, and values have been transmitted to the young as the individuals fulfill their biological potential for reproduction, growth, and development. The biosocial perspective takes into account the biological substrate and the social environment as determinants of patterns of behavior and pinpoints areas in which contemporary human parental behavior exhibits continuities with, and departures from, patterns evident throughout human history. Unless discontinuities in family behaviors and their overall costs and benefits are examined, we are not in a position to assess them objectively in comparison with modern circumstances. The biosocial perspective, therefore, extends our understanding of parental behavior by sensitizing us to the variety of patterns among current practices as well as by highlighting the full range of parent–child patterns that have been represented in the evolutionary or historical past. Both the spectrum of options and the basis for making judgments about these options are expanded.

The term biosocial was selected to emphasize the functional unity of both biological and socioenvironmental factors. The mutual influences of these factors are more than additive; indeed, they are interrelated through reciprocal influences that can significantly alter the characteristics of each other. The potential for change and variation in biological attributes is less well understood than is the potential for human learning and behavior change. There has been a tendency to perceive biological behaviors as being unlearned, independent of the environment and not readily susceptible to change. There also has been an expectation that there will be uniformity of response to a specific stimulus. For human beings, prior experience, motivation, and context will influence biological responses to all kinds of stimuli whether they be pathogenic bacteria or social interactions. For example, this biosocial perspective is now beginning to be applied to physical health. Behavioral medicine is an emerging area of research and clinical practice (Hamburg *et al.*, 1982). The recognition of the continuous, mutual, and inseparable interaction between biology and social environment is one of the two critical foundations of the biosocial perspective. This is a theme that recurs throughout the chapters of this volume. Armed with a commitment to a biosocial science perspective, 32 scientists from the disciplines of anthropology, sociology, history, psychiatry, developmental psychology, social work, pediatrics, primatology, human evolution, and public health contributed chapters to this volume discussing their own research and the knowledge of their respective disciplines about school-age pregnancy and parenthood.

THE HUMAN RANGE OF REACTION

The second foundation of the biosocial perspective is a commitment to understand how biosocial phenomena fit into the genetically determined "range of reaction" for human beings. The genetic inheritance (*genotype*) of each individual sets a range for defining the potential expression of biological and behavioral attributes. Environmental factors weigh very heavily in determining the actual expression that is attained—*phenotype*. For example, the genetic programming for such phenotypic characters as stature and body size includes a range of reaction in accordance with both caloric and protein intake during childhood. Chronic food stress or chronic overfeeding produce very different adult phenotypes from the same genetic programming. This range of reaction in the expression of genotype has been set by the variations in food abundance regularly experienced by human populations in time past. In assessing the genetic components of human behavior, differentiation must be made between the individual and a population. For populations, most biological attributes occur in a normal distribution curve. The "reaction range" of the human species refers to the spectrum of biological and behavioral expressions of genetic heritage that occur in the normal, expectable social and physical environment of a population. The normal, expectable environment too is defined not by the present but by the past evolutionary and historical experience of the species. Recognizing the normal, expectable environment from our human heritage and defining the resultant range of reaction, allows us to ask questions as to whether a phenomenon is really new and outside past experience or if it is simply one aspect of the expected variability of expression. In this volume, Section IV *(Comparative Dimensions: Species, History and Culture)* and Section V *(The Modern World)* comprise a collection of chapters that, taken together, incisively address the issue of whether adolescent pregnancy and parenthood is a phenomenon about which our species has accumulated both biological and cultural wisdom or whether we are being confronted with challenges about which we have no past experience.

THE CONTEMPORARY PROBLEM

There is no question that contemporary school-age pregnancy and parenthood is a very visible phenomenon that is viewed with alarm and has been described as a national epidemic (Guttmacher Institute, 1976). In response to national concern, in 1978 Congress passed the Adolescent Health Services and Pregnancy Prevention and Care Act. There was particular concern about the trend toward increasing numbers of adolescents 16 years and younger who become pregnant, carry the pregnancy to term and choose to rear their infants. After fifteen years of societal concern and substantial public and private support for research and service programs, progress has not been made. A fresh look with new perspectives on the problem is indicated.

In prior research, basic questions about the meaning of these disturbing behaviors have not been posed. Is teenage pregnancy really an epidemic? As Vinovskis (1981) noted, except for the very youngest adolescents, contraception and abortion have lowered the birthrates for adolescents since 1970 to levels that are somewhat lower than those of the 1920s or the 1950s. However, the rates of adolescent childbearing outside of marriage has shown steep increases. For adolescents 17 years and younger the number of out-of-wedlock births in 1960 was 48,300; it rose to 127,197 by 1981, the year for which the latest figures are available (Baldwin, 1984). Perhaps what is really new and outside the human range of reaction is school-age parenthood without support of cultural institutions as is the case of a single mother or a school-age mother married to a school-age father. A host of questions are raised. Have other ethnic groups or other cultures, at present or in times past, had experience with these problems? If so, what are the contextual similarities and differences? How can the adaptive strategies be assessed? Do isolation and social and economic stresses put adolescent mothers at very high risk in our society? How much are the unfavorable outcomes of pregnancy and parenthood related to the immaturity of the young mother as the primary factor? How much as a contributing factor? What have we learned from the interventions that have been tried? This volume does not answer but begins to address these important questions.

ETHNIC AND HISTORIC EXPERIENCE

The cross-cultural and historical records indicate that, although parenthood by young adolescent girls was relatively rare, when it did occur it was in a very different social context (Konner and Shostak; Vinovskis; Whiting, Burbank and Ratner, this volume). First, the young mother was likely to be married since pregnancy tended to function as a timer of marriage. Second, she was unlikely to find herself in an isolated household without a network of supportive and caring relatives and neighbors. Furthermore, she was highly unlikely to establish a household with a young adolescent boy but, instead, to have an adult, socially mature husband. The phenomenon of a school-age boy as social father and head of household is virtually unheard of in other cultures. In modern society the adolescent father appears to be just as much at risk as the school-age mother (Elster and Lamb, this volume). He experiences the same negative trajectory for his life course in terms of diminished educational and employment opportunities, poverty, early divorce, and frequent changes of marital partner. School-age fatherhood is a neglected area of research. Very little is known about the forces which attract or push young adolescent boys into fatherhood and household roles.

Several of the chapters in this volume discuss issues of ethnic differences. Some ethnic groups in our society have had a longer experience with school-age pregnancy than others. Rates of adolescent sexuality, pregnancy, and parenthood traditionally have been very much higher among blacks than other ethnic groups in the United States. While the levels of these behaviors continue to be highest among blacks, the trends since 1970 have been for the white rates to rise and for the black rates to be stable for the younger adolescents and declining among the oldest black adolescents. In this volume, B. Hamburg calls attention to an important subgroup of urban, poor, black adolescents who are choosing early childbearing as an alternate life course that promotes their social and cultural survival and enhances personal development. The prevailing trend among adolescent and young adult whites in the mainstream of society is to complete schooling, enter the work force promptly, and to delay childbearing until the late twenties or even the early thirties when time out for pregnancy and childbearing is taken. For blacks, however, adolescence and early adulthood is a time of the life cycle when unemployment is very high and the lack of job opportunities is predictable. Some black adolescents are able to benefit from a subcultural institutionalization of the extended family and informal networks of support. They rely on their mothers, neighbors, and relatives for economic aid and child care assistance in order to complete education and obtain job training during the adolescent years. These young, unmarried mothers and their children have good outcomes and their life options are not diminished. More can be learned about the factors that differentiate these successful, young black adolescents from those who have dismal outcomes. In general, research into coping competence, good outcomes, and successful negotiation of adolescent parenthood across all ethnic groups is a promising and neglected line of enquiry. Prior to 1976 systematic research on the phenomenon of school-age pregnancy was virtually nonexistent. Although the amount of research and programmatic attention to the problem has increased dramatically in recent years, it has been of rather limited scope, focusing on perinatal health outcomes for mother and child and long-term economic consequences for the "family". These are important issues and much has been learned. Klerman, in this volume, reviews the educational, employment, and social consequences of adolescent parenthood as represented in existing research.

Although hispanic groups are the fastest growing population in the United States, there has been little research attention to their pregnancy and fertility behavior or to ethnographic descriptions of their lives as subcultures in the United States. Field, et al. report, in this volume, some pioneering research that makes systematic comparisons between blacks and hispanics. It is generally accepted that cognitive and language development of infants and children is highly correlated with patterns of mother-child interaction. There is an extensive literature on black–white comparisons that show major differences. Little systematic data exists on child rearing attitudes or parenting styles among hispanics. This research details ethnic differences in patterns of verbal interaction. These studies underscore some important issues of methodology. Much of the black-white comparison literature confounds ethnicity and socioeconomic class. Middle class, affluent whites were often compared with lower-class, poor blacks. In the studies reported here,

the blacks and hispanics were matched for socioeconomic status. Differences were found between the ethnic groups. Initial assessment of
the children revealed differences in outcomes between ethnic groups.
However, these differences did not persist on long-term follow-up. These
studies report interesting data and the authors provide some guidelines
for rigorous methodology in pursuing research on ethnic differences.

METHODOLOGICAL ISSUES

The fact that adolescent pregnancy and parenthood has been identified chiefly as a major social problem in need of urgent attention has
shaped the prior research agenda. There has been emphasis on survey
studies of prevalence and on reports of interventions that often represent
social inventions rather than rigorous research designs. These studies
have been atheoretical and outside of the mainstream of research in
the biomedical or behavioral science disciplines. As a result, most of
those scientists failed to see the relationship of these issues to the mainstream of their disciplinary concerns or to be attracted to these issues
as areas of scientific interest.

Social problems are, by definition, behaviors that are viewed as
violating the social norms and are seen as negative. In the absence
of a broad knowledge base from relevant disciplines, conventional
wisdom and unsubstantiated reports have influenced scientific thinking.
For example, as Gelles (this volume) notes, the belief that teenage
mothers have a high risk of child abuse rests on data from reports by
hospitals and social agencies that already subscribe to that conviction,
making them much more likely to report a young mother with an injured
child as an abuser. Gelles discusses more comprehensive studies on
child abuse suggesting the young mothers may be no more likely to
abuse than mature mothers but that women who begin their reproductive careers as school-age mothers are more likely to become abusers of later children born after the mother is fully adult. Such data
suggest that school-age mothers may find themselves on a developmental trajectory that leads them to poor maternal behavior years later.
Furthermore, in spite of the fact that most samples report that children
are abused by fathers as much as by mothers, the question of school-
age status for the father is not regularly reported in standard child
abuse statistics as it is for the mother.

The failure to study both males and females has been a general
issue for adolescent research. With a few notable exceptions, the traditional adolescent literature is that males predominate as research
subjects. Adolescent pregnancy and parenthood is one of the few exceptions and represents an almost exclusively female emphasis. As
noted by B. Hamburg it is important to study both sexes and try to

understand the demonstrable convergences and contrasts in their responses.

Even where systematic research has been carried out, too often scientists have failed to relate their work to significant existing bodies of knowledge outside their own field. This has rendered scientists blind to sampling errors. For example, much of the otherwise excellent research on adolescent fertility and demographics of adolescent pregnancy is flawed because inappropriate age categories have been studied. Much useful data has been lost by pooling data for all adolescents 19 years of age and under without regard for the known developmental distinctiveness of the biosocial stages of early, middle, and late adolescence (B. Hamburg, this volume). The psychosocial and legal implications of age 18 and older as compared to school-age adolescents has also been ignored.

In a similar vein, the hazards of using chronologic instead of biologic age when studying pubertal and/or maturational effects has not been understood because of ignorance of the variations in normal biological development of adolescents. Garn, Pesick, and Petzold (this volume) suggest that many of the assumptions about the negative sequellae of pregnancy in school-age girls are founded on their presumed reproductive immaturity. Garn et al. demonstrate that school-age girls who get pregnant are taller and fatter than their peers because they have matured earlier. Ultimately, however, they are shorter than the mean for adult women because of their earlier cessation of growth. Under conditions of adequate nutrition, their negative sequellae regarding fetal and infant development and child birth are not different from those of mature women of the same, small body size. The biology of adolescents, except perhaps for the very youngest of girls, may not be universally negative for reproduction and many negative outcomes may come from what Super (this volume) refers to as "negative associated circumstances" such as stress from lack of social support, loss of educational and employment opportunities, and unhealthy teenage life styles. In any case the interactions of biological age, social age, and environmental impact is a fruitful area for further enquiry.

Perhaps the most important theme running through many chapters in this volume is a recognition that further research and successful interventions will not be formulated until unitary concepts such as "The Pregnant Teenager" and "The Adolescent Mother" are modified. The importance of defining the biosocial context in which early reproduction occurs is emphasized by many authors in the volume including: Gelles, B. Hamburg, Field et al., Klerman, Vinovskis, and Super.

The tradition of viewing adolescent pregnancy and parenthood as a social problem has fostered the tendency to search for negative outcomes and to accept information more readily that appears to confirm poor biological and social outcomes. Much of this data comes from clinicians and agencies that serve troubled adolescents. In addition, medical and psychiatric research has a long tradition of emphasis on studying pathology. A number of the chapters (Garn *et al.*; Gelles, B. Hamburg, and Super, this volume) discuss the various ways in which this bias toward pathology has impeded scientific progress. It is encouraging that across several behavioral science disciplines there is active research related to stress and coping responses to a range of challenges across the life span in which serious attention is being paid to studying good outcomes under conditions of adversity and seeking to understand the personal and socioenvironmental forces that can explain these good outcomes. This body of work has immediate relevance for studies of adolescent pregnancy and parenthood.

DEFINING THE NORMATIVE

A substantial portion of this volume is devoted to papers attempting to map the human range of reaction from biosocial perspectives: using animal models for precocious pregnancy and parenthood (Altmann), comparative anatomy and biology (Lancaster, Reiter), the cross-cultural and historical record (Eveleth; Konner and Shostak; Whiting, Burbank and Ratner; Vinovskis), and special circumstances in modern society (Elster and Lamb). Altmann and Lancaster present data that suggest that in spite of the fact that nonhuman primate females continue growth during their first pregnancy and lactation, except under situations of very restricted food supply, their higher rate of fetal and infant loss appears to come mainly from their social and psychological inexperience rather than a biological competition between mother and offspring for nutritional resources.

Papers by Eveleth, Lancaster, and Reiter point toward an evolved growth program for human females which in time past and in nonwestern societies established a temporal separation between the pubertal development of secondary sex characteristics and the onset of sexual behavior, resulting in a much later assumption of fertility and parenthood. In those programs, an intervening time period of perhaps two years passed in the slow accumulation of body fat which represents the stored energy reserves required to support a pregnancy and lactation. Modern improvements in diet and health lowered the age of reproductive maturation to what is probably the earliest biological limit based on data reporting the secular trend in age of menarche. The age of menarche has dropped 3 months per decade over the past 150 years. Menarche now occurs at a mean age of 12.8 years for girls in the United States as compared to about age 17 in the early 1800s. Perhaps even more significant than the earlier onset of both menarche and fertility may be a collapsing of the biological steps and social controls that prolonged the interval between puberty and parenthood.

At the same time that biology has hastened the onset of reproductive maturation in modern society, culture has delayed the onset of social maturity so that the end result is an adolescence greatly expanded at both its ends, now constituting a major period of the life cycle—equal in length to childhood. In spite of the fact that adolescence has expanded to as long as 10 years, society has found few meaningful activities for this period besides schooling. It would appear that the secular trend of early maturation is only a necessary precondition for the increase in school-age reproduction and the social changes dating from the 1960s were more significant factors. This would explain why, although the secular trend toward earlier menarche had levelled off by 1947 in the United States, it was not until major social changes such as the new roles for women, sexual permissiveness, blocked aspirations of youth, high divorce rates and the phenomenon of working mothers, both single and married, beginning in the 1960s, that we find a precipitous rise in school-age parenthood (Chilman, Eveleth, this volume).

The contributions by Worthman and by Peterson and Crockett focus on the stresses inherent in adolescent development even under the best of circumstances. Passage through puberty involves the maturation of numerous biological and behavioral systems including growth of the body and sex organs, development of secondary sex characteristics, maturation of the endocrine system, and intellectual, social, and psychological development. It appears that developmental asynchrony is a normative experience for adolescents and that it is not until the age of 18 to 19 that the various systems of the body and brain all appear to reach an adult state of development. For this reason, younger adolescents, even if they are years past menarche, may be at psychosocial risk because of their relative immaturity in terms of knowledge, social experience, and cognitive development.

The lack of communication between parents and their adolescents about matters of sexuality, pregnancy, and parenthood has persisted despite the societal change toward more openness about sex. There has been a popular but untested belief among many policymakers and practitioners that adolescent sexual and contraceptive behaviors would be effectively modified if parents were more actively involved with their adolescents in discussions and decision making concerning these matters. Furstenberg and colleagues in this volume report their systematic studies of the validity of these assumptions. Their results reveal that parental involvement has minimal, if any, influence on the effective use of birth control. Siblings and peers are found to have the major influence. This research raises issues about ways in which to help parents be more informed and effective communicators with their adolescents and points out the need for a broader, more comprehensive strategy for educating adolescents. These might include creative use of the mass media and more peer-mediated, school-based programs.

CONCLUSION

The biosocial perspective rests on a critical commitment to recognize the continuous, mutual, and inseparable interaction between biology and social behavior. To study aspects of a problem from conceptualizations which recognize the importance of only one of these factors or which set biology and social behavior in causal competition is useless. It is futile to study human behavioral systems involved with reproduction and parenthood without integration of all the significant levels of causation. To paraphrase Tinbergen (1963), an explanation of why individuals behave in a certain way involves addressing any or all of four equally legitimate types of "why" questions: questions about ultimate function (survival and reproductive value), questions about causation (internal and external proximate factors), questions about ontogenetic development (personal and social history), and questions about evolutionary history (genetics and phylogeny).

Exploring the range of reaction for adolescent pregnancy and parenthood for the human species and the complex interactions of biology and behavior helps one to recognize that many, but not all, aspects of these phenomena are novel. In contemporary industrial societies, both biological and cultural factors have interacted to establish the widest separation between biological and social maturation known in human history. Furthermore, the social context in which the adolescent mother finds herself is entirely new. In time past, the stresses and problems of adolescent motherhood, if they should occur, were handled by a variety of established cultural responses ranging from marriage to a mature husband, infant adoption by relatives or strangers, to infanticide or child abandonment. These culturally defined responses did not include the establishment of a household headed by either a single, school-age mother or by adolescent parents. Dramatic improvements in human diet and health have produced a large pool of reproductively mature adolescents at risk for pregnancy in a contemporary climate of sexual permissiveness. At the same time, society has minimized social and economic supports for a predictable outcome—adolescent parenthood. In the modern world there are, instead, increased demands for training and education before the assumption of adult roles.

REFERENCES

Alan Guttmacher Institute. *Eleven million teenagers: A national epidemic.* New York: Planned Parenthood, 1976.

Baldwin, W. *Adolescent childbearing today and tomorrow.* Statement to U.S. Senate Human Resources Committee, Washington, D.C., National Institute of Child Health and Human Development, 1984.

Hamburg, D.A., Elliott, G.R., and Parron, D.L. *Health and behavior: Frontiers of research in biobehavioral sciences.* Washington, D.C.: National Academy of Sciences, 1982.

Tinbergen, N. On aims and method of ethology. *Zeitschrift für Tierpsychologie,* 1963, *20,* 410-433.

Vinovskis, M.A. An "epidemic" of adolescent pregnancy? Some historical considerations. *Journal of Family History,* 1981, *6,* 205–230.

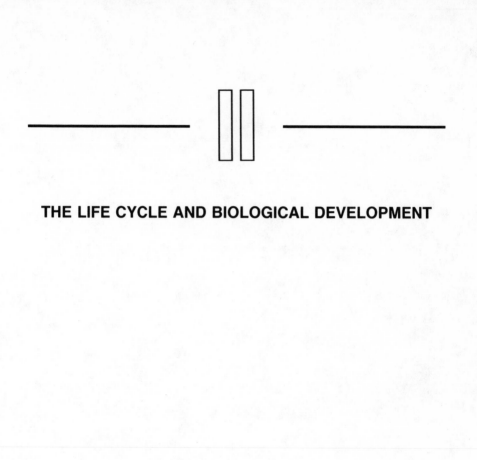

THE LIFE CYCLE AND BIOLOGICAL DEVELOPMENT

2

HUMAN ADOLESCENCE AND REPRODUCTION: AN EVOLUTIONARY PERSPECTIVE

Jane B. Lancaster

When the life cycle of the human female is viewed from the perspective of parenthood, its major features clearly support a uniquely human pattern of high levels of long-term parental investment and the dependency of multiple young of differing ages. For a variety of reasons, most modern cultures present poor models for the female life cycle during most of human history because of their wide range of variation in women's activities, health, nutrition, numbers of children born and reared, and the use of artificial techniques to alter fertility. A real understanding of the evolutionary pressures lying behind women's reproductive biology must currently start with a reconstruction of how it unfolds in the hunting-gathering life style in which it evolved: a life style representing fully 99% of human history. Such a model, based on data drawn from the few remaining hunter-gatherers of today, is fraught with distortions and confounds but, nevertheless, has already provided us with some important insights into major evolutionary novelties in the reproductive lives of modern women. Short (1976), relying heavily on Howell's (1979) careful work on !Kung hunter-gatherer demography, sketches the most striking features of women's biological legacy from the hunter-gatherer era. They include a long period of adolescent subfertility following menarche, late age for first birth, a pattern of nearly continuous nursing during the day, many years of lactation, low frequency of menstrual cycling during the life course, and early menopause. Figure 2.1 illustrates the contrasting patterns of reproductive life found in hunter-gatherer and modern women. Whereas a hunter-gatherer woman can expect nearly 15 years of lactational

17

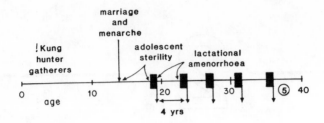

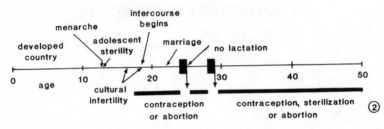

FIGURE 2.1. Changing patterns of human fertility. !Kung hunter-gatherers have a relatively late menarche and adolescent subfertility defers the birth of the first child until age 19. Lactational amenorrhea keeps births 4 years apart. Early menopause results in a completed family size of about 5 children, only 2 to 3 of which will survive into adulthood.

In developed countries menarche occurs at 12 to 13, cultural infertility breaks down in the late teens, and intercourse before marriage requires the use of contraception or abortion. Lactation is so short that birth spacing is dependent on contraception. If the desired family size is 2, contraception, sterilization, or abortion are necessary for a further 20 years. The result of this imposed sterility is a ninefold increase in the number of menstrual cycles (after Short 1976:16).

amenorrhea and just under 4 years each of pregnancy and menstrual cycling, the modern woman experiencing two pregnancies with little or no breast feeding is likely to spend over 35 years in menstrual cycling—a ninefold increase. The generality of this worldwide shift from lactation amenorrhea to menstrual cycling has been confirmed in a recent review of data from preindustrial and industrial societies (Harrell, 1981).

A basic human pattern emerges from such a perspective which emphasizes low fertility and extremely restrained reproduction based on the postponed development of fertility in the life cycle, an extremely high rate of embryonic mortality, and long lactational amenorrhea

(Short 1976, 1979b) supplemented by various cultural practices such as taboos on intercourse during lactation, infanticide, and birth control. In spite of what would seem to be an impressive array of biological and behavioral adaptations leading to late and low rates of fertility, the past 150 years has witnessed a period of radical population growth that appears to be associated with an increasingly earlier entrance into reproduction in the life cycle. Clearly, the presence of such evolutionary novelties in the modern human pattern of reproduction are important to provide insight into investigating the mechanisms involved and the search for possible remedies.

Following Short's lead, it is possible to gain major insights into the biology and behavior of modern adolescents by comparison with closely related species. Adolescence is a critical and expensive feature of the life cycle for any animal. Since its length postpones the adult phase of the life cycle but may also provide critical learning about the social and ecological setting of adult experience before undertaking reproduction, its course and duration must be shaped by conflicting evolutionary forces of intense measure. A cross-species perspective suggests that adolescence in the human species has its own unique set of characteristics—some of which are shared with our closest living relatives, the great apes, and others which may be found only in humans. Using an evolutionary and cross-species, comparative perspective, the remainder of this chapter will explore these major features of human adolescence: the sequencing of human pubertal events, the low fertility once characteristic of adolescence, the relationship between body fat and fertility, and the relationship between pregnancy and lactation to the growth of the human brain. The goals of such an exploration include an alerting function in recognizing evolutionary novelties, the identification of appropriate animal models for research into mechanism, and the development of a general appreciation of the adaptive features of human biology and behavior shaped by millions of years of evolution.

THE SEQUENCING OF PUBERTAL EVENTS: A COMPARATIVE PERSPECTIVE

Short (1976) reviews the milestones in human pubertal events and notes the interesting fact that boys and girls have very different programs (Fig. 2.2). For girls, the first external sign of puberty is the development of the breast bud. This is an odd and noteworthy feature of human development and one that is likely to go unnoticed without comparative mammalian data. The typical primate female will not begin to develop breasts until the later stages of pregnancy. The breasts of the human female are made conspicuous and stable with deposits

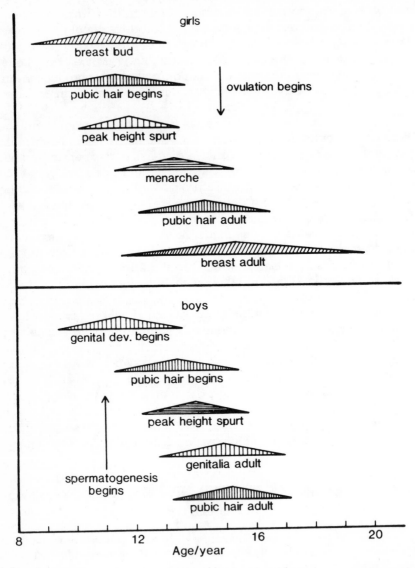

FIGURE 2.2. The sequence of pubertal events in boys and girls indicating a
major contrast in the timing of fertility compared to other growth
events (From Short 1976:7).

of fat, in contrast to other primates whose breasts experience an increase in glandular tissue that resorbs again after weaning if another pregnancy does not ensue. The deposition of fat during human adolescence on the breasts and buttocks is a unique feature of human sexual dimorphism that constitutes a continuous advertisement of an ability to lactate rather than a cyclic fertility advertised by estrous swelling, as do so many other higher primates (Lancaster, 1984; J.B. Lancaster and C.S. Lancaster, 1982).

It is also worth noting that menarche is a relatively late event in the sequence of human pubertal changes, but that it still usually precedes the establishment of regular patterns of ovulation by several years. Menarche itself is preceded by most of the essential features of physical development indicating adult status: the adolescent growth spurt, the attainment of nearly adult values for weight and stature, and the growth of breasts and pubic hair. It is interesting that one of the most crucial features of reproductive success for women, adult capacity of the pelvic inlet and birth canal, is not attained until the very end of the sequence of pubertal events, years after menarche. Even among well-nourished, middle-class girls in a modern sample whose menarche was 12 to 13 years, adult pelvic dimensions were not attained until ages 17 to 18 (Moerman, 1982). The adolescent growth spurt which precedes menarche does not involve the growth of the female pelvis which, if anything, continues its unique, slow trajectory for several years after adult stature is reached. This late attainment of adult pelvic capacity gives indirect evidence for a very recent historical separation by as much as six years in the maturation of reproductive capacity and the completion of pelvic growth. Considering the heavy pressure by natural selection on cephalopelvic disproportion leading to infant deaths in time past, it is reasonable to surmise that our species has only recently been confronted with this problem on a regular basis.

Another contrast in pubertal sequencing can be found when comparing the production of sex cells in boys and girls. As Short has noted (1976, 1979a), the onset of spermatogenesis for boys precedes virtually all other pubertal changes, whereas in girls ovulation occurs very late in the sequence. As Richardson and Short (1978:21) state, the boy becomes potentially fertile at the very beginning of pubertal development, passing through a phase of being a "fertile eunuch" before acquiring his male secondary sex characteristics, whereas the girl develops nearly all her secondary sex characteristics to their fullest extent before acquiring her fertility. This fact suggests some special evolutionary pressure to delay fertility for the human female, giving her a time when she can function both socially and sexually as an adult but not assume a maternal role.

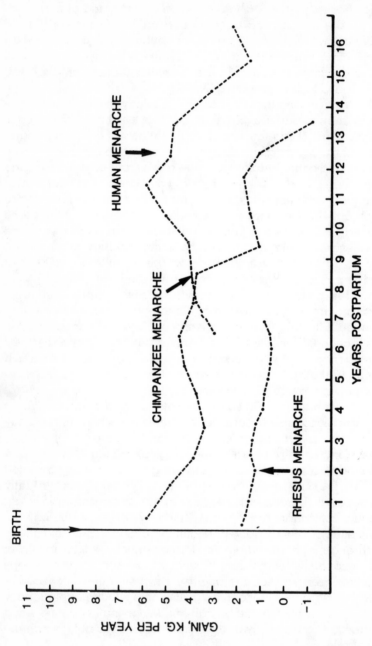

FIGURE 2.3. Comparative weight velocity curves for the rhesus monkey, chimpanzee, and humans. Major weight gain in the human and chimpanzee female occurs before menarche, whereas in the rhesus, it is nearly a year later (after Tanner, 1962).

A delay in the establishment of fertility until after the attainment of adult stature is not universal to female primates, many of which continue to grow not only after menarche but even during their first pregnancy and lactation. Gavan and Swindler (1966) and Watts and Gavan (1982) note differences among the higher primates in the location of menarche in the growth period (see Fig. 2.3). Rhesus monkey females have attained only 30% of their adult stature when they reach menarche in contrast to humans and chimpanzees who reached 70 and 80%, respectively. Altmann *et al.* (1981) note that female baboons in Kenya commence cycling at about $4\frac{1}{4}$ to 5 years of age, experience their first pregnancy at about 6 years, and give birth to their first infant at $6\frac{1}{2}$. Their attainment of full growth coincides with first pregnancy and birth, but not with menarche. Similarly, Froehlich *et al.* (1981) and Mori (1979) note a smoothly decelerating growth trajectory for wild monkeys in which females continue to gain weight for several years after their first pregnancy.

The adolescent growth spurt itself, so prominent in human development, may not be typical of other primates. In an early study, Gavan and Swindler (1966) concluded that while a growth spurt is so obvious for both human males and females, even on the basis of simple plots of annual increments in stature, nothing comparable could be demonstrated for nonhuman primates. However, in a follow-up study (Watts and Gavan, 1982) computer analysis of the same data base demonstrates that there is an adolescent growth spurt of much smaller magnitude than the human that can be discerned for the rhesus monkey and chimpanzee but only when compared to a predicted curve of growth. Such data suggest that an adolescent growth spurt comparable to the human may not occur at all in the monkey and ape females and whatever spurt that does occur is of minor magnitude. It is unlikely that this contrast is one that reflects dietary differences rather than species adaptation. Although Stini (1979) notes that humans growing under conditions of nutritional stress show an altered form of growth curve in both stature and weight which is more linear and has a more prolonged trajectory, the rhesus and chimpanzee data analyzed by Watts and Gavan came from well-fed laboratory populations. It is interesting that poor nutrition affects the growth patterns of a human male much more than it does a female. Frisch and Revelle (1969) found that in nutritionally growth-limited males there was a more rapid maturation, particularly in late growth, with a marked reduction in mature weight. For females, maturation rate was not particularly affected, and although there was a reduction in mature size, the growth pattern remained proportionate with adult size and weight 95% complete before menarche.

As noted in Fig. 2.3, mean age of puberty closely coincides with that of the peak of the adolescent spurt in the female chimpanzee, but in the female rhesus, menarche precedes the beginning of the adolescent acceleration and occurs, on the average, $1\frac{1}{2}$ years before the peak. Thus, sharp contrasts exist between the human condition with a prominent growth spurt in both height and weight preceding menarche and the nonhuman primate pattern in which an adolescent growth spurt is minor and follows (rhesus monkey) or is coincident with (chimpanzee) menarche.

It is possible that a pattern of female growth which allows for conflict between maternal growth and weight gain and fetal growth and lactation explains the poor figures for maternal success often reported for primiparous female monkeys and apes. For example, Drickamer (1974) for colony rhesus, Nadler (1975) for captive gorillas, Dazey and Erwin (1976) for colony pigtail macaques, Taub (1980) for colony squirrel monkeys, Glander (1980) for wild howler monkeys, and Mori (1979) for provisioned Japanese macaques, all report major contrasts in success in rearing infants between primiparous and multiparous mothers. Generally, when statistics are given, the mortality of infants born to primiparous primate mothers is more than double that of experienced and fully matured females. To date, only one study (Small and Rodman, 1981) reports no difference in reproductive success for first-time mothers observed in a laboratory colony of bonnet macaques. Several of the authors point to differences in fatness, body size, social rank, and food acquisition as keys to this differential in reproductive performance. Both Mori (1979) and Drickamer (1974), reporting on free-ranging but provisioned macaque colonies, note that females from high-ranking matrilines begin reproduction as much as a year earlier than other females, space their infants more closely, and are more successful in rearing young. Mori (1979) suggests the same and finds the maternal success is closely correlated with body weight and matrilineal status. Small-for-age females have poor reproductive success indicating that a reduction in body size in the face of restricted nutrition is a poor reproductive strategy for female primates. As Ralls (1976) states, bigger mothers are better mothers.

Finally, comparisons of life cycle events between wild and captive primates must be tempered with the recognition that primates raised in captivity show identical elements of a secular trend in growth described so fully for human populations during the past 150 years and for modern rural-urban comparisons. The major milestones of menarche, first birth, and completed growth are advanced in the laboratory and completed adult stature and weight are increased. According to Altmann et al. (1981), virtually all primates reported so far, which are healthy and well-fed in the laboratory or freely provisioned but free-ranging in the wild, show the secular trend in growth. Altmann et al.

demonstrate that the ages at which developmental milestones for baboons occur in the field as compared to those in captivity were advanced by a ratio of approximately 5:3. Similarly, Coe et al. (1979), in reviewing similar data for captive and wild chimpanzees, reported advances in developmental milestones on the order of 5:4.2 and 7:5.25. In the laboratory, chimpanzee females reach menarche around 8.5 years and first give birth at age 10–11, whereas wild chimpanzees reach menarche at 11–13 and first birth is at 13–15 years. It would be interesting to investigate how the secular trend in development affects psychosocial and cognitive development in laboratory-reared primates. Certainly, the secular trend leading to more rapid psychosexual development in humans does not seem to correlate with an advance in cognitive maturation. Perhaps primates might serve as useful experimental models in which the effects of cultural values, education, and training could be ruled out.

THE PERIOD OF ADOLESCENT SUBFERTILITY

At least 40 years ago, there was a general recognition that adolescent female primates, whether rhesus monkey, chimpanzee, or human, are not instantly fertile at the time of menarche (Montagu, 1979; Young and Yerkes, 1943). Data collected at that time suggested that a period of postmenarcheal subfertility lasted for about a year in the rhesus and up to two years for the chimpanzee and human. This information fits well with observations by anthropologists on tribal societies indicating that, although sexual activity almost invariably follows menarche, the likelihood of pregnancy is very low for the first few years. However, it is only very recently that the mechanism behind adolescent subfertility has been outlined (Lunenfeld et al., 1978; Reiter, this volume). It appears that rising ovarian estrogen secretion at puberty eventually triggers a reflex discharge of luteinizing hormone from the pituitary leading to ovulation. However, responsiveness of the pituitary and gonads is regulated by a progressive maturation of feedback regulatory centers in the hypothalamus. This positive feedback system takes time to mature: as Lunenfeld et al. noted, the ovary learns to ovulate. It appears that it takes nearly a year for this mechanism to develop in the rhesus monkey (Dierschke et al., 1974; Robinson and Goy, 1981). In a study of 8000 Finnish girls by Widholm and Kantero (1971: cited in Ryde-Blomqvist 1978:147) only 57% of the girls had established regular menstrual cycles by one year postmenarche and not until 6 years postmenarche were 80% cycling regularly. Similar data using basal body temperature changes to indicate ovulation suggest that not until age 18–20 are 75% of menstrual cycles ovulatory (Doring 1969). Short (1978) cites data on the sexual cycles of a wild female chimpanzee whose first estrous cycle began at age 11, followed 9 months later by menarche (a typical sequence for nonhuman primates). In spite of regular copulations, she did not conceive for nearly 3 more years. What is remarkable about this data is the extremely long time it takes in the higher primates for fertility to be established after regular sexual activity is assumed. According to Richardson and Short (1978), mammals such as sheep and rats have a first estrus associated with ovulation.For such species, the positive feedback mechanism regulating ovulation matures at birth, not years after menarche, so that for them, puberty equals instant fertility. One might speculate that the unusual demands placed on female primates for high levels of long-term parental investment based on experience in the social and physical environment has led to a delay in the maturation of the system regulating fertility but not in the one regulating the onset of sexual behavior.

The effect of the secular trend on the period of adolescent subfertility has not been fully explored. Papers by Lunenfeld et al. (1978) and Brown et al. (1978) make it clear that there is a wide range of variation in how soon after menarche an individual girl will establish regular ovulatory cycles. It is possible that not only is the mean age of menarche occurring earlier but that the timetable of developmental landmarks is collapsing; that is, fertility now follows menarche more rapidly in well-nourished, inactive girls.

FAT AND FERTILITY

A crucial factor in the fertility of human women relates to critical levels of fat storage. First proposed by Frisch (1978) and recently reviewed by Cohen (1980) and Huss-Ashmore (1980), the critical fatness hypothesis suggests that human women will not ovulate unless adequate stores of fat have been deposited. These fat deposits represent enough stored energy (around 150,000 calories) to permit a woman to lactate for a year or more without having to increase her prepregnancy caloric intake. Frisch believes that not only birth-spacing but also the timing of the onsets of menarche and menopause may rest on the storage of energy fat. Cohen (1980) notes the appeal of this hypothesis for explaining the secular trend in both the earlier onset of menarche and also the loss of a long period of adolescent subfertility in modern society. Sedentism combined with high levels of caloric intake lead to early deposition of body fat in young girls and "fool" the body into early biological maturation long before cognitive and social maturity are reached.

Skeptics of the critical fatness hypothesis have tended to focus on its critical threshold aspect but do not really undercut the important relationship between fertility and fatness. Ellison (1981a,b) demonstrates that the completion of the adolescent growth spurt in stature is a much better predictor of impending menarche than is a weight gain based on fat storage. This is not surprising when it is remembered that, in terms of evolutionary priorities, human growth of stature is programmed to virtually stop at menarche, whereas there should still exist something on the order of two more years before fertility will be established during which fat can be stored. Perhaps the critical fatness hypothesis would be a better predictor of onset of fertility than of menarche.

A second line of criticism focuses on the fact that populations suffering chronic malnutrition do not ordinarily cease reproduction and many such women will have children even though their ratio of fat to body weight is below the threshold proposed by Frisch (Bongaarts, 1980). Again, this is not an unexpected finding; an adaptive program for growth and reproduction would be one that hastens or slows growth and sexual maturation on the basis of food supply but only up to a point. The program should have limits on either end which prevent the establishment of reproduction in large juveniles or the indefinite delay of reproduction in the face of chronic food shortage. Evidence for just such a program in nonhuman primates is beginning to come from field studies. Mori (1979) investigated the relationship between population changes, food supply, body weight, and maturation in a group of Japanese macaques over a 25-year period. He found that daughters from high-ranking matrilines were larger in weight and stature than their peers and tended to give birth as soon as they had reached 6.5 kg, frequently a year before their peers and two years before the smallest and lowest-ranking females. Such females continued to gain weight during their early years of reproduction. Eventually, small females did become pregnant even if they weighed only 6 kg but their offspring showed a much higher mortality rate especially when the food supply was low. The relationship of rank to fat storage has been confirmed in the laboratory as well which suggests that even under conditions of ample food supply, low-status females may have problems of food access (Small, 1981).

In spite of the criticisms of Frisch's hypothesis, there is a growing body of evidence recently published by Garn (1980) demonstrating that early-maturing girls tend to be taller at puberty than their peers but ultimately shorter than the mean for adult women and fatter during their entire life course. Even at age 70, nearly 55 years after menarche, heavy rather than lean women report earlier menarcheal age. Both sons and daughters of such women tend to be faster growing; but reaching maturity earlier, they are ultimately shorter as well.

It is interesting that recent studies on the link between obesity and diabetes (Hartz et al., 1984; Kissebah et al., 1982) suggest that there may be two routes to fat deposition in the human. One route is influenced by androgens and tends to concentrate fat around the waist and upper body in fat cells that have the capacity to radically expand or shrink. The other route is via estrogens which concentrate fat that is very resistant to loss on the lower body. When obese women diet, there is a strong tendency for weight to be lost from the upper body but not from the lower. In fact, it appears to be much harder to shrink or kill normal-sized fat cells from the lower body, so that women who are fat only in these areas find it very hard to lose weight even if they diet faithfully. If concentrations of fat on the hips, buttocks, and thighs of women is "reproductive fat," it should not be surprising that these stores might be buffered against weight loss and accumulate under the influence of estrogens (Stini, 1979).

In spite of the fact that one of the most striking and uniquely developed features of human sexual dimorphism is fat deposition, very little significance has been attached to it. Reviews of sexual dimorphism in human and nonhuman primates (Alexander et al., 1979; Hamburg, 1978; Leutenegger, 1982; McCown, 1982) tend to focus on sex differences in body size and potential for aggression and do not note the extraordinary difference between men and women in fat storage or the lack of such conspicuous dimorphism in nonhumans primates. In fact, only Bailey (1982), Hall (1982), Huss-Ashmore (1980), and Stini (1979, 1982) give fat storage in women the emphasis it deserves. Sexual dimorphism in human body fat is much greater than in muscular tissue. Approximately 15% of body weight in the young adult male and about 27% of the female is adipose tissue, whereas muscle tissue represents an average of 52% for the male and 40% for the female (Bailey, 1982). When corrections are made for the smaller body size of the human female, women are indeed a great deal fatter than calculations of average sex differences would indicate. For instance, in comparing volume of body segments corrected for frame size, Bailey (1982) found that women are 40.2% larger than men for the gluteal (buttocks) segment. Huss-Ashmore (1980) argues that the distinctiveness of fat storage in women on breasts, buttocks, and thighs advertises healthy systemic function and the ability to reproduce and successfully rear children. As such, reproductive fat in women should be differentially located than fat in men, localized for more dramatic display and closely linked to the development of other secondary sex characteristics.

FAT RESERVES, LACTATION, AND GROWTH
OF THE HUMAN BRAIN

It is only very recently that evolutionary theorists have turned from such behavioral topics as aggression and sexual behavior to lactation as a key variable in understanding species' differences (Blurton-Jones, 1972; Daly, 1979; Pond, 1979). Perhaps one reason for this delayed interest was that few recognized the enormous interspecies variability in virtually all aspects of lactation: the constituents of milk, frequency of nursing, length of nursing bout, and duration of lactation. Blurton-Jones (1972) and more recently Anderson, (1983), Stini (1982), and Stini et al. (1980) profile the unusual features of human milk and lactation. One of the most striking of these is its exceedingly low protein content (46% that of the cow and 15% of the rabbit). At the same time, it is rich with lactose and lipids with values ranging 22 and 42% above those of the cow. The composition of human milk represents a balance of numerous other constituents as well, but it is clear from the ratios of protein, lactose, and lipids that it amply supplies the nutrients necessary for activity and growth of the brain and provides only low levels of nutrients necessary to develop lean muscle and tissue. This is not surprising when it is noted that even by age 10 a human reaches only 50% of adult body size but has reached virtually adult values for brain size by age 4 (Dobbing, 1974).

The pecularities and uniqueness of human milk can be best understood if the unusual program for human brain growth is taken into account. At birth, the brains of rhesus monkey infants are approximately 68% of the adult size, chimpanzees 45%, and humans 23% (Kerr et al., 1969; Passingham, 1975). The human infant's brain grows exceedingly rapidly after birth, but it does not reach 45% of the adult size until 6–7 months of age, and by the end of the first year, it has completed only 65% of its total growth (Figure 2.4). The human brain completes 93–95% of its growth in volume by the end of the fourth year, the usual age of weaning among human hunter-gatherers. There are other animal species which also have extensive postnatal growth of the brain but they are generally what zoologists have labeled as r-selected species; that is, they tend to rapidly produce litters of small embryonic young which grow very quickly after birth and are weaned within a few weeks or months (Dobbing and Sands, 1979). With the exception of the great apes and humans, most animals with single young and large adult body size produce precocial infants with well-developed brains, able to sense the world and locomote at birth. Figure 2.5 illustrates the extremely long duration of brain growth in the human, the nutrients for which cannot be ensured by the timing of births to an optimal season of the year.

Dobbing (1974) and Frisancho (1978), in reviewing the most critical and vulnerable periods of brain growth in humans, focus on the last trimester of fetal life and the first postnatal year as crucial. Although the adult number of nerve cells develops during the first trimester of

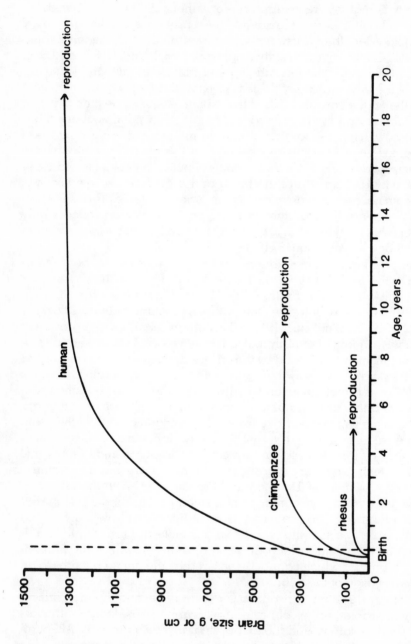

FIGURE 2.4. Growth of the brain in humans, chimpanzees, and the rhesus monkey (after Passingham, 1975; Kerr et al., 1969).

30

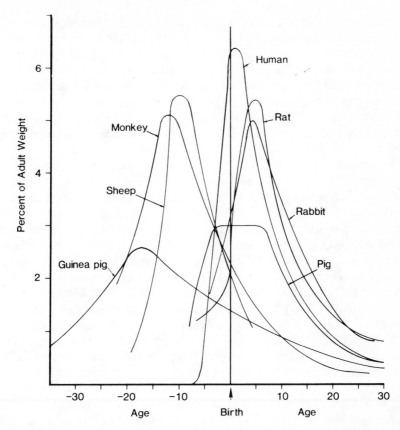

FIGURE 2.5. The brain growth spurts of 7 mammalian species expressed as first-order velocity curves of the increase in weight with age. The units of time for each species are: guinea pig, 1 day; rhesus monkey, 4 days; sheep, 5 days; pig, 1 week; human, 1 month; rabbit, 2 days; rat, 1 day. Rates are expressed as weight gain as a percentage of adult weight for each unit of time (from Dobbing and Sands, 1979).

pregnancy, the energetically demanding stages for the production of the brain's packing cells (oligodendroglia, glial cells) followed by synaptic arborization of the nerve cells and by the production of insulating material (myelin) which coats the long fibers through which nerve cells send messages, occur in the three months just before birth and the subsequent year. The vulnerable nature of brain growth for such a long period postpartum may explain one recently described feature of maternal weight gain and fetal growth. According to Winick (1981), preparations for lactation are so important that, if the mother is inadequately nourished, they will take place at the expense of fetal growth.

The pregnant woman will continue to deposit fat during pregnancy even it is means that fetal growth in body size will be reduced below optimal levels for neonate survival. Winick recommends that women should gain at least 25 pounds in pregnancy to ensure that the fetus will not have to compete for nutrients with maternal fat storage processes. The energetic greed of the human infant's brain is truly impressive. During the first year of life, up to 65% of its total metabolic rate is devoted to the brain and only 8% to muscle tissue (Holliday, 1978).

The question remains as to why human beings are committed to such a potentially vulnerable program of brain growth, one that is so dependent on maternal lactation over such a long time period. Schultz (1941) and, more recently, Lindburg (1982) have laid to rest what is known as the obstetrical dilema theory which argues that, when humans evolved bipedal locomotion and a pelvis in the shape of a bony ring, the dual demands of efficient bipedalism and an intelligent, large brain were in direct conflict. The supposed solution to this conflict was the birth of an immature, helpless infant with major (75%) brain growth programmed for outside the womb. The only problem with this thesis is that it fails to explain the immaturity of the great ape infant whose brain grows 55 to 64% after birth even though maternal pelvic capacity is nearly one-third larger than needed. Lindburg turns to a work by Mason (1968) that suggests that the immaturity of great ape and human infants may best be understood as an adaptation for transition into a social, learning environment at an early stage of neural development. This might help to explain why we find similarities in the great ape and human pattern of slow growth in the juvenile period but the attainment of adult stature and weight before first pregnancy in contrast to the macaque mother whose infant's brain grows little after birth but who still may be growing herself during her early reproductive years.

CONCLUSION

The timing of growth, development, and the onset of reproduction within the life cycle has always been under heavy selective pressure from natural selection. The result of this procedure is a special program for each species which provides a range of variation for each event which is appropriate to conditions ranging from optimal to suboptimal habitat. The basic evolutionary pattern for human females is one of slow growth during a prolonged period of juvenile dependency followed by a rapid completion of growth in stature, and sometimes body weight as well, before menarche. Menarche is followed by several years of sexual activity with very low probability of impregnation during which a young woman can gain experience about her social and physical environment before undertaking the demands of motherhood. During this period of adolescent subfertility, a substantial store of body fat will be deposited in the human female at the same time that her male peer is using energy surpluses to grow greater stature and lean muscle tissue. This differential in male and female growth patterns leads to the major element of human dimorphism in secondary sex characteristics: fat storage. The evolutionary pressure for the development of such an unusual degree of dimorphism in nutrient reserves is the unique demands of the developing human brain which grows 2/3 of its total size in the first four years postpartum. It is not noteworthy that the great ape pattern appears to be intermediate and foreshadows the human pattern. Great apes also have a long, 4-year period of lactation and bear relatively helpless infants with brains that will grow at least 55-64% between birth and the end of the second year.

The critical factor in adjusting this program to the environment, allowing it to take advantage of differences in habitat optimality, appears to be an interaction of diet and exercise, energy acquisition, and expense. Recent changes in human life styles including diets higher in simple carbohydrates and fats in combination with lowered energy demands appear to signal optimal habitat conditions, thereby speeding up sexual and physical maturation. Today, we may be witnessing a maximal lowering of the mean age for menarche and fertility to the lowest point within the range of variation established long ago by evolutionary processes. For most of human history, for most individuals, and under most conditions, the human pattern of growth and development was expressed in such a way as to allow social, physical, psychological, and sexual development to unfold at a more leisurely pace with first birth in the late teens preceded by several years of adolescent subfertility. Today, the earlier onset of adolescence and more rapid assumption of fertility by age 12–14 means that humans can no longer count on the evolved mechanisms of time past for appropriate timing of reproductive events. It is abundantly clear that only culturally based systems can ensure that a child will not become a mother.

ACKNOWLEDGMENTS

The stimulus for writing this article came from several years of planning and discussion with members of the Social Science Research Council's Committee for Biosocial Science Perspectives on Parent Behavior and Offspring Development. The support and encouragement of the Social Science Research Council is gratefully acknowledged. Partial funding of the activities of the committee was granted by the

National Institute for Child Health and Human Development (Grant No. 5R13-HD11777-02) and by the William T. Grant Foundation. Data on reproduction, parental investment, and the human life cycle was developed during a Summer Research Fellowship awarded by the Faculty Research Council of the University of Oklahoma. Special thanks are due to LaDon Deatherage for her help in the collection of data and library references and to Carri Swope and Darlene Thornton for assistance in preparing the manuscript. The helpful comments on an earlier version of the manuscript are gratefully acknowledged to Judith K. Brown, Mildred Dickemann, Patty Gowati, James Gavin, Barbara King, Ron Nadler, and S. L. Washburn.

REFERENCES

Alexander, R. D., Hoogland, J., Howard, R., Noonan, K., and Sherman, P. Sexual dimorphisms and breeding systems in pinnipeds, ungulates, primates, and humans. *In* N. Chagnon and W. Irons (Eds.), *Evolutionary biology and human social behavior*. North Scituate, Mass.: Duxbury Press, 1979, pp. 402-435.

Anderson, P. The reproductive role of the human breast. *Current Anthropology*, 1983, *24*, 25-46.

Altmann, J., Altmann, S., and Hausfater, G. Physical maturation and age estimates of yellow baboons, *Papio cynocephalus*, in Amboseli National Park, Kenya. *American Journal of Primatology*, 1981, 1389-399.

Bailey, Stephen M. Absolute and relative sex differences in body composition. *In* R. Hall (Ed.), *Sexual dimorphism in Homo sapiens*. New York: Praeger, 1982, pp. 363-390.

Blurton-Jones, Nicholas. Comparative aspects of mother-child contact. *In* N. Blurton-Jones (Ed.), *Ethological studies of child behaviour*. Cambridge: Cambridge University Press, 1972, pp. 305-329.

Bongaarts, John. Does malnutrition affect fecundity? *Science*, 1980, *208*, 564-569.

Brown, J. B., Harrisson, Patricia, and Smith, Margery A. Oestrogen and pregnanediol excretion through childhood, menarche, and first ovulation. *Journal of Biosocial Science, Suppl.*, 1978, *5*, 43-62.

Coe, C. L., Connolly, A. C., Kraemer, H. C., and Levine, S. Reproductive development and behavior of captive female chimpanzees. *Primates*, 1979, *2*, 571-582.

Cohen, Mark N. Speculations on the evolution of density measurement and population in *Homo sapiens*. *In* M. N. Cohen, R. S. Malpass, and H. G. Klein (Eds.), *Biosocial mechanisms of population regulation*. New Haven: Yale University Press, 1980, pp. 275-304.

Daly, Martin. Why don't male mammals lactate? *Journal of Theoretical Biology*, 1979, *78*, 325-345.

Dazey, J., and Erwin J. Infant mortality in *Macaca nemestrina*. *Theriogenology*, 1976, *5*, 267-279.

Dierschke, D. J., Weiss, G., and Knobil, E. Sexual maturation in the female rhesus monkey and the development of estrogen-induced gonadotrophic hormone release. *Endocrinology*, 1974, *94*, 198-206.

Dobbing, John. The later development of the brain and its vulnerability. *In* J. A. Davis, and J. Dobbing (Eds.), *Scientific foundations of paediatrics*. Philadelphia: W. B. Saunders, 1974, pp. 565-577.

Dobbing, J. and Sands, J. Comparative aspects of the brain spurt. *Early Human Development*, 1979, *3*, 79-83.

Doring, G. K. The incidence of anovular cycles in women. *Journal of Reproductive Fertility, Suppl.*, 1969, *6*, 77.

Drickamer, L. C. A ten-year summary of reproductive data for free-ranging *Macaca mulatta. Folia primatologica*, 1974, *21*, 61-80.

Ellison, P. T. Threshold hypotheses, developmental age, and menstrual function. *American Journal of Physical Anthropology*, 1981, *54*, 337-340.(a)

Ellison, P.T. Prediction of age at menarche from annual height increments. *American Journal of Physical Anthropology*, 1981, *56*, 71-75.(b)

Froehlich, J. W., Thorington, R. W. Jr., and Otis, J.S. The demography of Howler monkeys *(Alouatta palliata)* on Barro Colorado Island, Panama. *International Journal of Primatology*, 1981, *2*, 207-237.

Frisancho, A. R. Nutritional influences on human growth and maturation. *Yearbook of Physical Anthropology*, 1978, *21*, 174-191.

Frisch, Rose. Population, food intake, and fertility. *Science*, 1978, *199*, 22-30.

Frisch, R., and Revelle, R. Variation in body weights and the age of the adolescent growth spurt among Latin American and Asian Populations, in relation to caloric supplies. *Human Biology*, 1969, *41*, 185-212.

Garn, S. M., Jr. Continuities and change in maturational timing. *In* O. Brim and J. Kagan (Eds.), *Constancy and change in human development*. Cambridge: Harvard University Press, 1980, pp. 113-162.

Gavan, J. A., and Swindler, D. R. Growth rates and phylogeny in primates. *American Journal Physical Anthropology*, 1966, *24*, 181-190.

Glander, K. Reproduction and population growth in free-ranging mantled howling monkeys. *American Journal of Physical Anthropology*, 1980, *53*, 25-36.

Hall, R. L. (Ed.). *Sexual dimorphism in Homo sapiens*, 1982, New York: Praeger.

Hamburg, B. A. The biosocial bases of sex difference. *In* S. L. Washburn and E. R. McCown (Eds.), *Human evolution: Biosocial perspectives*. Menlow Park, Ca.: Benjamin/Cummings, 1978, pp. 155-214.

Harrell, B. B. Lactation and menstruation in cultural perspective. *American Anthropologist*, 1981, *83*, 796–823.

Hartz, A. J., Rupley, D. C., & Rimm, A. R. The association of girth measurements with disease in 32,856 women. *American Journal of Epidemiology*, 1984, *119*, 71-80.

Holliday, M. A. Body composition and energy needs during growth. *In* F. Falker and J. M. Tanner (Eds.), *Human growth*. New York: Plenum, 1978, Vol. 2, pp. 117-139.

Howell, Nancy. *Demography of the Dobe !Kung*, 1979, New York: Academic Press.

Huss-Ashmore, R. Fat and fertility: Demographic implications of differential fat storage. *Yearbook of Physical Anthropology*, 1980, *23*, 65-91.

Kerr, G. R., Kennan, A. L., Waisman, H. A., and Allen, J. R. Growth and development of the fetal rhesus monkey. I. Physical growth. *Growth*, 1969, *33*, 201-213.

Kissebah, A. H., Vydelingum, N., Murray, R., Evans, D. J., Hartz, A. J., Kalkhoff, R. K., and Adams P. W. Relation of body fat distribution to metabolic complications of obesity. *Journal of Clinical Endocrinology and Metabolism*, 1982, *54*, 254-260.

Lancaster, Jane, B. Evolutionary perspectives on sex difference in the higher primates. In A. S. Rossi (Ed.), Gender and the life course. New York: Aldine, 1984, pp. 3-27.

Lancaster, J. B. and Lancaster, Chet S. Parental investment: The hominid adaptation. In D. Ortner (Ed.), How humans adapt: A biocultural odyssey. Washington, D. C.: Smithsonian Institution Press, 1983, pp. 33-66.

Leutenegger, Walter. Sexual dimorphism in nonhuman primates. In R. Hall (Ed.), Sexual dimorphism in Homo sapiens. New York: Praeger, 1982, pp. 11-36.

Lindburg, D. G. Primate obstetrics: The biology of birth. American Journal of Primatology. Suppl., 1982, 1, 193-199.

Lunenfeld, F., Kraiem, Z., Eshkol, A., and Werner-Zodrow, I. The ovary learns to ovulate. Journal of Biosocial Science, Suppl., 1978, 5, 43-62.

McCown, E. R. Sex differences: The female as baseline for species description. In R. Hall (Ed.), Sexual dimorphism in Homo sapiens. New York: Praeger, 1982, pp. 37-84.

Marshall, W. A. and Tanner, J. M. Puberty. In J. A. Davis and J. Dobbing (Eds.). Scientific foundations of paediatrics. Philadelphia: W. A. Saunders, 1974, pp. 124-152.

Mason, W. A. Scope and potential of primate research. Science and Psychoanalysis, 1968, 12, 101-118.

Moerman, Marquisa L. Growth of the birth canal in adolescent girls. American Journal of Obstetrics and Gynecology, 1982, 143, 528-532.

Montagu, M. F. Ashley. The reproductive development of the female: A study in the comparative physiology of the adolescent organism. 3rd ed. Littleton, Mass.: Wright PSG, 1979.

Mori, Akio. Analysis of population changes by measurement of body weight in the Koshima troop of Japanese monkeys. Primates, 1979, 20, 371-399.

Nadler, R. D. Determinants of variability in maternal behavior of captive female gorillas. In S. Kondo, M. Kawai, A. Ehara, and S. Kawamura (Eds.), Proceedings, Symposia of the 5th Congress of the International Primatological Society. Tokyo: Japan Science Press, 1975, pp. 207-216.

Passingham, R. E. Changes in the size and organization of the brain in man and his ancestors. Brain, Behavior and Evolution, 1975, 11, 73-90.

Pond, Caroline M. The significance of lactation in the evolution of mammals. Evolution, 1977, 31, 177-199.

Ralls, Katherine. Mammals in which females are larger than males. Quarterly Review of Biology, 1976, 51, 245-276.

Richardson, D. W., and Short, R. V. Time of onset of sperm production in boys. Journal of Biosocial Science Suppl., 1978, 5, 15-26.

Robinson, J. A., and Goy, R. W. The pubescent rhesus monkey: Characteristics of the menstrual cycle and effects of prenatal androgenization. Biology of Reproduction, 1981, 24 (Suppl. 1), abstract 90.

Ryde-Blomqvist, Elsa, Contraception in adolescence: A review of the literature. Journal of Biosocial Science Suppl., 1978, 5, 129-158.

Schultz, A. H. The relative size of the cranial capacity in primates. American Journal of Physical Anthropology, 1941, 28, 273-287.

Short, R. V. The evolution of human reproduction. Proceedings of Royal Society, 1976, B195, 3-24.

Short, R. V. Discussion: Hormonal patterns in childhood and adolescence. Journal of Biosocial Science Suppl., 1978, 5, 58-61.

Short, R. V. Sexual selection and its component parts, somatic and genital selection, as illustrated by man and the great apes. Advances in the Study of Behavior, 1979, 9, 131-158.(a)

Short, R. V. When a conception fails to become a pregnancy. *Maternal Recognition of Pregnancy, Ciba Foundation Series*, 1979, *64*, 377-394.(b)

Small, Meredith F. Body, fat, rank, and nutritional status in a captive group of rhesus monkeys. *International Journal of Primatology*, 1981, *2*, 91-95.

Small, Meredith F. and Rodman, Peter. Primigravidity and infant loss in bonnet macaques. *Journal of Medical Primatology*, 1981, *10*, 164-169.

Stini, William A. Adaptive strategies of human populations under nutritional stress. *In* W. A. Stini (Ed.), *Physiological and morphological adaptation and evolution*. Mouton: The Hague, 1979, pp. 387-407.

Stini, William A. Sexual dimorphism and nutrient reserves. *In* R. Hall (Ed.), *Sexual dimorphism in Homo sapiens*. New York: Praeger, 1982, pp. 391-419.

Stini, W. A., Weber, C., Kemberling, S., and Vaughan, L. Lean tissue growth and disease susceptibility in bottle-fed versus breast-fed infants. *In* E. S. Green and F. E. Johnston (Eds.), *Social and biological predictors of nutritional status, physical growth, and neurological development*. New York: Academic Press, 1980, pp. 61-79.

Tanner, J. M. *Growth at adolescence*, 1962, London: Blackwell.

Taub, D. M. Age at first pregnancy and reproductive success among colony-born squirrel monkeys *(Saimiri sciureus, Brazilian)*. *Folia primatologica*, 1980, *33*, 262-272.

Watts, E. S., and Gavan J. A. Postnatal growth of nonhuman primates: The problem of the adolescent spurt. *Human Biology*, 1982, *54*, 53-70.

Winick, Myron. Food and the fetus. *Natural History*, 1981, *90*, 76-81.

Young, W. C., and Yerkes, R. M. Factors influencing the reproductive cycle in the chimpanzee: The period of adolescent sterility and related problems. *Endocrinology*, 1943, *33*, 121-154.

3

TIMING OF MENARCHE: SECULAR TREND AND POPULATION DIFFERENCES

Phyllis B. Eveleth

INTRODUCTION

Menarche is probably the best indicator a girl has of "growing up." This developmental milestone signifies the change from child to woman. This significant event is caused by heightened activity of the sex hormones. However, menarche does not mean that the reproductive system is functionally mature since many of the first menstrual cycles may occur without ova or the ova may be abnormally developed (Treloar, 1974). In fact, Vollman (1966) has shown that 45% of menstrual cycles in the first year are anovulatory or abnormal, and not until 23 years of age, on average, did he find that 97% of the cycles were normal. There is also some evidence that girls who have early menarche (12 years of age) have more anovulatory cycles and lower ketosteroid urinary levels than girls who experience delayed menarche (Cristesçu et al., 1966).

To the investigator in child development, menarche is also considered a major event, since it is the clearest indicator of sexual maturation. Thus, many studies of adolescent development have recorded age of menarche along with height, weight, and other body size data.

Menarche does not by any means indicate the beginning of puberty, for in 99–100% of girls, menarche occurs after the period of greatest acceleration in height growth, that is, when height growth is slowing down.

METHODOLOGY

Studies to determine median age of menarche in a population are easy and inexpensive to carry out. However, in order to obtain reliable

TABLE 3.1. Status Quo Study

Need: Large, representative sample
       Sufficiently broad age range
Ask: When were you born?
      Have you begun your menstrual periods?
Record: Percentage "YES" and "NO" at each age
Analyze: Probits or logits
Result: Median age of menarche
        Standard deviation

results, certain methodologies must be followed. Recall studies (asking a group of women when they reached menarche) are fraught with problems of poor memory and even deliberate falsification, so that we can not place as much confidence in the results as we can in the other two types of studies. These are the *status quo* and the prospective study (Table 3.1). The *status quo* is the more common of the two and involves asking a sample of girls two questions: (1) when they were born and (2) whether or not they have begun their menstrual periods. The sample must be sufficiently large and representative of the population, and the age range must be broad to include young girls who have not menstruated. The ages of eight to sixteen years would be an ideal range for a study of American girls. However, since mean age varies among different populations, the age range of the sample needs to be adjusted accordingly when studying other populations.

From these data, a table is constructed giving the percentage of "YES" and "NO" answers at each age. Using either probit or logit transformation, the median age and standard error and standard deviation of the age of menarche in the population is then estimated (Tanner and Eveleth, 1975).

The prospective method can be employed in longitudinal growth studies. Girls are asked at each visit whether they have begun their menstrual periods. This method will give reliable results if the visits are not over 1 year apart.

POPULATION DIFFERENCES

There is a wide age range for reaching menarche in present-day populations. *Within* any population, there is considerable individual variation of the age when girls begin their menstrual periods, and *among* populations the range is equally as great (Table 3.2). When speaking of populations, of course, the median or average age of menarche is being considered.

Different European countries are actually quite similar in average

TABLE 3.2. Median Age of Menarche

Place	Age ± S.E.	Place	Age ± S.E.
Hongkong (well-off) (Low et al., 1982)	12.4 ± 0.18	London (Tanner, 1973)	13.0 ± 0.03
United States (blacks) (MacMahon, 1973)	12.5	Stockholm (M. Furth and G. Lindgren unpublished data, 1972)	13.1 ± 0.08
La Plata, Argentina (Lejarraga et al., 1980)	12.5 ± 0.05	Ibadan, Nigeria (Oduntan et al., 1976)	13.7 ± 0.03
Naples (rural) (Carfagna et al., 1972)	12.5 ± 0.02	India (urban) (Indian Council of Medical Research, 1972)	13.7
Merida, Venezuela (Limongi et al., 1979)	12.6 ± 0.09	Maya Indians (Sabharwal et al., 1966)	15.1 ± 0.25
United States (whites) (MacMahon, 1973)	12.8	New Guinea, Megiar (Wark and Malcolm, 1969)	15.5 ± 0.20
Madrid (well-off) (Marin, 1971)	12.8 ± 0.12	Rwanda, Tutsi (Heintz, 1963)	16.5 ± 0.16
Cuba (national) (Jordan, 1979)	12.9 ± 0.07	Rwanda, Hutu (Heintz, 1963)	17.0 ± 0.30
Japan (urban) (Yanagisawa and Kondo, 1973)	12.9 ± 0.01	New Guinea, Bundi (Malcolm, 1970)	18.0 ± 0.19

age of menarche, although Mediterranean populations tend to be somewhat earlier than English, Dutch, or Scandinavians (Eveleth and Tanner, 1976). The data from American and French Canadian girls of European descent are very similar to the data of girls from southern and eastern Europe (12.8 and 12.9 years). Some of the Latin American countries such as Cuba, Chile, Venezuela, and Argentina, also have reported menarcheal ages comparable to those of southern Europe (Eveleth and Tanner, 1976; Lejarraga et al., 1980). European populations in relatively underdeveloped rural areas experience menarche later, more like European populations of 100 years ago. American blacks experience menarche somewhat earlier than American whites (12.5 years versus 12.8 years) (MacMahon, 1973) but, with the exception of Cuban mulatto girls (13.0 years), other black populations are later than whites living in the same geographic area (Eveleth and Tanner, 1976). Nigerian urban girls who are considered to be well-off reached menarche at 13.5 years (Uche and Okorafor, 1979); in Ibadan, the average age was 13.7 years (Oduntan et al., 1976). However, a trend toward earlier ages can be seen: Girls with university-educated parents had earlier menarche (13.2 years) than other urban girls, and Nigerian Ibo girls in private schools had an average age of menarche of 13.4 years in 1978, which was earlier than the age of 14.1 years reported in 1960 (Uche and Okorafor, 1979).

Both Chinese and Japanese girls experience early menarche. Well-off girls from Hong Kong reach menarche as early as American blacks, at about the youngest age in the world (Chang, 1969). More traditional Melanesian populations from New Guinea have the latest record menarche, ranging from 15.5 years for the Megiar to 18.0 years for the Bundi. Other traditional (village) groups reporting late menarche are the Hutu and Tutsi of Rwanda (Heintz, 1963), and Maya Indians of Yucatan (Sabharwal et al., 1966).

INDIVIDUAL DIFFERENCES

In any population, 95% of the girls will experience menarche anywhere from 2.5 to 3 years before to 2.5 to 3 years after the average age of menarche for the population. If the average age is 12.5 years, as it is among American black girls, and since the distribution is normal, we should expect to find some girls beginning their menstrual periods at 9.5 and many more beginning at 10.5 years. By 13.5 years, 75% of the girls should have begun menarche.

Individual variation in menarcheal age within a population is a reflection of both heredity and environment. Monozygotic twin sisters experience menarche at about the same age (differing only about 2 to 3 months), whereas dizygotic sisters differ by an average of 9 months (Fischbein, 1977).

TABLE 3.3. Age at Menarche in Athletes and Dancers[a]

	N	Mean age ± S.E.
Nonathlete control	30	12.2 ± 0.3
Shotputters	9	13.4 ± 0.6
Sprinters	24	13.5 ± 0.3
Distance runners	12	13.6 ± 0.3
Discus and javelin	10	13.6 ± 0.5
Jumpers and hurdlers	11	13.7 ± 0.4
Ballet dancers	67	13.7 ± 0.1

[a] After Malina et al., 1973; Frisch et al., 1980.

Individual differences in age at menarche may be influenced by physical training for sports. Malina and his colleagues (1973, 1978) have reported consistently later menarche (from recall data) for female athletes than for the nonathlete controls (Table 3.3). Hypotheses as to why this should occur vary. One explanation is that physique in late maturers is more suitable for success in athletic performance. Another is that socialization of early maturers is away from sports. Ballet dancers also have been reported to reach menarche later than the population average (Frisch et al., 1980). Frisch's explanation for this is a high level of activity coupled with restricted food intake resulting in a low weight for height. Girls who are overweight or who have more fat than normal tend to reach menarche earlier (Frisch, 1972; Johnston et al., 1975). Similarly, menstrual cycles temporarily cease in girls who are losing weight or who are anorectic (Frisch and McArthur, 1974). Since adipose tissue is a significant extragonadal source of estrogen (Frisch, 1980), a link between obesity and menarche can be hypothesized.

SECULAR TREND

The average age of menarche has been decreasing in Europe and North America for the last 150 years. Maturation is not only earlier, but a related secular change is seen in body size: children and adults are taller now than they were in the 1880s (Tanner, 1969). The fact is that today children reach puberty earlier. Adolescents attain adult stature and also stop growing earlier than they did 150 years ago.

Although the age of menarche has been decreasing in the last 150 years, I do not think we should assume that menarche has been getting progressively earlier throughout the history of mankind. Classical and medieval writings indicate that menarche might have occurred at around 13 to 14 years of age in classical Greece and Rome (Amundsen and Diers, 1969) and from 12 to 15 years from the sixth through the fifteenth centuries (Amundsen and Diers, 1973; Herlihy, 1978). Tanner (1981) thinks average age of menarche in classical and medieval times might have been somewhat later since the medieval writers were probably considering the better-off girls, and we do know that poorer girls generally have menarche later than the well-off. As shown in Fig. 3.1, for the nineteenth to the late twentieth century in Europe, we have considerable evidence of a trend toward earlier menarche.

Recently, a question has been raised regarding the magnitude of the secular decrease in the average age of menarche in the nineteenth and twentieth centuries (Bullough, 1981). This criticism is based on the fact that the nineteenth-century data are not perfect. Namely, they are from small and preselected samples, such as obstetrical patients, and most of them are based on retrospective recall, often from older women. Despite these shortcomings, the consistency of the results points to a marked trend toward earlier menarche that outweighs the possible errors in the old studies (Tanner and Eveleth, 1975; Tanner, 1981). Tanner's (1981) recent comprehensive survey of historical data from northwestern Europe shows a clear decline in average age of menarche throughout the nineteenth century to present times.

A recent report of mid-nineteenth-century data outweighs some of the criticisms of the older studies (Manniche, 1983). A large number of women (3385) from various rural and urban areas in Denmark, grouped by socioeconomic status, were estimated to have an average age of menarche of 16 years 3 months. The averages ranged from 14 years 3 months for urban, upper-class women to 16 years 8 months for rural,

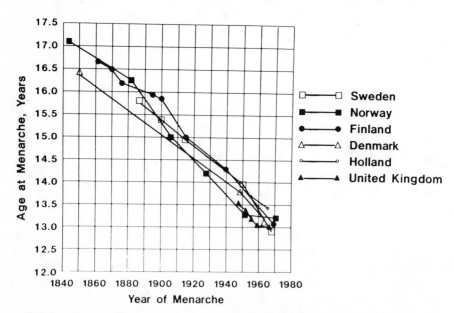

FIGURE 3.1. Secular decrease in average age at menarche in Europe. (Redrawn from Eveleth and Tanner, 1976.)

lower-class women. In 1980, the average menarcheal age in Denmark was a little under 13 years, which indicates an average reduction in menarcheal age of 2–3 months per decade since 1980.

The problem is more complex than is perceived by Bullough. When we speak of a decline of 2–3 months per decade, we are speaking of an average over a long period of time. Some regions and some populations, such as the upper socioeconomic groups or urban populations, may demonstrate quite different rates from low-income or rural groups. The improvement in health and nutrition leading to earlier menarche may have little effect on the upper socioeconomic or urban groups since these girls already were well-nourished and, as discussed below, had an earlier mean age of menarche than girls from the lower socioeconomic groups. An example of this comes from Poland from where it has recently been reported that the trend from the mid-1960s to the mid-1970s was a decrease in menarcheal age of 0.25 years per decade in Warsaw but 0.64 years per decade in rural areas (Laska-Mierzejewska et al., 1982).

Further insight into how the decline occurred in one population is provided by some new evidence from Norway (Brudevoll et al., 1979). Medical records found in some clinic cellars in Olso dating back to 1873 showed a decline in mean menarcheal age from 15.6 to 14.6 years from 1860 to 1900. After leveling off from 1900 to 1920, menarche declined

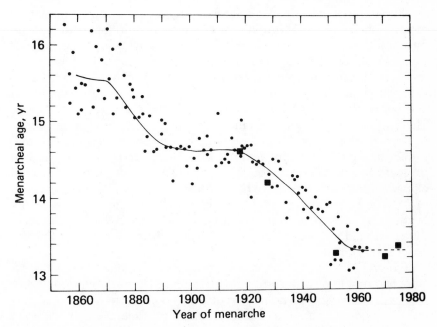

FIGURE 3.2. Secular decrease in age at menarche in clinic patients in Oslo from 1860 to 1980. (Redrawn from Brudevoll et al., 1979.)

again until 1960, when it again leveled off at 13.4 years. These data are shown in Figure 3.2 (each point represents about 50 maternity clinic patients).

Wyshak and Frisch (1982) recently have reported on their review of 218 reports on age of menarche in Europe from 1795 to 1981. They found an average rate of decline of 2–3 months per decade, with varying rates and varying ages for different countries. In the United States, they reported a decline in about 2 months per decade from 1877 to 1947, at which time the average age leveled off at 12.8 years.

Most investigators are agreed that improved nutrition is the major cause of earlier maturation (see Eveleth and Tanner, 1976 for review). There are other factors as well that influence the timing of menarche, and these will be discussed below. Because of the many influences on timing of maturation, there is no reason why we should expect changes to occur at a regular rate over the decades or to be the same in all countries. Just as we see variability among populations for secular increase in height, we see variability in secular decrease in menarcheal age. Furthermore, there is now evidence from some countries (i.e., Norway, England, and the United States) that the decline has leveled off (Eveleth, 1979).

FACTORS INFLUENCING THE TIMING OF MENARCHE

The timing of menarche is influenced by a considerable number of factors, one of the most important of which is nutrition. Many of the other factors are influenced, or are concomitant with, good or poor nutritional status. For example, chronic undernutrition delays menarche in the poor rural areas of Appalachia in the southern United States. A longitudinal study of 30 girls reported a mean menarcheal age of 14.4 years versus 12.4 for well-nourished controls (Dreizen et al., 1967). These girls were also delayed in skeletal maturation and were shorter during childhood, although there was no difference in adult height.

Similarly, an improvement in nutritional status may lead to a decline in average age at menarche. The establishment of a new industrial city in Poland also improved the nutrition of the population. Girls born of parents who had migrated from poor, rural villages to the new city had earlier menarche than their peers who were born and raised in the rural villages. They were also taller and heavier (Panek and Piasecki, 1971).

In many other populations, we find a similar picture related to socioeconomic status and rural living (Fig. 3.3): The well-off, and, therefore (we assume) better-nourished girls in a population showed an earlier age of menarche than the poor, although exceptions to this have been reported from Sweden, Chile, and Montreal, where no differences between socioeconomic groups were seen (Eveleth and Tanner, 1976).

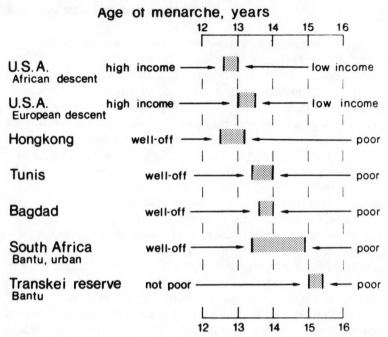

FIGURE 3.3. Difference in some socioeconomic groups in average age at menarche. (From Eveleth and Tanner, 1976. Reproduced by permission of the publisher.)

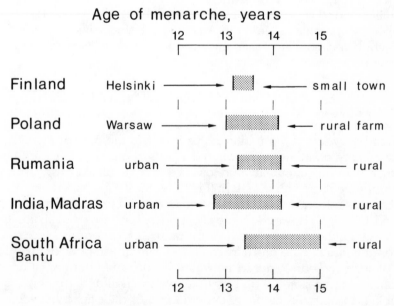

FIGURE 3.4. Difference in some urban and rural groups in average age of menarche. (From Eveleth and Tanner, 1976. Reproduced by permission of the publisher.)

In regard to the urban–rural differential, mean menarcheal age is lower in the cities today than in the country (Fig. 3.4) (Eveleth and Tanner, 1976). It is believed that nutrition plays a large role in this, but other factors such as medical care, sanitation, and better living conditions in the city than in the country may be involved.

Family size has been reported to influence timing of menarche, so that girls from smaller families matured earlier than those from larger families (Malina, 1979; Roberts et al., 1975). In a large sample of girls from northeast England, Roberts and his colleagues (1975) found that the larger the family in which the girl grew up, the later her age at menarche, and that this was independent of social class. In fact, it would appear that in Britain today family size is a more sensitive indicator of general care variables that have biological relevance than are the traditional socioeconomic groups.

Genetic factors also play a substantial role in the timing of menarche. Some evidence of this was given earlier in the comment of the similarity of menarcheal age in twins. Additional evidence from populations comes from migrants to Australia. As we have seen, girls in northwest and central Europe reach menarche at a later average age than those from southeast Europe. Interestingly, among migrant groups to Australia, those girls born in Australia to immigrants from northwest and central Europe had a later median menarcheal age (13.1 years) compared to those born of immigrants from southeast Europe who had an earlier median age (12.5 years) (Jones et al., 1973). The difference is significant and is confirmed by the menarcheal ages of children born before the parents migrated to Australia. This seems to indicate that the northwest–southeast difference is due to genetic differences rather than to nutritional or climatic ones.

INTERRELATIONSHIPS AMONG EVENTS AT PUBERTY

It is important not only to clinicians but also to caregivers and teachers to be aware of the relationships between the appearance of the first menses and other maturational events at puberty. Menarche is a rather late event of puberty and, as stated above, almost always occurs after the peak growth in height (Fig. 3.5). Most girls experience menarche when their breasts are close to achieving adult size and shape (breast stage 4). However, there is considerable individual variability, with menarche occurring at the fully mature breast stage (breast stage 5) or at a less mature one (Marshall, 1977). In British girls, an average of almost 2.5 years elapsed between the beginning of breast development (breast stage 2) and menarche (Marshall and Tanner, 1969). Pubic hair normally appears either before or after the breasts begin to develop. The two usually neither occur simultaneously nor do they progress in unison (Marshall, 1977, 1978). The interrelationship among

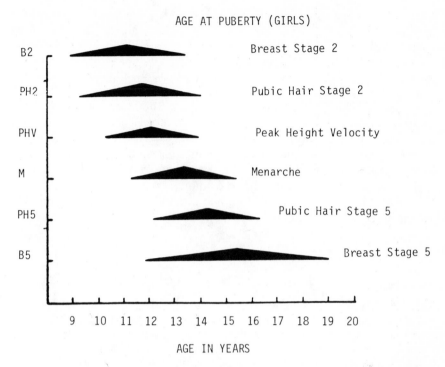

AGE AT PUBERTY (GIRLS)

FIGURE 3.5. Relationship among events of puberty in girls. (After W. A. Marshall, and J.M. Tanner, 1969.)

these events of puberty is more important when assessing normal development than is the chronological age at which they occur.

There is only very little information on population differences in the events of puberty other than menarche. Chinese girls tend to experience menarche and develop breasts earlier than English, Dutch, Parisian, or Indian girls (Eveleth, 1979).

The decline in the age of menarche can be assumed to be a precondition to the current increase in adolescent sexuality and pregnancy. Girls who have reached menarche will be taller, heavier, and more mature in secondary sexual characteristics than those who have not. This, at least, would biologically permit mature sexual relationships if other social and behavioral conditions encouraging them were present. A median age of menarche in the United States of 12.5 to 13 years and an occurrence of first menses in some girls at 9.5 years, even though many of the first menstrual cycles are abnormal in the first years, means that pregnancy is biologically possible as early as 13 or 14 years of age. On the other hand, no secular decrease in menarcheal age has been reported from traditional societies where caloric intake is restricted: menarche still occurs late, and the birth of the first child occurs even later.

SUMMARY

Menarche, or the onset of menstruation, is a major event in adolescent development. There is a wide range among populations of average age at menarche as well as a considerable individual variation. The mean age of menarche among populations ranges from 12.4 to 18.0 years; the individual variation, among American black girls, for example, is 9.5–15.5 years, with a mean age of 12.5 years. In the last 150 years, the mean age of menarche has been declining in Europe and the United States. Factors influencing this secular change are improved nutrition and health. On the average, rural populations and lower socioeconomic groups have a later menarche than urban and upper socioeconomic groups. Genetic factors also play a substantial role in timing of menarche.

REFERENCES

Amundsen, D. W., and Diers, C. J. The age of menarche in classical Greece and Rome. *Human Biology*, 1969, *41*, 125-132.

Amundsen, D. W., and Diers, C. J. The age of menarche in medieval Europe. *Human Biology*, 1973, *45*, 363-370.

Brudevoll, J. E., Liestol, K., and Walloe, L. Menarcheal age in Oslo during the last 140 years. *Annals of Human Biology*, 1979, *6*, 407-416.

Bullough, V. L. Age at menarche: A misunderstanding. *Science*, 1981, *213*, 365-366.

Carfagna, M., Figurelli, E., Matarese, G., and Matarese, S. Menarcheal age of schoolgirls in the District of Naples, Italy, in 1969-70. *Human Biology*, 1972, *44*, 117-125.

Chang, K. S. F. Growth and Development of Chinese Children and Youth in Hong Kong. University of Hong Kong. 1969.

Cristesçu, M., Petrovici, D., and Onofrei, M. Sur l'acceleration du developpement des caracteres sexuels secondaires. *Annuaire Roumain d'Anthropologie*, 1966, *3*, 65-70.

Dreizen, S., Spirakis, C. N., and Stone, R. E. A comparison of skeletal growth and maturation in undernourished and well-nourished girls before and after menarche. *Journal of Pediatrics*, 1967, *70*, 256-264.

Eveleth, P. B. Population differences in growth: Environmental and genetic factors. *In* F. Falkner and J. M. Tanner (Eds.), *Human growth* (Vol 3). New York: Plenum Press, 1979, pp. 373-394.

Eveleth, P. B., and Tanner, J. M. *Worldwide variation in human growth*. Cambridge: Cambridge University Press, 1976.

Fischbein, S. Onset of puberty in MZ and DZ twins. *Acta Genetica Medica Gemellology* (Roma), 1977, *26*, 151-158.

Frisch, R. E. Weight at menarche: Similarity for well-nourished and undernourished girls at differing ages, and evidence for historical constancy. *Pediatrics*, 1972, *50*, 445.

Frisch, R. E. Pubertal adipose tissue: Is it necessary for normal sexual maturation? Evidence from the rat and human female. *Federation Proceedings*, 1980, *39*, 2395-2400.

Frisch, R. E., and McArthur J. W. Menstrual cycles: Fatness as a determinant of minimum weight for height necessary for their maintenance or onset. *Science*, 1974, *185*, 949-951.

Frisch, R. E., Wyshak, G., and Vincent, L. Delayed menarche and amenorrhea in ballet dancers. *New England Journal of Medicine*, 1980, *303*, 17-19.

Heintz, N. Petit-Maire Croissance et puberte feminines au Rwanda. *Memoires Academie Royale des Sciences Naturelles et Medicales*, 1963, *12*, 1-143.

Herlihy, D. The natural history of medieval women. *Natural History*, 1978, *87*, 56-67.

Indian Council of Medical Research (ICMR). *Growth and physical development of Indian infants and children*. Technical Report Series No. 18, ICMR, New Delhi, 1972.

Johnston, F.E., Roche, A.F., Schell, L.M., and Wettenhall, N.B. Critical weight at menarche. *American Journal of Diseases in Children*, 1975, *129*, 19-22.

Jones, D. L., Hemphill, W., and Meyers, E.S.A. Height, weight and other physical characteristics of New South Wales Children. Part I. Children aged five years and over. New South Wales Department of Health, G-96543-a K 5705, 1973.

Jordan, J.R. *Desarrollo humano en Cuba*. Ediciones Cientifico-Tecnica, Ministerio de Cultura, La Habana, 1979.

Laska-Mierzejewska, T., Milicer, H., and Piechaczek, H. Age at menarche and its secular trend in urban and rural girls in Poland. *Human Biology*, 1982, *9*, 227-233.

Lejarraga H., Sanchirico, F., and Cusminsky, M. Age of menarche in urban Argentinian girls. *Annals of Human Biology*, *1980*, 7, 579-582.

Limongi, I. Villarroel, A., Villarroel, V., Ramirez, M., Gonzales M., Arata, G., and Bishop, W. *Variabilidad en el desarrollo puberal de escolares femeninos Venezolanos*. Paper presented at the International Congress of Human Auxology, Havana, Cuba, 1979.

Low, W. D., Kung, L. S., and Leong, J. C. Y. Secular trend in sexual maturation of Chinese girls. *Human Biology*, 1982, *54*, 539-551.

MacMahon, B., *Age at menarche: United States*. U.S. Department of Health, Education and Welfare Publication No. (HRA) 74-1615, NHS, Series 11, No. 133. National Center for Health Statistics, Rockville, Md., 1973.

Malcolm, L. A. Growth and development of the Bundi child of the New Guinea highlands. *Human Biology*, 1970, *42*, 243-328.

Malina, R. M. Secular changes in size and maturity: Causes and effects. *Monographs of the Society for Research in Child Development*, 1979, *179*, 59-102.

Malina, R. M., Harper, A. B., Avent, H. H., and Campbell, D. E. Age at menarche in athletes and nonathletes. *Medicine and Science in Sports*, 1973, *5*, 11-13.

Malina, R. M., Spirduso, W. W., Tate, C., and Baylor, A. M. Age at menarche and selected menstrual characteristics in athletes at different competitive levels and in different sports. *Medicine and Science in Sports*, 1978, *10*, 218-222.

Manniche, E. Age at menarche: Nicolai Edvard Ravn's data on 3385 women in mid-19th century Denmark. *Annals of Human Biology*, 1983, *10*, 79-82.

Marin, B. Edad actual de la menarquia en escolares espanolas. *Archivos de la Facultad de Medicina*, 1971, *5*, 355-362.

Marshall, W. A. *Human growth and its disorders*. New York: Academic Press, 1977.

Marshall, W. A. Puberty. *In* F. Falkner and J. M. Tanner (Eds.), *Human growth* (Vol. 2). New York: Plenum Press, 1978, pp. 141-181.

Marshall, W. A., and Tanner, J. M. Variations in pattern of pubertal changes in girls. *Archives of Diseases in Childhood*, 1969, *44*, 291-303.

Oduntan, S. Olu, Ayeni, O., and Kale, O. O. The age of menarche in Nigerian girls. *Annals of Human Biology*, 1976, *3*, 269-274.

Panek, S., and Paisecki, E. Nowa Huta: Integration of the population in the light of anthropological data. *Materialy: Prace Antropologiczne*, 1971, *80*, 1-249.

Roberts, D. F., Danskin, M. J., and Chinn S. Menarcheal age in Northumberland. *Acta Paediatrica Scandinavia*, 1975, *64*, 845-852.

Sabharwal, K. P., Morales, S., and Mendez, J. Body measurements and creatinine excretion among upper and lower socio-economic groups of girls in Guatemala. *Human Biology*, 1966, *38*, 131-140.

Tanner, J. M. *Trend towards the earlier physical maturation of children, 1850–1965*. Paper presented at the Second Foneme International Convention on Human Formation from Adolescence to Maturity, Milan, Italy, 1969.

Tanner, J. M. Trend toward earlier menarche in London, Oslo, Copenhagen, The Netherlands and Hungary. *Nature*, 1973, *243*, 95-96.

Tanner, J. M. *A history of the study of human growth*. Cambridge: Cambridge University Press, 1981.

Tanner, J. M., and Eveleth P. B. Variability between populations in growth and development at puberty. *In* S. R. Berenberg (Ed.), *Puberty: Biological and psychosocial components*. Leiden: Stenfert Kroese, 1975.

Treloar, A. E. Fecundity potential of the human female, from menarche to menopause. *Human Biology*, 1974, *46*, 89-108.

Uche, G. O., and Okorafor, A. E. The age of menarche in Nigerian urban school girls. *Annals of Human Biology*, 1979, *6*, 395-398.

Vollman, R. F. The length of the premenstrual phase by age of women. *Excerpta Medica*, 1966, series *133*, 1171-1175. (Proceedings of the Fifth World Congress on Fertility and Sterility.)

Wark, M. L., and Malcolm. L. A. Growth and development of the Lumi child of the Sepik district of New Guinea. *Medical Journal of Australia*, 1969, *2*, 129-136.

Wyshak, G., and Frisch, R. E. Evidence for a secular trend in age of menarche. *New England Journal of Medicine*, 1982, *306*, 1033-1035.

Yanagisawa, S., and Kondo, S. Modernization of physical features of Japanese with special reference to leg length and head form. *Journal of Human Ergology*, 1973, *2*, 97-108.

THE NEUROENDOCRINE REGULATION OF PUBERTAL ONSET

Edward O. Reiter

INTRODUCTION

Puberty is the transitional period between the juvenile state and adulthood during which the adolescent growth spurt occurs, secondary sexual characteristics appear, fertility is achieved, and profound psychological changes take place. It is presumed that the metabolic, psychologic, and behavioral modifications ensure the ability not only to bear offspring but also to nurture them within a family setting. The events characterizing pubertal maturation of the reproductive endocrine system are part of a continuum extending from sexual differentiation and ontogeny of the hypothalamic–pituitary gonadotropin–gonadal system in the fetus to senescence (Grumbach, 1980; Reiter and Grumbach, 1982). Two independent processes, controlled by different mechanisms but closely linked temporally, are involved in the increase of sex steroid secretion in the peripubertal and pubertal periods. Adrenarche, the increase in adrenal androgen secretion (in some way related to sex hair growth), precedes by about 2 years the second event, gonadarche, the activation of the hypothalamic–pituitary gonadotropin-gonadal apparatus that had been active at a low level during childhood. We focus here on the latter process.

The regulatory systems that control human male and female reproduction comprise the following fundamental components:

1. The arcuate nucleus of the medial basal hypothalamus and its transducer neurosecretory neurons translate neural signals into a periodic, oscillatory chemical (a decapeptide) signal, gonad-

otropin-releasing hormone (GnRH). GnRH, synthesized by the neurosecretory peptidergic neurons and released from their axon terminals at the median eminence into the primary plexus of the hypothalamic–hypophyseal portal circulation, is transported by this private conduit to the anterior pituitary gland. A growing body of evidence in primates indicates that catecholaminergic, dopaminergic, and opioid neuronal networks, as well as sex steroids, modulate the release of GnRH. The relative importance of these neurotransmitter pathways remains to be established in humans.

2. The pituitary gonadotropes (cells in the pituitary gland secreting the gonadotropins) that, in response to the GnRH rhythmic signal, release LH and FSH in a pulsatile manner at periodic intervals.

3. The gonads (testis, ovary).

This control mechanism, with its three principal components (the arcuate GnRH neurosecretory neurons, the pituitary gonadotropes, and the gonadotropin-responsive elements of the gonad) is common to all mammalian species. It is at each of these loci that modulating factors exercise their effect. Further, at each of the latter two levels, the target cells contain specific cell-surface receptors for the peptide hormones that mediate the cellular response to the signal.

The hypothalamic–pituitary–gonadal system in the human differentiates and functions during fetal life and early infancy, is suppressed to a low level of activity for almost a decade during childhood, and is reactivated during puberty (Grumbach, 1980; Kaplan et al., 1976). In this light, puberty represents not the initiation of pulsatile secretion of GnRH and, thus, of pituitary gonadotropins, but the reactivation, after a protracted period of quiescent or absent activity, of the GnRH neurosecretory neurons in the arcuate nucleus and their endogenous, apparently self-sustaining oscillatory secretion. This system initially is operative in the fetus. Experimental and clinical studies support the hypothesis that the CNS, not the pituitary gland or gonads, restrains the activation of the hypothalamic–pituitary gonadotropin–gonadal system in prepubertal children. This inhibition appears to be mediated through the suppression of GnRH synthesis and its pulsatile secretion (Grumbach, 1980; Conte et al., 1981).

TIMING OF THE ONSET OF PUBERTY

The specific mechanisms involved in the timing of puberty are complex and poorly understood. The average age at onset of puberty shows a secular trend over the past century toward earlier occurrence, cutting across geographic and ethnic lines (Tanner, 1981; Zacharias and Wurtman, 1969). This progressive decline in the age at puberty is thought to be due to improvements in socioeconomic conditions, nutrition, and general health; in developed nations, such a trend appears to have slowed or ceased over the last 20 years (Tanner, 1981).

Influences other than socioeconomic also affect the age at puberty. The association of a minimal percentage of body fat with menarche and the initiation of the pubertal growth spurt and the suggestion of a "critical" factor in altering metabolic rate and hypothalamic function have been widely debated (Frisch and Revelle, 1970; Ojeda et al., 1980). An effect of nutritional factors and body composition upon the time of onset of puberty is supported by the earlier age of menarche in moderately obese girls (Zacharias et al., 1970), by delayed maturation of the reproductive endocrine system in states of malnutrition and chronic illness (McArthur 1976; Reiter et al., 1981, 1982), following early athletic or ballet training (Frisch et al., 1981; Warren, 1980), and by the relationship of amenorrhea to such states of diminished body fat as anorexia nervosa (Sherman et al., 1975), voluntary weight loss (McArthur et al., 1976), and vigorous physical conditioning (Frisch et al., 1981; McArthur et al., 1980; Warren, 1980). When increments in excretion of urinary gonadotropin were correlated with changes in body composition at puberty, however, both developmental events appeared to occur simultaneously rather than sequentially (Penny et al., 1978). Although menarche is a relatively late pubertal event and is removed from those neural factors that influence both the gonadotropin–gonadal sex steroid and physical changes at the initiation of puberty, the possibility exists that some alteration of body metabolism, including the ratio of fat to lean body mass, may affect CNS restraints of pubertal onset. In humans, the pineal gland and melatonin do not appear to have an important inhibitory influence on this control system (Fevre et al., Boyar 1979; Lenko et al., 1981; Sklar et al., 1981) despite a contrary unconfirmed report (Silman et al., 1979).

In the United States, the mean age of menarche is approximately 12.5 chronologic years (Frisch and Revelle, 1970; Grumbach, 1980; Ojeda et al., 1980; Styne and Grumbach, 1978). Another cardinal event of pubertal maturation, considerably less well studied, namely the age of the first conscious ejaculation, has recently been reported to be 14.3 chronologic years in Israel (Laron et al., 1980).

THE PATTERNS OF GONADOTROPIN SECRETION

There are two patterns of gonadotropin secretion: tonic and cyclic (Grumbach, 1980; Reiter and Grumbach, 1982; Styne and Grumbach, 1978). Tonic or basal secretion is regulated by negative or inhibitory feedback mechanisms: Changes in the concentration of circulating sex steroids, and possibly "inhibins" (putative nonsteroidal regulators of FSH secretion produced by germinal tissue), result in reciprocal changes in secretion of pituitary gonadotropins. This is the general pattern of secretion in males and one of the control mechanisms in females. Cyclic secretion involves positive or stimulatory feedback mechanisms: An increment in circulating estrogens to a critical level for a sufficient duration initiates a synchronous, pulsatile burst of LH and FSH (the midcycle surge), which is characteristic of the pattern in normal adult females prior menopause. FSH and LH are probably always secreted in a pulsatile or episodic manner at periodic intervals, irrespective of whether the secretion is tonic or cyclic.

In adult males, pulsatile release of LH has a periodicity of about 90 minutes; the periodicity of the LH secretory episodes is similar in adult females except during the mid- and late-luteal phases of the menstrual cycle, when the LH pulses are diminished to every 3-4 hours. The pulsatile secretion of FSH in normal adults is less prominent; this has been attributed, in part, to the longer half-life of FSH than LH, to differences in the factors that modulate the action of GnRH on FSH and LH release, and to fundamental differences in the secretory pattern for the two gonadotropins.

The physiologic implications of this new concept of gonadotropin secretion was unclear until the classic observations of Knobil and his associates (Knobil, 1980; Knobil et al., 1980; Pohl and Knobil, 1982) in the rhesus monkey. They described the inhibition of gonadotropin secretion by the continuous infusion of GnRH via desensitization or down-regulation of gonadotrope GnRH receptors (Clayton and Catt, 1981; Nett et al., 1981). Discontinuous or pulsatile stimulation (e.g., 1 μg/min) by GnRH restores pulsatile release of gonadotropin in adult monkeys with hypothalamic lesions that had obliterated arcuate nuclei and thus extinguished endogenous GnRH secretion. These studies provided evidence that the GnRH input to the pituitary gonadotropes is frequency-coded. Intermittent abrupt rises of GnRH levels in portal blood occur at intervals of 2 to 3.5 hours. In a single patient whose portal blood was sampled during surgery, over 100-fold variation in GnRH levels was demonstrated (Carmel et al., 1979).

GONADOTROPIN LEVELS FROM FETAL LIFE THROUGH PUBERTY

The changing pattern of gonadotropin and sex steroid secretion according to age and level of maturation has been discussed and are shown schematically in Fig. 4.1 (Grumbach, 1980; Ojeda et al., 1980; Reiter and Grumbach, 1982; Styne and Grumbach, 1978). Kaplan and her associates (1976); (see Table 4.2, this chapter for review) described development of pituitary gonadotropin secretion in the fetus from the third month of gestation. The pattern of changes of FSH and LH concentrations in fetuses is consistent with a sequence of increased syn-

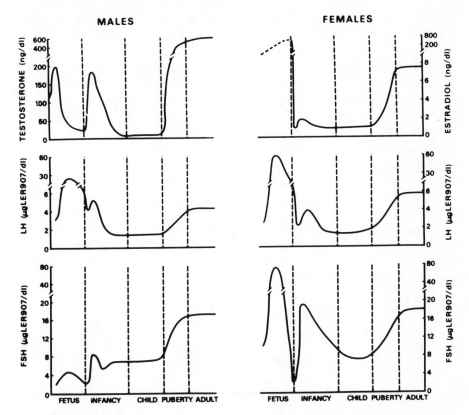

FIGURE 4.1. Schematic representation of changes in gonadotropin and sex steroid levels in males and females from fetus to adulthood (Winter et al., 1975, 1976).

thesis and secretion in which peak serum concentrations reach adult castrate levels at midterm followed by a decline that persists to delivery.

After the fall in sex steroids, especially estrogens, during the first days after birth, the concentration of FSH and LH increases and exhibits wide perturbations during the first months of life; intermittent high gonadotropin concentrations are associated with increased testosterone values in male infants and estradiol levels in females (Winter et al., 1975, 1976). By about 6 months in males and 1–2 years in females, concentrations of gonadotropins decrease to the low levels present during childhood until the onset of puberty.

In the peripubertal period, gonadotropin concentrations rise. In girls, FSH levels rise during the early stages of puberty and then plateau, whereas LH levels tend to rise in later stages; in boys, FSH concentrations rise progressively during puberty, whereas LH levels increase sharply in early pubertal development and then gradually rise throughout the remainder of pubertal maturation. In addition to these changes in immunoreactive gonadotropins, serum concentrations of biologically active LH have been quantified throughout life (Dufau et al., 1977; Reiter et al., 1982). In human studies, bioactive LH concentrations are usually undetectable during prepubertal years, then rise dramatically during pubertal maturation (Reiter et al., 1982). The increment in mean LH levels between pubertal and prepubertal states has generally been greater using bioassays than standard immunoassay techniques, perhaps because of methodologic problems but possibly related to qualitative changes in the LH molecule.

EPISODIC RELEASE OF GONADOTROPINS AND THE DEVELOPMENT OF CIRCADIAN RHYTHMS

In adult men and in women during the follicular and early luteal phases, discrete episodic or pulsatile bursts of LH occur about once very 90 minutes (Judd, 1979; Rebar and Yen, 1979) (see Fig. 4.2). In prepubertal children, some, but not all, investigators have found se-

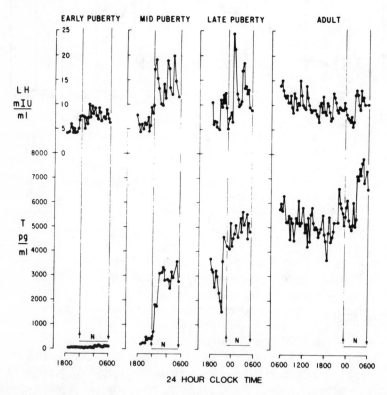

FIGURE 4.2. Changes in pulsatile release in LH and testosterone from prepubertal to adult years in normal males (Judd, 1979).

cretory episodic bursts of LH (Judd, 1979; Penny et al., 1977); the pulses are of lower amplitude than in pubertal children or adults. Penny et al. (1977) pointed out that the increase in the plasma concentration of LH during puberty changes in frequency. In such studies, concentrations of gonadotropins are low, and it is often difficult to demonstrate episodic release for methodologic and statistical reasons. Mainly sleep-associated pulsatile release of LH occurs in early and midpuberty; only late in puberty are prominent LH pulses noted during the day (Boyar et al., 1972). In addition, pulsatile release of FSH occurs in pubertal individuals, although the spikes are smaller than those of LH (Judd, 1979).

In addition to ultradian (episodic) fluctuations of gonadotropin release, a circadian rhythm (with nocturnal peaking) develops during late childhood and adolescent years. In prepubertal boys, Parker et al. (1975), but not Boyer et al. (1972), reported significant LH increments in some sleeping children. When a larger group of prepubertal subjects were studied, the discrepancies appear to have been resolved (Judd, 1979). In boys younger than 10.5 years, LH concentrations rose significantly in only 22% of nights, while in the older prepubertal boys, LH levels were greater during sleep in 78% of nights. Generally similar, although somewhat less striking, nocturnal increments have been described in serum FSH levels in prepubertal and late prepubertal children. During puberty, there is further maturation of sleep-enhanced LH secretion, presumably related to alterations in CNS restraint of the hypothalamic GnRH pulse generator that leads to increased activity initially, mainly during sleep. In early and mid-pubertal subjects, pulsatile LH release occurs largely during sleep; in late puberty, pulsatile release is demonstrable throughout the whole day and simulates the adult pattern. The factors that lead to the initiation and development of this circadian rhythm remain unclear; patients with early sexual maturation as in idiopathic precocious puberty, who have early onset of true puberty, exhibit the same pattern of LH secretion as normal pubertal children (Boyar et al., 1973a). The pattern of enhanced sleep-associated LH secretion occurring in agonadal patients during the pubertal period suggests that this pattern does not depend upon gonadal function (Boyar et al., 1973b).

Such sleep-associated LH release appears to correlate with increased sensitivity of pituitary gonadotropes to administration of GnRH in the peripubertal period and during puberty (Beck and Wuttke, 1980; Corley et al., 1981).

CENTRAL NERVOUS SYSTEM AND THE ONSET OF PUBERTY

In both human and nonhuman primates, the increased LH and FSH secretion in the fetus and during infancy is followed by a long period,

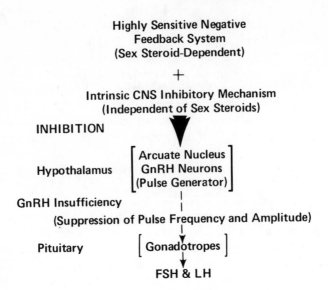

FIGURE 4.3. Dual mechanism of restraints of puberty (Reiter and Grumbach, 1982).

approximately one decade, in which the reproductive endocrine system is suppressed (Grumbach, 1980; Grumbach et al., 1974; Reiter and Grumbach, 1982; Styne and Grumbach, 1978). The factors involved in this restraint of the onset of puberty are not well understood. Two mechanisms have been involved to explain the prepubertal impediment by the CNS of gonadotropin secretion. One is a sex steroid-dependent mechanism, a highly sensitive hypothalamic–pituitary–gonadal negative feedback system. The other is a sex-steroid-independent mechanism that can be ascribed to "intrinsic" CNS inhibitory influences (Grumbach, 1980; Conte et al., 1975, 1981) (Figure 4.3).

NEGATIVE FEEDBACK MECHANISM (SEX STEROID-DEPENDENT)

Hohlweg and Dohrn (1932) suggested 50 years ago that at puberty a CNS "sexualzentrum" that regulates gonadotropin secretion changed its sensitivity to circulating sex steroids. Studies in the fetal sheep, which has a pattern of fetal pituitary gonadotropin secretion similar to that of the human fetus, describe a decrement in GnRH-evoked gonadotropin release after midgestation with advancing gestational age (Mueller et al., 1981). The inhibition of hypothalamic–GnRH release and lowered pituitary gonadotropin secretion appear to be consequences of the progressive acquisition of increased sensitivity of the hypothalamic "gonadostat" (the arcuate GnRH neurosecretory neurons), and probably the pituitary gland, to inhibitory effects of high concentrations of sex steroids in the fetal circulation. This hypothalamic–

regulatory mechanism is not fully developed at birth. During childhood, this tonic control mechanism is exquisitely sensitive to the suppressive effect of small amounts of circulating sex steroids. Coincident with the onset of puberty, the hypothalamic–gonadostat (the arcuate nucleus), and possibly the pituitary gland, becomes progressively less sensitive to inhibitory effects of sex steroids upon GnRH release, which results in increased release of GnRH in a pulsatile pattern and enhanced secretion of gonadotropins. In adults, the hypothalamic–pituitary negative feedback mechanism is less sensitive to feedback by sex steroids, and adult levels of gonadotropins and sex steroids are present.

Evidence for an operative and highly sensitive negative feedback mechanism in prepubertal children has been summarized (Grumbach et al., 1974; Reiter and Grumbach, 1982): (1) The pituitary gland in the prepubertal child secretes small amounts of FSH and LH, suggesting that the hypothalamic–pituitary, gonadotropin–gonadal complex operates during childhood, but at a low level of activity. (2) The low level of gonadotropin secretion in childhood is rapidly shut off by administration of sex steroids. When small amounts of estrogens are administered to prepubertal children, a quick and significant decrease in gonadotropin secretion ensues (Kelch, et al., 1972); in contrast, considerably higher levels of estrogen are required to suppress gonadotropin secretion in the adult (Kulin and Reiter, 1972). The elevated gonadotropin concentration in infancy and early childhood in agonadal patients is evidence that hormones secreted by the normal prepubertal gonad, despite their low level, inhibit gonadotropin secretion.

"INTRINSIC" CNS INHIBITORY MECHANISM (SEX STEROID-INDEPENDENT)

The diphasic pattern of basal and GnRH-induced FSH and LH secretion from infancy to adulthood (i.e., higher in the first year of life than in the next 8–10 years) is qualitatively similar in normal individuals and in patients with gonadal dysgenesis, but in the latter, gonadotropin levels are strikingly higher except during the mid-childhood nadir (Conte et al., 1975). The striking fall in gonadotropin secretion and reserve (Conte et al., 1981) in agonadal children 4–11 years old (mid-childhood nadir) suggests the presence of CNS inhibitory influences independent of gonadal sex steroid secretion that restrain gonadotropin production and delay of the onset of puberty. Such a pattern cannot be explained by gonadal sex steroid feedback since functional gonads are lacking, or by increased secretion of adrenal sex steroids, since concentrations are low and suppression of the adrenal does not augment serum levels of gonadotropins. The nature of this postulated intrinsic CNS inhibitory system during infancy and childhood remains uncertain (Figure 4.4). Suppression of this neural inhibitory mechanism would lead to reactivation of gonadotropin secretion at puberty. In pa-

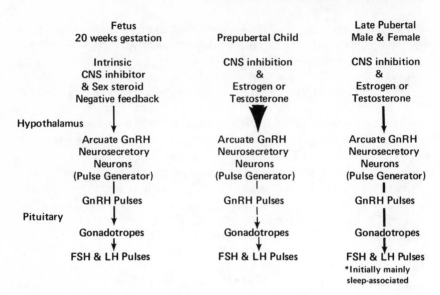

FIGURE 4.4. Scheme illustrating the changes in the activity of the arcuate GnRH
pulse generator during development and the effect on pituitary
gonadotropes and the hypothesis that the functional GnRH insufficiency of the prepubertal child is a consequence of CNS restraint by sex steroid-dependent and sex steroid-independent
mechanisms (Reiter and Grumbach, 1982).

tients who develop true precocious puberty due to hypothalamic lesions, the intrinsic CNS inhibitory system is impaired and results in the
premature appearance of the augmented, pulsatile gonadotropin secretion characteristic of puberty.

Whether the possible inhibitory effects of opioids (Morley et al., 1980;
Moult et al., 1981; Quigley et al., 1980; Quigley and Yen, 1980) and
dopamine (Huseman et al., 1980; Quigley et al., 1980) on gonadotropin
secretion can be translated to the prepubertal period remains to be
established. Preliminary studies administering opiate and dopamine
inhibitors have yielded inconclusive results in childhood. The location
of the negative feedback mechanism is not defined. Present evidence
suggests that estrogen-induced gonadotropin suppression occurs at
both the hypothalamic and pituitary levels (Knobil, 1980; Pohl and
Knobil, 1982).

INTRINSIC MATURATIONAL CHANGES IN THE CONTEXT OF ENVIRONMENTAL INFLUENCE

As indicated in the earlier discussion relating the timing of the onset
of puberty to various factors, there appear to be many influences upon
the age of onset of pubertal development. Nutritional factors and the

body fat composition, levels of activity and energy utilization, psychosocial phenomena, and such climatic events as seasonality (e.g., photoperiodicity) have all been implicated as controlling factors. In the context of the discussion that has just been completed, one must consider these varied influences as affecting the hypothalamic GnRH pulse generator, which alters the character of LH secretory patterns that stimulate gonadal tissue. With the exception of humans, some higher primates, and domesticated species that humans have protected from the pressures of annual environmental change, most other mammals confine sexual activity to a breeding season. At other times, they are anovulatory and do not exhibit mating behavior (Foster and Ryan, 1982). The primary external controlling factor for this type of behavior is photoperiod, providing the environmental cue on a yearly basis. In addition, as studied in the developing lamb, adequate nutritional status must be achieved before the effect of the appropriate photoperiod may be expressed (Karsch and Foster, 1981; Foster and Ryan, 1982). These external cues, namely photoperiod and nutritional status, alter feedback sensitivity, not only to govern the onset of fertility in the lamb but to then regulate the reproductive seasonality in the adult.

The neuroendocrine modulators of this alteration of estradiol sensitivity are not known. In lower animals, the pineal gland has been considered as a photoneuroendocrine mediator of seasonal reproduction, although its role in higher species is obscure. As noted earlier, its role in primates has certainly been open to question, with recent studies suggesting limited influence.

Although elegant studies in young and adult sheep have examined the influence of photoperiod, nutritional status and even pheromones upon the maturation of the hypothalamic–pituitary–gonadal axis, their significance for primate reproductive behavior and neuroendocrine regulation is not obvious. Although considerable experimental energy has been devoted to examine the effects of a so-called "critical weight" or associated metabolic activity upon the events of puberty, a mechanistic relationship of altered body composition or metabolic rate and a change in function of the GnRH pulse regulator is not available. In general terms, the need to achieve adequate nutritional growth status is true in the primate, but full sexual development and reproductive function with adult-level activity of the reproductive endocrine system may occur in the child of several years of age. The premature activation of the hypothalamic pulse generator in the syndrome of idiopathic precocious puberty demonstrates that CNS dysfunction may override environmental cues such as the body weight, fat composition, or socioeconomic conditions. It may be that the varied extraneuroendocrine influences upon puberty do not, in fact, regulate the process but merely serve to modulate a genomically determined neuroendocrine activity and to affect its expression (Foster and Ryan, 1982).

THE INTERACTION OF SYNTHETIC GnRH WITH PITUITARY GONADOTROPIN SECRETION

If increased secretion of gonadotropins with the approach of puberty is a consequence of a change in neural and hormonal restraints on synthesis and pulsatile secretion of GnRH, the disinhibition of the arcuate GnRH oscillator should lead to increased GnRH pulses (frequency and amplitude) initially, followed by increased gonadotropin secretion by the pituitary and, finally, to augmented output of sex steroids by the gonad. GnRH secretion is not readily measured directly in the human being; however, endogenous release can be assessed indirectly and qualitatively by the gonadotropin response to exogenous GnRH (Grumbach et al., 1974). With the availability of synthetic GnRH, the pituitary sensitivity to GnRH and the dynamic reserve or readily releasable pool of pituitary gonadotropins have been examined during different stages of pubertal maturation and in many disorders involving the hypothalamic–pituitary–gonadal system. The results support the concept that the prepubertal state is characterized by functional GnRH insufficiency (Grumbach, 1980; Grumbach et al., 1974; Reiter and Grumbach, 1982).

The release of LH following the administration of GnRH is minimal in prepubertal children beyond infancy, increases strikingly during the peripubertal period and puberty, and is still greater in adult males and females. The change in the maturity-related patterns of FSH release after administration of GnRH is quite different from that of LH and results in a striking reversal of the FSH/LH ratio of gonadotropin release. Prepubertal and pubertal females release much more FSH than males at all stages of sexual maturation. Prepubertal girls, in fact, have a larger readily releasable pool of pituitary FSH than pubertal girls or prepubertal or pubertal males. Because basal levels of serum FSH and LH are similar in prepubertal children, the dramatic difference in secretion of FSH and LH evoked by GnRH administration demonstrates clearly the difference between pituitary sensitivity and the actual basal secretory rate of FSH and LH.

The heightened LH response of pituitary gonadotropes to exogenous GnRH in peripubertal children who do not yet exhibit physical signs of sexual maturation provides further evidence that the self-priming effect (Grumbach et al., 1974; Reiter and Grumbach, 1982) of endogenous GnRH augments pituitary responsiveness to exogenous GnRH. The degree of previous exposure of gonadotropes to endogenous GnRH appears to affect both the magnitude and quality of LH responses to a single dose of GnRH. Before puberty, the low setpoint of the hypothalamic gonadostat to inhibitory feedback effects of low concentrations of plasma sex steroids as well as intrinsic CNS factors suppress secretion of GnRH. As a result, the prepubertal pituitary gland has a small pool of releasable LH and, thus, decreased responsiveness to acute administration of synthetic GnRH. With the approach of puberty, increased release of endogenous GnRH increases the number of LH receptors on the gonadotrope (Clayton and Catt, 1981), augments pituitary sensitivity to exogenous GnRH, and enlarges the reserve of LH in the gonadotrope. The explanation for the discordance of FSH and LH release during maturation is not clear, but recent studies by Knobil (1980) with differing modes of administration of GnRH suggest that the pulse frequency of the pattern of secretion of endogenous GnRH is a major factor. Reducing GnRH pulse frequency from one every hour to one every 3 hours strikingly increased the ratio of FSH to LH. Further, endogenous sex steroids may affect this ratio (e.g., differential inhibitory effects of testosterone and estradiol on FSH and LH release).

These findings and the above-noted phenomenon of gonadotrope desensitization by chronic GnRH administration led to the administration of GnRH by intermittent intravenous infusion (Knobil, 1980). When GnRH was given intermittently, gonadotropin secretion did not show refractoriness and was fully reestablished in animals with lesions of the medial basal hypothalamus in which the arcuate nucleus (and its GnRH neurons) was obliterated. When GnRH was administered to prepubertal monkeys in a pulsatile manner, spontaneous menstrual cycles were established (Knobil, 1980; Pohl and Knobil 1982). These data dramatically demonstrated the importance of the pattern of GnRH administration and stimulated a series of investigations in humans.

When GnRH was administered by varying routes to patients with hypogonadotropic hypogonadism, immature responses to standard GnRH tests were normalized. Treatment of males with LH and FSH deficiency with hourly subcutaneous pulses of GnRH on 10 successive nights led to increased mean gonadotropin levels, the appearance of pulsatile LH secretion, and a greater augmentation of LH than FSH secretion (Jacobson et al., 1979). In other series of patients with hypogonadotropic hypogonadism due to primary hypothalamic dysfunction or to anorexia nervosa, a 5-day low-dose program of intermittent intravenous GnRH achieved a maturation of gonadotrope function (Marshall and Kelch, 1979; Valk et al., 1980). These studies suggest that administration of GnRH in a pulsatile manner, presumably comparable to that which occurs in the normal individual, leads to reversal of the FSH/LH ratio, as is commonly seen during spontaneous pubertal development. The data provide further indirect support for the reawakening of augmented pulsatile GnRH release by the arcuate nucleus oscillator (rather than basic changes at the level of the gonad or anterior pituitary) as the first hormonal change in the onset of puberty.

MATURATION OF THE POSITIVE FEEDBACK MECHANISM

In normal women, the midcycle surge in LH and FSH secretion is attributed to the positive feedback effect of an increased, critical concentration of estradiol for a sufficient length of time during the latter part of the follicular phase. This stimulatory effect of estradiol upon gonadotropin secretion has not been demonstrated in prepubertal or early pubertal girls; it is a later maturational event and does not occur before midpuberty (Grumbach et al., 1974; Reiter et al., 1974). Development of positive feedback action of estradiol requires: (1) ovarian follicles primed by FSH to secrete sufficient estradiol to reach and maintain a critical level in the circulation; (2) a pituitary gland that is sensitized by estrogen to amplify and augment the effect of GnRH and that contains a large enough pool of releasable LH to provide an LH surge; and (3) in addition to the usual adult pattern of pulsatile LH–RH secretion, sufficient GnRH stores for GnRH neurosecretory neurons to respond to estradiol stimulation with an acute increase in GnRH release, though this last requirement has not been firmly established in primates.

Estrogen-induced positive feedback seems to occur directly at the pituitary level so long as the gonadotropes are being or have been recently exposed to GnRH (Knobil, 1980). Moreover, Knobil et al. (Knobil, 1980; Knobil et al., 1982) reestablished menstrual cyclicity in lesioned monkeys by chronic intermittent administration of GnRH. Pulsatile GnRH treatment at a fixed dose led to sufficient gonadotropin secretion to stimulate estradiol synthesis and release by ovarian follicles and to induce an ovulatory LH surge in the absence of an endogenous hypothalamic GnRH secretory surge. Hence, an increase in neither frequency nor amplitude of GnRH pulse is required to induce a midcycle LH surge. However, the data do not exclude the possibility that, in the normal adult female, estrogen also induces an increase in GnRH release and, thus, has a positive feedback effect on both the pituitary gland and the hypothalamic GnRH neurons.

Even though gonadotropin cyclicity and estrogen-induced positive feedback have been demonstrated by midpuberty and prior to menarche, the positive feedback loop does not appear to be complete at that time (Grumbach et al., 1974; Reiter et al., 1974). Indeed, the modulating action of the pubertal ovary in its output of estradiol on the hypothalamic–pituitary–gonadotropin unit appears insufficient to induce an ovulatory LH surge even when there are adequate pituitary stores of readily releasable LH and FSH. The ovary, from either lack of sufficient gonadotropin stimulation or decreased responsivity, does not secrete estradiol in sufficent amount or duration to induce the ovulatory LH surge.

The hormonal patterns of postmenarchal adolescents reflect the

TABLE 4.1. Ovulatory and Anovulatory Cycles in Postmenarchal Years[a]

Age (years postmenarchal)	Ovulatory	Anovulatory	Ovulatory (%)
0–0.9 ($N = 28$)[b]	2	24	14
1–1.9 ($N = 29$)	8	18	38
2–2.9 ($N = 20$)	9	10	50
3–3.9 ($N = 21$)	7	11	48
4–4.9 ($N = 25$)	14	9	64
5–6.3 ($N = 15$)	12	2	87

[a] Modified from D. Apter (1980).
[b] Number of cycles studied.

transition from anovulatory to ovulatory cycles, showing changes in cyclic secretion of gonadotropins, estrogens, androgens, and progesterone; the latter has generally been used as a marker of development of a corpus luteum, providing evidence for ovulation (Apter et al., 1978; Apter, 1980). The incidence of ovulatory cycles is shown in Table 4.1. Not only are there cycles in which ovulation has or has not occurred, but the duration of luteal activity only gradually evolves to the "adult" length. Thus, development of fertility of female adolescents must be considered as a continuous process of variable duration. Not only is the percentage of ovulatory cycles increasing with postmenarchal years, but also the attainment of the proper hormonal milieu for implantation of a fertilized ovum (i.e., an appropriate progesterone-secreting corpus luteum) is occurring.

Similar extensive studies have not been undertaken in males to relate presence of viable spermatozoa to hormonal changes. As cyclicity is not a prerequisite for germinal maturation in the testes, it would appear that quantitative and progressive hormonal changes (as have been noted above) rather than further qualitative hypothalamic disinhibition determine fertility.

Table 4.2 summarizes the proposed development of the hypothalamic–pituitary gonadotropin–gonadal apparatus.

ADRENARCHE (CONTROL OF ADRENAL ANDROGENESIS)

The adrenal component of adolescent maturation, with a characteristic late pre- and early pubertal increase in adrenal androgen secretion is not well understood (Cutler and Loriaux, 1980; Grumbach et al., 1978; Parker and Odell, 1980). Both cross-sectional and longitudinal studies have shown a significant increment in adrenal androgen secretion by 8 years of age in both boys and girls. A progressive rise in plasma concentrations of adrenal androgens occurs during late childhood and adolescence, correlated with the growth and development of the zona reticularis of the adrenal cortex, reaching adult levels in late adolescence. Gonadotropin and gonadal steroid concentrations

TABLE 4.2. Postulated Ontogeny of Hypothalamic–Pituitary Gonadotropin–Gonadal Circuit

A. Fetus
   1. Hypothalamic arcuate GnRH neurosecretory neurons (pulse generator) operative by 80 days gestation
   2. Episodic secretion of FSH and LH by 80 days gestation
   3. Initially unrestrained secretion of GnRH (100–150 days)
   4. Maturation of negative sex steroid feedback mechanisms after 150 days gestation—sex difference
   5. Low level of GnRH secretion at term

B. Early infancy
   1. Arcuate GnRH pulse generator highly functional after 12 days of age
   2. Prominent RSH and LH episodic discharges until about age 6 months in males and 12 months in females with transient increase in plasma levels of testosterone and estradiol in males and females, respectively

C. Late infancy and childhood
   1. Negative feedback control of FSH and LH secretion becomes highly sensitive to sex steroids (low setpoint), maximum sensitivity attained by age 2–4 years
   2. Intrinsic CNS inhibition of arcuate GnRH pulse generator operative, maximum sensitivity by about 4 years
   3. Arcuate GnRH pulse generator inhibited; amplitude and probably frequency of GnRH discharges low
   4. Secretion of FHS, LH, and sex steroids is low

D. Late prepubertal period
   1. Decreasing sensitivity of hypothalamic–pituitary unit to sex steroids (increased setpoint) and decreasing effectiveness of intrinsic CNS inhibitory influences
   2. Increased amplitude and frequency of GnRH pulses; initially most prominent with sleep (nocturnal)
   3. Increased sensitivity of gonadotropes to GnRH
   4. Increased secretion of FSH and LH
   5. Increased responsiveness of gonad to FSH and LH
   6. Increased secretion of gonadal hormones

E. Puberty
   1. Further decrease in CNS restraint of arcuate GnRH neurons including the sensitivity of negative feedback mechanism to sex steroids
   2. Prominent sleep-associated increase in episodic secretion of GnRH gradually changes to adult pattern of pulses every 90–120 minutes
   3. Pulsatile secretion of LH follows pattern of GnRH
   4. Progressive development of secondary sex characteristics
   5. Mid- to late puberty–maturation of positive feedback mechanism and capacity to exhibit an estrogen-induced LH surge
   6. Spermatogenesis in male; ovulation in female

do not begin to increase until approximately 2 years after the adrenarche. It appears, therefore, that activation of adrenal androgen-secreting mechanisms normally precede activation of a hypothymic–pituitary gonadotropin-gonadal axis. This temporal relationship between the adrenarche and maturation of gonadal function has suggested that adrenal androgens may play an important role in the onset of gonadarche.

Considerable information, however, suggests that adrenarche and gonadarche are independent events, apparently controlled by separate mechanisms, and that adrenarche is not essential for the onset of gonadarche (Grumbach et al., 1978; Sklar et al., 1980). In support of this hypothesis has been the demonstration that onset of puberty and the age of menarche occur within the normal range in patients with primary adrenal insufficiency as well as in patients with premature adrenarche, thus either in absence of adrenal androgens or in presence of modestly elevated levels (Grumbach et al., 1978). In further studies, in patients with idiopathic precocious puberty, functional agonadism, and precocious adrenarche, a dissociation between adrenarche and gonadarche were again described (Sklar et al., 1981).

The control of adrenal androgen secretion has not been well defined. Three different mechanisms have been discussed: (1) an intrinsic alteration in the activity of enzymes involved in adrenal androgenesis; (2) secretion of an extrapituitary factor, such as an estrogen; and (3) a pituitary androgen-stimulating hormone, as yet uncharacterized. None of these hypotheses has been buttressed by sufficient experimental data to make them acceptable. The most recent, and perhaps most attractive, hypothesis is that a putative and elusive adrenal–androgen stimulating hormone (AASH), in the presence of ACTH, induces differentiation of the zona reticularis and synthesis and secretion of adrenal androgens and adrenarche, an event that occurs independently of activation of the hypothymic–pituitary gonadotropin–gonadal axis.

SUMMARY

The events that characterize the maturation of the reproductive endocrine system during the time of puberty and that culminate in the attainment of fertility have been considered largely from the neuroendocrinologic point of view. In this context, hypothalamic neurosecretory cells integrate neuronal input from higher cortical centers to develop an oscillatory program of stimulation of pituitary gonadotropin secreting cells. Throughout early childhood years, this hypothalamic system is largely dormant; a poorly understood process of temporal and maturational events leads to activation of the arcuate nucleus pulse generator at puberty. Socioeconomic conditions, nutritional status, and altered degrees of energy expenditure seem to be factors in determining the time of pubertal events that lead to the intricate and subtle orchestration of the adult menstrual cycle.

The maturational events that culminate in ovulation and spermatogenesis have been detailed, with greater emphasis placed on studies in the female where more data are available. Of major significance to this discussion is the ability of the adolescent ovary not only to ovulate but also to maintain an environment in which a fertilized ovum may be implanted in a receptive uterine endometrium. The hormonal milieu necessary for that environment requires an appropriately functioning corpus luteum. The preovulatory ovary initiates its own ovulatory stimulus by producing sufficient estrogen to trigger the release of pituitary LH which leads to rupture of the follicle and release of the ovum. Thus, the ovary must produce enough estrogen to elicit an ovulatory LH spike. In addition, growth and development of the postovulatory follicle, namely the corpus luteum, depends upon hormonal events that occurred prior to the ovulatory event. An adequate interaction between intraovarian estrogen and stimulatory gonadotropins in cells of the preovulatory follicle is needed to create a corpus luteum with life span and steroidogenic capacity adequate to produce sufficient progesterone to nurture the uterine endometrium, the site at which the fertilized ovum fulfills its destiny. It seems, therefore, that the complex neuroendocrine maturational changes that we have discussed and that lead to increasing gonadotropin stimulation of the ovaries must initiate extremely complex intraovarian events which result not only insufficient estrogen to trigger ovulation but also permit the postovulatory follicle to exist as a progesterone-secreting uterothrophic organ adequate to sustain the early stages of pregnancy.

Although the neuroendocrine control of the gonadotropin secretory process that results in ovulation in adult women has now been studied in great detail (though many questions remain), the maturational process that extends from the first ovulation and postmenarchal ovulatory frequency of less than 15 to a 90% ovulatory frequency in the sixth postmenarchal year is not understood. Further, the adequacy of corpus luteum function during teenage years has been examined less thoroughly so that such questions as the relationship of an adequate luteal progesterone secretory system to body energy stores, lipid composition, and general nutritional and health status remains elusive. The temporal relationship between age of menarche and the time of onset of ovulatory cycles has been assessed. This indirectly may provide some answer to the question as to whether there is a secular trend in the establishment of fecundibility. Vihko and Apter (Endocrine Society Proceedings, 1983) further refined their longitudinal studies of the onset of ovulatory menstrual cycles in adolescent years: Early menarche was associated with early onset of ovulatory cycles. The times from menarche until the presence of ovulatory cycles in 50% of cycles studied related directly to the ages of menarche: Girls with menarchal age below 12 developed ovulatory cycles about 1 year later, those with menarche between 12 and 13 years, and those greater with menarche after 13 in 4.5 years. Thus, in view of the already established relationships between the age of menarche and the multiple factors included in Frisch's "Critical Fatness Hypothesis," one could draw a further conclusion that there is an association between ovulatory cycles and body composition; but this conclusion is complex, especially when one realizes that merely 2 years difference in age of menarche is associated with over a fourfold difference in the menarche–fecundity interval.

The ovary must "learn" not only to interact with a maturing neuroendocrine apparatus (to ovulate) but, as importantly, to function as an early pregnancy sustenance organ. Although the reasonability of a relationship between many nonendocrine events (which would determine the ability of the organism to succeed in pregnancy, delivery, and parenthood) and the neurohumoral and ovarian secretory capabilities must seem obvious, no quantitative experimental data substantiate the notion.

The relationship of the adrenarche to a circular trend, or more generally to a nutritional/energy expenditure model, is not clearly established. Certainly, in simple terms, the first appearance of pubic hair, as a marker of early puberty in many studies in the past, in all likelihood would correlate with early adolescent growth and thus with the surge in weight or body fat. Young obese girls tend to have an earlier appearance of pubic hair growth, but these observations are not substantiated by careful measurement of adrenal androgen secretion. Further, the delay in pubic hair growth was less than that of breast development and menarche in studies of ballet dancers (and in young female athletes), suggesting that the neuroendocrine or local adrenal mechanisms that control the onset of production of adrenal androgens are less susceptible to the maturation-inhibiting effects of extreme energy expenditure or diminished total body fat content. Clearly, the association of the adrenarche with nutritional status awaits careful examination utilizing modern biochemical techniques in a prospective manner.

REFERENCES

Apter, D. Serum steroids and pituitary hormones in female puberty: A partly longitudinal study. *Clinical Endocrinology*, 1980, *12*, 107–120.

Apter, D., Viinikka, L., and Vihok, R. Hormonal pattern of adolescent menstrual cycles. *Journal of Clinical Endocrinology and Metabolism*, 1978, 47, 944–954.

Beck, W., and Wuttke, W. Diurnal variations of plasma luteinizing hormone, follicle-stimulating hormone, and prolactin in boys and girls from birth to puberty. *Journal of Clinical Endocrinology and Metabolism*, 1980, 50, 635–639.

Boyar, R., Finkelstein, J., Roffwarg, H., Kapen, S., Weitzman, E., and Hellman, L. Synchronization of augmented luteinizing hormone secretion with sleep during puberty. *New England Journal of Medicine*, 1972, *287*, 582–86.(a)

Boyar, R., Finkelstein, J.W., David, R., Roffwarg, H., Kapen, S., Weitzman, E.D., and Hellman, L. Twenty-four hour patterns of plasma luteinizing hormone and follicle stimulating hormone in sexual precocity. *New England Journal of Medicine*, 1973, *289*, 282–286.(a)

Boyar, R.M., Finkelstein, J.W., Roffwarg, H., Kapen, S., Weitzman, E.D., and Hellman, L. Twenty-four hour luteinizing hormone and follicle stimulating hormone secretory pattern in gonadal dysgenesis. *Journal of Clinical Endocrinology and Metabolism*, 1973, *37*, 521–525.(b)

Carmel, P.W., Antunes, J.L., and Ferin, M. Collection of blood from the pituitary stalk and portal veins in monkeys, and from the pituitary sinusoidal system in monkey and man. *Journal of Neurosurgery*, 1979, *50*, 75–80.

Clayton, R.N., and Catt, K.J. Gonadotropin-releasing hormone receptors: Characterization, physiologic regulation and relationship to reproductive function. *Endocrine Review*, 1981, *2*, 186–209.

Conte, F.A., Grumbach, M.M., and Kaplan, S.L. A diphasic pattern of gonadotropin secretion in patients with the syndrome of gonadal dysgenesis. *Journal of Clinical Endocrinology and Metabolism*, 1975, *40*, 670–74.

Conte, F.A., Grumbach, M.M., Kaplan, S.L., and Reiter, E.O. Correlation of LRF-induced LH and FSH release from infancy to 19 years with the changing pattern of gonadotropin secretion in agonadal patients. *Journal of Clinical Endocrinology and Metabolism*, 1981, *50*, 1163–68.

Corley, K.P., Valk, T.W., Kelch, R.P., and Marshall, J.C. Estimation of GnRH pulse amplitude during pubertal development. *Pediatric Research 15*, 157–62.

Cutler, G.B., and Loriaux, D.L. Adrenarche and its relationship to the onset of puberty. *Federation Proceedings 39*, 2384–90.

Dufau, M.L., Beitins, I.Z., McArthur, J., and Catt, K. Bioassay of serum LH concentrations in normal and LH-RH stimulated human subjects. *In* P. Trom and H.R. Nankin (Eds.), *The testis in normal and infertile men*. New York: Raven Press, pp. 309–325.

Fevre, M., Boyar, R.M., and Rollag, M.D. Dosage radioimmunologique de la melatonine au cours du nycthemere chez le garcon pubere. *Annales of Endocrinology Paris* 1979, *40*, 555–56.

Foster, D.L., and Ryan, K.D. Puberty in the lamb: Sexual maturation of a seasonal breeder in a changing environment. *In* M.M., Grumbach, P. Sizonenko, and M. Aubert (Eds.), *The control of the onset of puberty II*. Serono Symposium, 1986, in press.

Frisch, R.E., and Revelle, R. 1970. Height and weight at menarche and a hypothesis of critical body weights and adolescent events. *Science*, 1970, *169*, 397–99.

Frisch, R.E., Gotz-Welbergen, A.V., McArthur, J.W., Albright, T., Witschi, J., Bullen, B., Birnholz, J., Reed, R.B., and Hermann, H. Delayed menarche and amenorrhea of college athletes in relation to age of onset of training. *Journal of the American Medical Association*, 1981, *246*, 1559–1563.

Grumbach, M.M. The neuroendocrinology of puberty. *In* D.T. Krieger and J.C. Hughes (Eds.), *Neuroendocrinology*. Sunderland, Mass: Sinauer Associates, 1980, pp. 249–258.

Grumbach, M.M., Roth, J.C., Kaplan, S.L., and Kelch, R.P. Hypothalamic–pituitary regulation of puberty in man: Evidence and concepts derived from clinical research. *In* M.M. Grumbach, G.D. Grave, and F.E. Mayer (Eds.), *The control of the onset of puberty.* New York: Wiley, 1974, pp. 115–166.

Grumbach, M.M., Richards, G.E., Conte, F.A., and Kaplan, S.L. Clinical disorders of adrenal androgen function and puberty: An assessment of the role of the adrenal cortex in normal and abnormal puberty in man and evidence for an ACTH-like pituitary adrenal androgen stimulating hormone. *In* V.H.T. James, M. Serio, G. Giusti, and L. L. Martini (Eds.), *The endocrine function of the human adrenal cortex.* London/New York: Academic Press, 1978, pp. 583–612.

Hohlweg, W., and Dohrn, M. Uber die Beziehungen zwischen Hypophysenvorderlap und Keimdrusen. *Klinische Wochenschrift*, 1932, *11*, 233–235.

Huseman, C.A., Kugler, J.A., and Schneider, I.G. Mechanism of dopaminergic suppression of gonadotropin secretion in men. *Journal of Clinical Endocrinology and Metabolism*, 1980, *51*, 209–214.

Jacobson, R.I., Seyler, L.E., Tamborlane, W.V., Gertner, J.M., and Genel, M. Pulsatile subcutaneous nocturnal administration of Gn–RH by portable infusion pump in hypogonadotropic hypogonadism: Initiation of gonadotropin responsiveness. *Journal of Clinical Endocrinology and Metabolism*, 1979, *49*, 652–654.

Judd, H.L. 1979. Biorhythms of gonadotropins and testicular hormone secretion. *In* D.T. Krieger (Ed.), *Endocrine rhythms.* New York: Raven Press, 1979, pp. 299–324.

Kaplan, S.L., Grumbach, M.M., and Aubert, M.L. The ontogenesis of pituitary hormones and hypothalamic factors in the human fetus: Maturation of the central nervous system regulation of anterior pituitary function. *Recent Progress in Hormone Research*, 1976, *32*, 161–243.

Kelch, R.P., Kaplan, S.L., and Grumbach, M.M. Suppression of urinary and plasma follicle-stimulating hormone by exogenous estrogens in prepubertal and pubertal children. *Journal of Clinical Investigation*, 1973, *52*, 112–28.

Knobil, E. The neuroendocrine control of the menstrual cycle. *Recent Progress in Hormone Research*, 1980, *36*, 53–88.

Knobil, E., Plant, T.M., Wildt, L., Belchetz, P.E., and Marshall, G. Control of the rhesus monkey menstrual cycle: permissive role of the hypothalamic gonadotropin-releasing hormone. *Science*, 1980, *207*, 1371–1373.

Kulin, H.E. and Reiter, E.O. Gonadotropin suppression by low dose estrogen: differential responses of FSH and LH. *Journal of Clinical Endocrinology and Metabolism*, 1972, *35*, 836–39.

Laron, Z., Arad, J., Gurewitz, R., Grunebaum, M., and Dickerman, Z. Age at first conscious ejaculation: milestones in male puberty. *Helvetica Paediatrica Acta*, 1980, *35*, 13–20.

Lenko, H.L., Lang, U., Aubert, M.L., Paunier, L., and Sizonenko, P.C. Melatonin in plasma and urine before and during puberty. *Pediatric Research*, 1981, *15*, 74. (Abstr.)

McArthur, J.W., O'Loughlin, K.M., and Alonso, C. Endocrine studies during the refeeding of young women with nutritional amenorrhea and infertility. *Mayo Clinic Proceedings*, 1976, *51*, 607–16.

McArthur, J.W., Bullen, B.A., Beitens, I.Z., Pagano, M., Badger, T.M., and Klibanski, A. Hypothalamic amenorrhea in runners of normal body composition. *Endocrine Research Communications*, 1980, *7*, 13–25.

Marshall, J.C., and Kelch, R.P. Low dose pulsatile gonadotropin releasing hormone in anorexia nervosa: A model of human pubertal development. *Journal of Clinical Endocrinology and Metabolism*, 1979, *49*, 712–718.

Morley, J.E., Baranetsky, N.G., Wingert, T.D., Carlson, H.E., Hershman, J.M., Melmed, S., Levin, S.R., Jamison, K.R., Weitzman, R., Chang, R.J., and Varner, A.A. Endocrine effects of naloxone-induced opiate receptor blockage. *Journal of Clinical Endocrinology and Metabolism*, 1980, *50*, 251–257.

Moult, P.J.A., Grossman, A., Evans, J.M., Rees, L.H., and Besser, G.M. The effect of naloxone on pulsatile gonadotropin release in normal subjects. *Clincial Endocrinology*, 1981, *14*, 321–324.

Mueller, P.L., Sklar, C.A., Gluckman, P.D., Kaplan, S.L., and Grumbach, M.M. Hormone ontogeny in the ovine fetus. IX. Luteinizing hormone and follicle stimulating hormone releasing factor in mid- and late gestation and in the neonate. *Endocrinology*, 1981, *108*, 881–886.

Nett, T.M., Crowder, M.E., G.E., and Duello, T.M. GnRH-receptor interaction. V. Down-regulation of pituitary receptors for GnRH in ovariectomized ewes by infusion of homologous hormone. *Biology of Reproduction*, 1981, *24*, 1145–1155.

Ojeda, S.R., Andrews, W.W., Advis, J.O., and White, S.S. Recent advances in the endocrinology of puberty. *Endocrine Review*, 1980, *1*, 228–257.

Parker, D.C., Judd, H.L., Rossman, L.G., and Yen, S.S.C. Pubertal sleep-wake patterns of episodic LH, FSH and testosterone release in twin boys. *Journal of Clinical Endocrinology and Metabolism*, 1975, *40*, 1099–1109.

Parker, L.N., and Odell, W.D. Control of adrenal androgen secretion. *Endocrine Review*, 1980, *1*, 392–410.

Penny, R., Olambiwonnu, N.O., and Frasier, S.D. Episodic fluctuations of serum gonadotropins in pre- and post-pubertal girls and boys. *Journal of Clincial Endocrinology and Metabolism*, 1977, *45*, 307–311.

Penny, R.; Goldstein, I.P., and Frasier, S.D. Gonadotropin excretion and body composition. *Pediatrics*, 1978, *61*, 294–300.

Pohl, C.R., and Knobil, E. The role of the central nervous system in the control of ovarian function in higher primates. *Annual Review of Physiology*, 1982, *44*, 583–594.

Quigley, M.E., and Yen, S.S.C. The role of endogenous opiates on LH secretion during the menstrual cycle. *Journal of Clinical Endocrinology and Metabolism*, 1980, *51*, 179–181.

Quigley, M.E., Sheehan, K.L., Caspar, R.F., and Yen, S.S.C. Evidence for increased dopaminergic and opioid activity in patients with hypothalamic hypogonadotropic amenorrhea. *Journal of Clinical Endocrinology and Metabolism*, 1980, *50*, 949-954.

Rebar, R.W., and Yen, S.S.C. Endocrine rhythms in gonadotropins and ovarian steroids with reference to reproductive processes. In D.T. Krieger (Ed.), *Endocrine rhythms*. New York: Raven Press, pp. 259–298.

Reiter, E.O., and Grumbach, M.M. Neuroendocrine control mechanisms and the onset of puberty. *Annual Review of Physiology*, 1982, *44*, 595–613.

Reiter, E.O., Kulin, H.E., and Hamwood, S.M. The absence of positive feedback between estrogen and luteinizing hormone in sexually immature girls. *Pediatric Research*, 1974, *8*, 740–745.

Reiter, E.O., Stern, R.C., and Root, A.W. The reproductive endocrine system in cystic fibrosis: 1. Basal gonadotropin and sex steroid levels. *American Journal of Diseases of Children*, 1981, *135*, 422–426.

Reiter, E.O., Stern, R.C., and Root, A.W. The reproductive endocrine system in cystic fibrosis: 2. Changes in gonadotrophins and sex steroids following LH-RH. *Clinical Endocrinology*, 1982, *16*, 127–137. (a)

Reiter, E.O., Beitens, I.Z., Ostrea, T., and Gutai, J.P. Bioassayable luteinizing hormone during childhood and adolescence and in patients with delayed pubertal development. *Journal of Clinical Endocrinology and Metabolism,* 1982, *54,* 155–166. (b)

Sherman, B.M., Halmi, K.A., and Zamudio, R. LH and FSH response to gonadotropin-releasing hormone in anorexia nervosa: Effect of nutritional rehabilitation. *Journal of Clinical Endocrinology and Metabolism,* 1975, *41,* 135–142.

Silman, R.E., Leone, R.M., Hooper, R.J.L., and Preece, M.A. Melatonin, the pineal gland and human puberty. *Nature (London)* 1979 *282,* 301–3.

Sklar, C.A., Conte, F.A., Kaplan, S.L., and Grumbach, M.M. Human chorionic gonadotropin-secreting pineal tumor: Relation to pathogenesis and sex limitation of sexual precocity. *Journal of Clincial Endocrinology and Metabolism,* 1981, *53,* 656–660.

Sklar, C.A., Kaplan, S.L., Grumbach, M.M. Evidence for dissociation between adrenarche and gonadarche: Studies in patients with idiopathic precocious puberty, gonadal dysgenesis, isolated gonadotroph deficiency, and constitutionally delayed growth and adolescence. *Journal of Clinical Endocrinology and Metabolism,* 1980, *51,* 548–556.

Styne, D.M., and Grumbach, M.M. Puberty in male and female: Its physiology and disorders. *In* S.S.C. Yen and R. Jaffe (Eds.), *Reproductive endocrinology.* Philadelphia: W.B. Saunders, 1978, pp. 189–240.

Tanner, J.M. *A history of the study of human growth.* Cambridge: Cambridge University Press, 1981, pp. 286–298.

Valk, T.W., Corley, K.P., Kelch, R.P., and Marshall, J.C. Hypogonadotropic hypogonadism: Hormonal responses to low dose pulsatile administration of gonadotropin-releasing hormone. *Journal of Clinical Endocrinology and Metabolism,* 1980, *51,* 730–737.

Vihko, R. and Apter, D. Early menarche indicates early onset of ovulatory cycles. *Proceedings of the 65th Endocrine Society,* San Antonio, Abstr. 933, 1983.

Warren, M.P. The effects of exercise on pubertal progression and reproductive function in girls. *Journal of Clinical Endocrinology and Metabolism,* 1980, *51,* 1150–1157.

Winter, J.S.D., Faiman, C., Hobson, W.C., Prasad, A.V., and Reyes, F.I. Pituitary–gonadal regulations in infancy. I. Patterns of serum gonadotropin concentrations from birth to four years of age in man and chimpanzee. *Journal of Clinical Endocrinology and Metabolism,* 1975, *40,* 545–551.

Winter, J.S.D., Hughes, I.A., Reyes, F.I., and Faiman, C. Pituitary–gonadal relations in infancy: 2. Patterns of serum gonadal steroid concentrations in man from birth to two years of age. *Journal of Clinical Endocrinology and Metabolism,* 1976, *42,* 679–686.

Zacharias, L., and Wurtman, R.J. Age at menarche. *New England Journal of Medicine,* 1969, *280,* 868–875.

Zacharias, L., Wurtman, R.J., and Schatzoff, M. Sexual maturation in contemporary American girls. *American Journal of Obstetrics and Gynecology,* 1970, *108,* 833–846.

5

THE BIOLOGY OF TEENAGE PREGNANCY: THE
MOTHER AND THE CHILD

Stanley M. Garn
Shelly D. Pesick
Audrey S. Petzold

INTRODUCTION

After reviewing 197 papers on teenage pregnancy that were abstracted by the National Library of Medicine in 1982, it is instructive to enumerate their contents by areas of emphasis or major concern.

The largest proportion of those papers (46%) had to do with intervention in teenage pregnancy (i.e., contraception and abortion). A smaller proportion (32%) of the "Medlar" abstracts related to the social, psychological, and economic consequences of teenage pregnancy. A still smaller proportion of those papers (17%) described the dimensional and developmental characteristics of the teenage mothers. A mere 5% of the papers reviewed considered the relevance of these characteristics to the conceptus and to the infant in postnatal time.

There is no longer any question that we need to know the family situations that lead to teenage pregnancy and the mind-sets of the girls who elect to become pregnant. There is no question of the economic cost of teenage pregnancy, even to the WIC (Womens-Infants-Children) program alone. Yet it is obvious that we need to know more about the developmental biology of teenage pregnancy and the characteristics of the teenage mother that bear on the quality of her conceptus.

There is great ignorance, even among pediatricians, about the body size of teenage mothers. Indeed, there is a tacit assumption that they are developmentally advanced (which is true) and, therefore, large for their age—which is false (cf. Forbes, 1981). There is the assumption,

77

not well founded, that the conceptus is at risk simply because of the tender age of the mother and (to use a dreadful term) her limited "gynecological age." There is the assumption that teenage pregnancy inevitably carries with it developmental risk to the mother and markedly increased risk of damage to the fetus as well (cf. Frisancho, et al., 1984).

Yet teenage pregnancies have long been the norm in most of the world. This remains so today even in populations far less well nourished than ours and where sexual maturity is delayed by several years. Thus, we cannot deal with teenage pregnancy as a recent historical abberation or as a byproduct of the secular trend to earlier maturation.

To answer some of these questions, we have turned to the data tapes of the National Collaborative Perinatal Project (NCPP) of the National Institute of Neurological and Communicative Disorders and Stroke (NINCDS) as originally described by Niswander and Gordon (1972). We have assumed the conventional chronological definition of teenager (i.e., age 13–19), since we have so few subteen mothers to study. However, we have examined the NCPP data year by year as well as by broader age groupings. Certain of the "teenage" effects are most evident in the youngest of the mothers and decline with advancing age, but in some situations they are detectable even into the third decade. Moreover, we have analyzed blacks and whites separately. Black neonates are smaller than white neonates, although developmentally more mature, however, black mothers are generally heavier than white mothers for reasons that go beyond socioeconomic status itself.

MATURATIONAL AND DIMENSIONAL CHARACTERISTICS OF TEENAGE MOTHERS

When we investigate pregnant teenagers age by age rather than lumped in a broad age group, three findings immediately attract our attention. First is their advanced sexual maturity, not only for the youngest of the teenage mothers but also throughout the pregnant teenage sample. Second is their small size, particularly for the youngest of the teenage mothers. Third, clearly, is their excessive weight gain during pregnancy (especially in the youngest subgroup, those pregnant by 15).

In a way, advanced sexual maturity in pregnant American teenagers is not surprising, especially for those who become pregnant before the average age of menarche. The extensive data of the NCPP show an increase in age at menarche with increasing age at first pregnancy from the earliest teens well into the third decade (Fig. 5.1). The indication is that sexual activity begins later in the later-to-mature, and this generalization extends beyond the immediate teenage period.

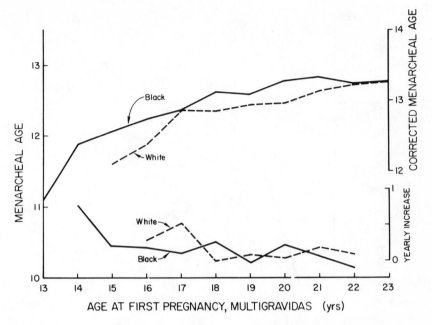

FIGURE 5.1. Relationship between age at menarche and age at first pregnancy. As might be expected, the youngest of the teenage mothers attained menarche well ahead of the national average. The age at menarche arranged with respect to age at pregnancy continues to increase into the third decade.

If we then plot prepregnancy weight against age at pregnancy, as in Fig. 5.2, we find an increase in prepregnancy weight through the teens amounting to 10 lb (4.5 kg) or more. The youngest of the teenage mothers are especially low in weight, as seen in the graph. This finding came as a considerable surprise to us.* We had assumed, as so many of our colleagues had assumed, that the young pregnant teenagers (being early maturing) would have achieved a more considerable weight before they became pregnant. That they have not done so is obvious, and, as we shall see, it bears on the low birth weights and increased incidence of prematurity in their offspring (Garn and Petzold, 1983).

In Fig. 5.3, we show both weight and stature arranged by age at

*We hastened to verify this observation with reference to equally mature but nonpregnant girls in two additional data bases. In both the Ten-State Nutrition Survey and in the Tecumseh, Michigan Community Health Survey, the postmenarcheal, nonpregnant girls evidenced the same dimensional trends documented above.

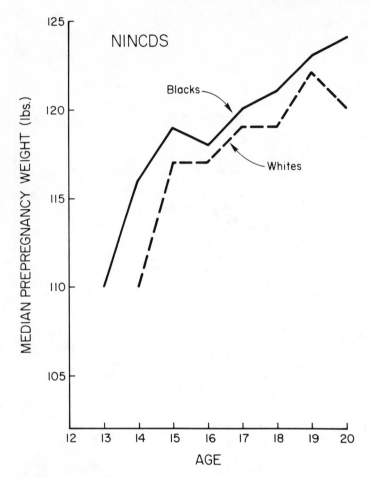

FIGURE 5.2. Prepregnancy weight by age at registration in the NCPP for blacks
(solid line) and whites (dashed line). In the youngest of the teenage
mothers prepregnancy weights are especially low, actually below
104 lb (47 kg) in 20% of cases.

pregnancy in the National Collaborative Perinatal Project. Both weight
and stature recapitulate the trend just mentioned toward increased size
with later age at pregnancy. Both parallel the trends for nonpregnant
participants in the Ten-State Nutrition Survey of 1968–1970, as shown
by the dashed lines on the graph. The youngest of the pregnant teenagers in the NCPP are both shorter and lighter in weight than their
third-decade peers. Both dimensional variables relate to pregnancy
outcomes in teenage pregnancies, as we shall soon see.

Last, in these descriptions of the teenage mothers we come to weight

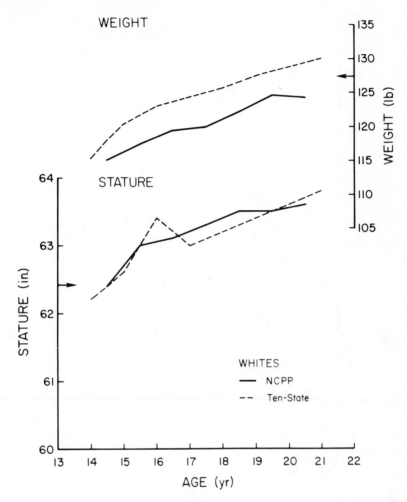

FIGURE 5.3. Weight (above) and stature (below) arranged by age at registration in the NCPP. As shown, both weight and stature increase with increasing maternal age. The youngest of the teenage mothers are exceptionally short and of low weight.

gain during pregancy, and in this respect there is a very dramatic age effect. Weight gain during pregnancy is considerably greater in the younger teenage mothers, by 3.5 kg or so (nearly 8 lb). This is a considerable difference, amounting to one-third of the average pregnancy weight gain in older mothers. Some investigators, of course, have attributed the larger weight gain in younger mothers to the accretion of maternal tissues that would ordinarily take place during 0.75 years of

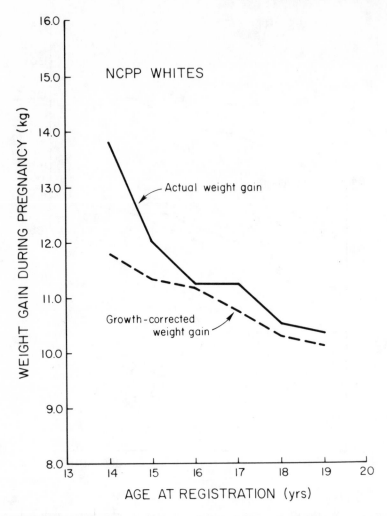

FIGURE 5.4. Decreasing weight gain during pregnancy with increasing age
at registration. Correcting for 0.75 years normal growth as shown
in the dotted line does not eliminate the systematically greater
weight gains in the youngest of the pregnant teenagers (cf. Garn
and Petzold, 1983, but see Hoff *et al.*, 1985).

normal nonpregnant growth. We have attempted to make growth
"corrections" by various calculations, one of which is also shown in
Fig. 5.4. Even after correcting (for 0.75 years) for normal growth, the
decreasing weight gain with increasing age is still there. Excess weight
gain is not limited to the early teens, and its decrease with increasing
age at pregnancy is not just a "growth" phenomenon.

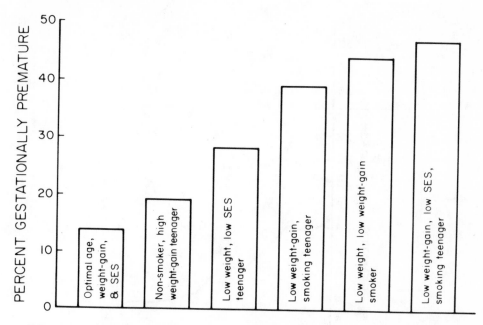

FIGURE 5.5. Additive effects of low age and other risk factors on the incidence of prematurity in blacks. As shown, low-income teenagers who smoke and who have a low weight gain during pregnancy have a threefold greater incidence of prematurity than that found in higher income nonsmoking women. For additional risk factors see Naeye and Peters (1982), Garn et al. (1977; 1981), and Garn (1986).

In short, early pregnancy is associated with (1) advanced maturity, (2) small size, (3) low weight, and (4) markedly increased weight gain during pregnancy.

THE CONCEPTUS

Teenage pregnancies are commonly viewed as "bad" for the conceptus on the basis of two commonly used measures—prematurity and low birth weight. By both of these measures, one gestational and one dimensional, teenage pregnancy greatly increases risks by 25, 50% and even more depending on the age grouping used and the number of risk factors included (see Fig. 5.5).

This point is very well demonstrated in the massive data of the National Collaborative Perinatal Project, first using the (conventional) <37-week cut-off for prematurity and restricting the sample to the fully "normal" neonates (lacking even minor abnormalities and requiring no as-

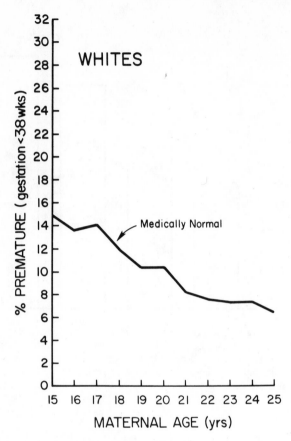

FIGURE 5.6. Decreased incidence of prematurity with advancing age. As shown here for the "medically normal" progeny of white mothers, short gestation lengths are nearly twice as common when the mother is 15 as when she is 25 years old.

sistance in breathing). Even by these rigid standards, it is seen that the incidence of "prematurity" is greatest at age 15 and below, and that the incidence of prematurity declines through the mid-twenties. As shown in Fig. 5.6, therefore, the incidence of prematurity declines from 15% at registration age 15 to less than 8% at registration age 25. Even if we use a more vigorous 34-week cut-off (extreme prematurity), the curve similarly declines, although it is, then, lower overall.

If we use birth weight as our criterion, instead of gestational prematurity, the teenage effect is of comparable magnitude. Moreover, the incidence of low birth weights increases as we add other risk factors (as we did in Fig. 5.5). However, when we next plot low birth weights

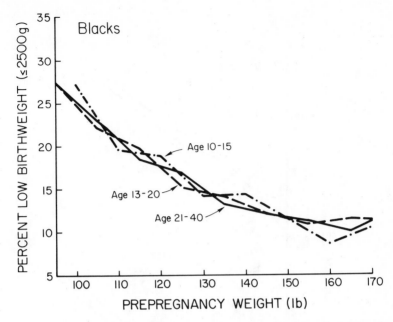

FIGURE 5.7. Relationship between prepregnancy weight and the incidence of low birth weight in younger and older girls and women. Whether for subteens, all teens, or older women, the lower the prepregnancy weight the higher the incidence of low birth-weight infants (cf. Garn and Petzold, 1983).

against prepregnancy weight, as in Fig. 5.7, for different age groups, we discover that the teenage effect is very much a maternal weight effect! Whether for subteens, all teens, or for older women, low birth weights are clearly a function of maternal prepregnancy weight and not of maternal age. Indeed weight-for-weight, subteens and third- and fourth-decade women yield the same incidence of low birth-weight neonates (see also Garn and Petzold, 1983; Garn, 1986).

While teenage pregnancies, therefore, result in an increased incidence of short gestation lengths, prematurity, and decreased size for duration of gestation (i.e., size-for-date), data on other disadvantages are more difficult to come by and to analyze, partly because of the sample sizes necessary. By way of example, it takes tens of thousands of pregnancies to ascertain the true incidence of placental abnormalities. Of course, there are some adverse conditions (such as Down's syndrome) that are far less common in the progeny of teenagers than in the progeny of mothers of older ages, as is well known.

It is relevant, therefore, to present our data on fetal deaths arranged

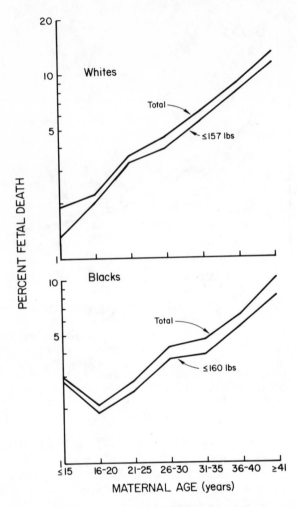

FIGURE 5.8. The increasing incidence of fetal death with advancing maternal age in whites and in blacks. The incidence of fetal death in the NCPP increases from the teenage period through age 40. The lowest incidence is found among teenage pregnancies. See Garn (1986).

by maternal age as shown in Fig. 5.8. Whether in the total NCPP series or in women below 157–160 lb (i.e., 72 kg), the incidence of fetal deaths actually increases from the early teens right through the fifth decade. In fact, the incidence of fetal death increases more than threefold, being least (≤3%) in teenagers and increasing to ≥10% or more in the oldest maternal age group considered.

So the major risks associated with teenage pregnancy have to do with the length of gestation (i.e., how long the fetus is carried) and to the size attained. In other respects, the disadvantages of teenage pregnancies may be minimal or at least not fully confirmed. In still other respects, the fetus of a teenager may be at a positive advantage, a point rarely made until now but of considerable practical importance.

Moreover, the question arises as to whether the gestational and dimensional disadvantages associated with teenage pregnancies are a direct product of the low reproductive age or whether they simply result from the smaller body size of the teenage mothers.

PREPREGNANCY WEIGHT AND WEIGHT GAIN IN TEENAGE AND OLDER MOTHERS

Two maternal variables bear a direct and directly linear relationship to the size of the infant at birth. These variables are, first, the maternal prepregnant weight (PPW) and, second, the weight gain during pregnancy. Their effects, moreover, are additive. A low PPW combined with a low weight gain yields a far smaller neonate than a high PPW and a high weight gain. The difference, at the extremes, is more than a kilogram in birth weight!

The relationship between prepregnancy weight (PPW) and the size of the infant at birth is much the same whether the mother is a teenager or a women in her twenties or thirties. This can also be documented by regressing birth weight against prepregnancy weight throughout the entire PPW weight range, as in Fig. 5.9. Teenagers and older women show virtually identical relationships to size of the infant at birth as do the younger teenagers ($\leq$ age 15) and those in the 16–20 age group. It follows, therefore, that the smaller size of teenage pregnant mothers is one explanation for the smaller size of their conceptuses.

If we use these regressions to compare the PPW–birth weight relationship in teenage and older mothers, black and white separately, we obtain two sets of lines. At all prepregnancy weights, the birth weights are higher for whites. At all prepregnancy weights, the birth weights are much the same for the teenage and older mothers.

If we next plot birth weight against weight *gain*, we do find a major difference between the teenagers and the older mothers. At any given weight gain, the older mothers yield a larger neonate. At any given weight gain, the teenage mothers yield a smaller neonate (Fig. 5.10). Especially for the youngest of the teenage mothers, birth weight for weight gain is dramatically less. Thus, we now can identify two reasons why teenage mothers yield a higher incidence of low birth-weight neonates. The first reason is their smaller PPW. PPW for PPW, younger and older women yield equally small or equally large babies. The

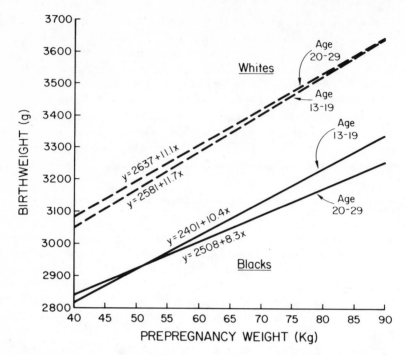

FIGURE 5.9. Birth weight by prepregnancy weight in blacks (below) and whites (above). As in Figure 5.7, there is little effect of maternal age on birth weight once prepregnancy weight is taken into account. However, at all prepregnancy weights from 40 to 90 kg whites yield consistently larger neonates than do blacks. See Garn (1986).

second reason is the smaller "yield" of conceptus for a given weight gain in the teenagers. This is truly a teenage effect.

One part of the "teenage effect," therefore, is not a result of lower age, developmental immaturity, or reproductive inefficiency. It is a maternal-size effect, relating to the smaller mass of the teenage mothers. It can be duplicated in low-weight older women. Another part of the "teenage effect" is a true age effect, inexplicably linked to developmental immaturity. Teenagers and especially younger teenagers yield a smaller neonate per unit of pregnancy weight gain (Fig 5.11).

Prepregnancy weight is scarcely mutable once pregnancy has begun, and it is impossible to change retroactively. Weight gain during pregnancy, however, may be susceptible to modification during pregnancy. Accordingly a larger weight gain by, for example, 4 kg or more may, in theory, be advocated for pregnant teenagers, consistent with their generally larger weight gain and the lesser impact on the fetus.

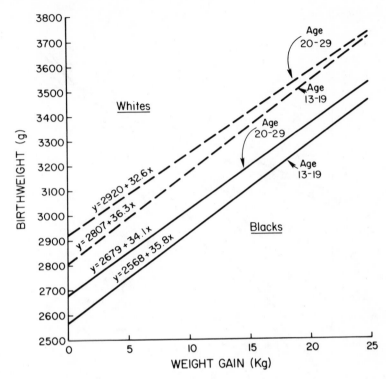

FIGURE 5.10. Relationship between weight gain during pregnancy and birth weight in older and younger mothers. As shown, older mothers yield a slightly larger infant for the same weight gain consistent with the notion that a larger portion of teenagers' weight gain during pregnancy goes to other products of conception or is retained by the mother herself. See Garn and Petzold (1983) and Garn et al. (1984).

DISCUSSION

As we have documented here, teenage pregnancies (and especially pregnancies in the early teens) carry with them a markedly increased risk of premature births and low birth weights. Moreover, for any given length of conception, the progeny of the teenage mother tends to be smaller (i.e., small-for-date, using the language of the specialist). Yet the fetus of the teenager, although smaller, is at less than average risk in many other respects, and grows better in the earlier years of life.

We discover that the smaller size of the teenagers' conceptus is in accordance with the smaller size of the mother herself. As we can show by weight-matching with older mothers in the third decade of life, there is very little difference in the size of the newborn when weight-matched

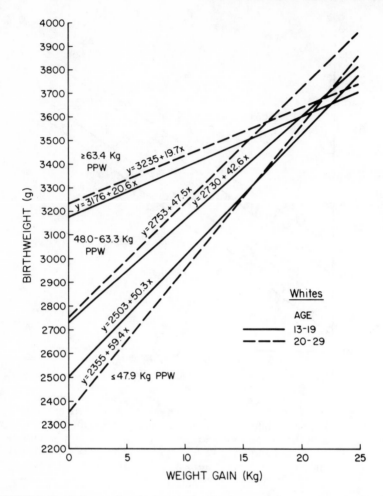

FIGURE 5.11. Relationship between pregnancy weight gain and birth weight in teenagers and older women at three different prepregnancy weight levels. As shown, there is at best a slight size advantage accruing to the progeny of older women at the higher levels of prepregnancy weight but not necessarily for those in the lowest prepregnancy weight category.

teenagers and older women are compared. So it is the small size of the teenage mothers, particularly those in the early teens, that appears to be chiefly responsible for low birth weights of teenage progeny.

However, it is also true that a given weight gain during pregnancy yields a smaller conceptus when the mother is in her earlier teens than when she is in her later teens and in her twenties. More of the pregnancy weight gain either goes to other products of conception when the mother is young or is added to the maternal tissue stores. Less of the maternal weight gain is reflected in the size of the neonate in the case of a teenage pregnancy.

It is useful and important to emphasize the small maternal stature and low weight in early teenage pregnancies, for it is too often assumed that such mothers are both early maturing *and* large for their age. Although they are early to mature (a biological necessity), 13-, 14-, and 15-year-old primiparous and multiparous girls are small. Corrections for "gynecological age" (i.e., years since menarche) are not effective in "explaining" or removing the teenage small-size effect.

While the term *gynecological age* is objectionable to anyone with a knowledge of etymology, it also turns out that years-since-menarche (which the term is intended to mean) bears little relationship to the size or developmental status or the quality of the conceptus. Only to the teenager is it important, since girls who have been postmenarcheal longer are somewhat heavier.

Now it has been suggested that teenage mothers produce smaller neonates because they (the mothers) are still growing and are therefore in active competition with their conceptuses for calories and nutrients. This is a reasonable explanation, but it may not be the correct one. The growth of the teenage mother, during and after pregnancy tends to be small, and her growth needs may also be small, even for additions to the skeletal mass (Garn *et al.*, 1984). Given the small size of the pregnant early teenagers, a more reasonable explanation for the maternal size effect is that small women are simply smaller reservoirs of calories and nutrients.

It has been suggested that teenage pregnancy is detrimental to the mother by diverting calories and nutrients to the fetus and the products of conception, thereby restricting growth in her size, growth of her fat-free mass, and growth of her mineral mass. This, also, is a reasonable suggestion, but extremely difficult to substantiate. For a girl who reaches menarche at 10.5–11.5 years [two standard deviations (S.D.) and one S.D. before the national average] and who delivers at 13.5 and 14.5 years, respectively, pregnancy demands (which peak late in pregnancy) may not represent a major diversion of nutrients, especially if associated with a 30-lb (14 kg) weight gain during pregnancy. On the other hand, a 20-lb (9 kg) weight gain during pregnancy does result in a long-term weight *loss* in pregnant teenagers, both black and white.

Yet in making these statements, it is very important to emphasize the paucity of data and the limitations of existing studies in teenage pregnancies, even including the NCPP. While 8000 pregnancies may appear to constitute a very ample sample *(N)* by conventional standards, the NCPP sample is approximately one-half black and one-half white, or 4000 each. It is moreover limited in the number of early teen whites. Moreover, as we have learned, we cannot lump 13-year-old girls (who show the teenage pregnancy effect to a maximum) and 18-year-old girls (who differ from 28-year-old women only to a slight degree) together (cf. Naeye, 1981).

There are, moreover, socioeconomic effects that complicate data sets and the results of data analyses. Girls of low socioeconomic status tend to be of smaller size but, as they progress through the teens, become fatter. Teenage girls of high socioeconomic status tend to be taller and with a larger fat-free mass, yet they are leaner. If the poorer, smaller, lower socioeconomic status teenager accepts a larger pregnancy weight gain and the taller, higher socioeconomic status primapara restricts pregnancy weight gain, analysis of both pregnancy outcomes and their interpretation become confusing indeed.

There have been various suggestions as to nutritional modification of the teenage effect. Indeed, as the data here clearly show, larger weight gains (in excess of 14 kg) are indeed normal in the younger pregnant teenagers and should be accepted as such. However, beyond that, weight gain may be of little benefit to the fetus in teenage pregnancies. Moreover, the greater weight gain will surely be retained as fat by the mother and, therefore, a step toward adult obesity.

SUMMARY

As shown in 8000 teenage pregnancies arranged by age at conception, three developmental and dimensional characteristics emerge that bear on their reproductive performance and the status of their progeny at birth. Teenage mothers tend to be early maturing, especially for the subteen at conception. They tend to be small, consistent with their early age at maturity, and they tend to high levels of weight gain during pregnancy.

When teenagers are matched with older women of comparable weight, their progeny are of comparable size at birth. Thus, the teenage effect has to do with maternal size and not age. Yet for a given weight gain during pregnancy, the conceptus of a teenage mother is smaller—more of the weight gained goes to the mother or to other products of conception. The teenage mothers do produce an excess of low birthweight and prematurely born neonates. In some respects (such as fetal death), however, the conceptus of a teenage mother is at lower risk. The progeny of teenage mothers also grow faster than the average during the preschool years, being (like their mothers) early maturers themselves.

Although increased weight gain during pregnancy is characteristic of the younger teenager and although an increased weight gain is associated with a larger neonate, weight gains in excess of 14 kg may lead to obesity on the part of the teenage mother and may be of little additional benefit to the conceptus.

ACKNOWLEDGMENTS

Work described in this chapter was supported by Contract N01-NS-5-2308 with the National Institute of Neurological and Communicative Disorders and Stroke, Contract No. 200-80-0501 with the Center for Disease Control and was completed under Grant HD13823 from the National Institutes of Health.

The manuscript was completed by Robert M. Leib.

REFERENCES

Forbes, G.B. *In* E. McAnarney and G. Strickle (Eds.), *Pregnancy in the teenager: Biological aspects.* New York: Alan Liss, 1981, pp. 84–90.

Frisancho, A.R., Matos, J., and Bollettino, L.A. Influence of growth status and placental function on birth weight of infants born to young still-growing teenagers. *American Journal of Clinical Nutrition*, 1984, *40*, 801–807.

Garn, S.M. *Prenatal antecedents of postnatal growth.* Ann Arbor: University of Michigan Press, 1986.

Garn, S.M. and Petzold, A.S. Characteristics of the mother and child in teenage pregnancy. *American Journal of Diseases of Children*, 1983, *137*, 365–368.

Garn, S.M., Johnston, M., Ridella, S.A., and Petzold, A.S. Effect of maternal cigarette smoking on Apgar scores. *American Journal of Diseases of Children*, 1981, *135*, 503–506.

Garn, S.M., Shaw, H.A., and McCabe, K.D. Effects of socioeconomic status and race on weight-defined and gestational prematurity in the United States. *In* S. Reed and F. Stanley (Eds.), *The epidemiology of prematurity.* Baltimore: Urban and Schwarzenberg, 1977, pp. 127–143.

Garn, S.M., LaVelle, M., Pesick, S.D., and Ridella, S.A. Are pregnant teenagers still in rapid growth? *American Journal of Diseases of Children*, 1984, *138*, 32–34.

Hoff, C., Wertelecki, W., Zansky, S., Reyes, E., Dutt, J., and Stumpe, A. Earlier maturation of pregnant black and white adolescents. *American Journal of Diseases of Children*, 1985, *139*, 981–986.

Naeye, R.L. Teenaged and pre-teenaged pregnancies: Consequences of the fetal maternal competition for nutrients. *Pediatrics*, 1981, *67*, 146–150.

Naeye, R.L. and Peters, E.C. Working during pregnancy: Effects on the fetus. *Pediatrics*, 1982, *69*, 724–727.

Niswander, K.R. and Gordon, M. *The women and their pregnancies.* U.S. Department of Health, Education and Welfare publication No. (NIH) 73–379.

DEVELOPMENTAL DYSSYNCHRONY AS NORMATIVE EXPERIENCE: KIKUYU ADOLESCENTS

Carol M. Worthman

INTRODUCTION

One of the more notable features of adolescence is the broad range of interindividual variation in the timing, rate, and pattern of physical maturational events (Tanner, 1962; Marshall, 1978). Even on the level of general experience and casual observation, it is readily apparent that adolescent peers differ markedly in appearance with regard to degree of physical maturation. Studies have identified developmental sequences of individual parameters at puberty (e.g., genital growth, gonadal steroid hormone production), but have consistently found wide interindividual variability in the timing and overall pattern of physical and sexual development (Harlan et al., 1979; Marshall and Tanner, 1969, 1970; Thorner et al., 1977). In a British sample, for instance, the ranges of variation in age at entering puberty and at reaching menarche overlap by over 2 years: about 15% of girls would already have reached menarche while the same proportion had not yet entered puberty (Marshall and Tanner, 1969).

Such findings characterize a life stage for which broad ranges must be recognized in order to accommodate the diversity of normal development in a population. Given this degree of variance, how does the individual going through puberty conceptualize the process? It is quite likely that any given individual will at some point deviate from his or her perception of the average experience. Indeed, normative crises appear to be endemic to this period.

However, the perception of individual developmental differences depends on the opportunity for comparison among peers or with a developmental model. Further, the consequences of perceived or actual differences are partly determined by the social structuring of adolescent experience, which may generate or ameliorate potentials for cognitive dissonance and conflict: tensions which seem inevitable in the Western context may not be so in another. Outcomes of early or late maturation for females, for example, would be quite different in a society where marriage occurs at menarche and age is not closely reckoned, than in one prescribing a long, chaste adolescence (see Whiting, this volume, Chapter 14). Distribution of individual and social costs of puberty is therefore largely determined by the social structure of adolescent experience, depending on what is optimized (e.g., cooperativeness, competitiveness) and what the constraints are in that structure.

The attainment of mature form and functioning in puberty is of importance to society on many levels, including that it determines lower limits on age at entry into reproductive career and affects entry age and degree to which adult tasks and roles can be performed. It is important to the maturing individual for similar reasons. Hence, social management of adolescence is necessary to canalize developmental changes to socially desirable outcomes. The process of normal physical development at puberty and its inherent variability, then, place meaningful, though broad, constraints on the social modelling of adolescents. In turn, outcomes on the individual level are shaped by that modelling. The relationships between individual ontogeny and social structure of experience at puberty will be explored in this chapter, using primarily material from a study of adolescent development in a Kenyan population. A preliminary framework for characterizing various social structures of adolescence and their outcomes is presented, drawing on data from other societies where relevant.

KIKUYU ADOLESCENTS

MATERIALS AND METHODS

Data on contemporary adolescents are taken mainly from a mixed longitudinal study of physical, social, and behavioral-psychological development of 9- to 17-year olds in a Kikuyu (Bantu) community conducted 1979–1981 under the auspices of the Department of Pediatrics, University of Nairobi Medical School. The study community, Ngecha, is a largely rural agrarian Southern Kikuyu population of 6900 inhabitants, located in central highland Kenya (1950 m alt.) about 35 km northwest of Nairobi. Subjects were drawn from a group that had been studied from infancy through mid-childhood by members of the Child Development Research Unit (CDRU), initiated by Beatrice and John Whiting. The CDRU collected a large body of ethnographic, socioeconomic, behavioral, and developmental data on the community, and on focal samples of households and individuals (Whiting and Whiting, 1975), which forms a vital basis for the later research. Information on traditional practice is drawn from Kikuyu ethnographies by Jomo Kenyatta (1938) and L.S.B. Leakey (1977).

Data on physical development is provided from a mixed longitudinal study of 84 boys and girls, six each of seven birth years, 1964–1970. Anthropometry and ratings of secondary sex character development were performed in the context of a clinical examination and general interview. Anthropometric measures were taken monthly by a single investigator, using the Harpenden (Holtain) survey set and an Avery hanging scale, applying standard techniques (Weiner and Lourie, 1969). Ratings of secondary sex character development were made separately for breasts (females) or genitals (males), pubic hair, and axillary hair (Tanner, 1962). Each sex was rated by a single investigator of the same sex.[1] Among other items in the clinical interviews, subjects were questioned by the same investigators about occurrence of menarche or, in the case of boys, emissions. We are fairly confident of this data, as the two investigators involved knew the respondents quite intimately.

Status quo data on menarche (for girls) and circumcision (both sexes), as well as separate residency (for boys), were obtained by questionnaire both from the core study group, and on a wider cross-sectional sample. A total of 867 responses were obtained, roughly one-half from each sex, of which 233 were repeat responses after a six-month interval. Median age of menarche, or circumcision (omitting, in girls, those who expected not to be circumcised), and of shifting residency to a boy's house were determined by probit analysis (Burrell et al., 1961). Formal and informal ethnographic interviews were also conducted, usually individually, with community members of both sexes, ages 9 to approximately 81.

TRADITIONAL AND CONTEMPORARY ADOLESCENCE

Social change and modernization proceeded rapidly in Ngecha during the British colonial and post-Independence periods, and has brought the cash crop, wage-earning economy, Christianity, schooling, and central government among other nontraditional elements. As has been detailed elsewhere,[2] these changes have especially altered the structure of adolescent experience. Traditionally, Kikuyu were an age-

[1] A collaborating physician, Dr. Julius Meme, of the Department of Pediatrics, University of Nairobi, performed the ratings of pubertal maturity for boys, and drew all blood samples.

[2] Worthman, C. M., and Whiting, J. W. M. *Social change in adolescent sexual behavior and mate selection in a Kikuyu community.* Manuscript submitted for publication, 1985.

grade, age-set society (Murdock, 1959). Each life state was ritually bounded and designated with a specific age-grade name. At puberty, circumcision of males and females marked initiation into a named circumcision-year cohort of classificatory sibs. Girls were to be circumcised just before menarche; the boys were initiated later, at around 18. The operation consisted, for boys, of cutting the prepuce, and for girls, of removing the very tip of the clitoris. As part of the initiation process, explicit teaching was provided, largely by senior warriors and maidens, concerning reproductive function and appropriate social and sexual behavior.

Initiates changed age-grades (circumcised young man = *mwanake*, young woman = *mūirītu*) and entered periods of bachelor warriorhood and maidenhood of several years' duration. Boys moved into young men's huts; girls remained at home. Warriorhood ended with the changeover of the regiment after a seven-year tenure; maidenhood ended with marriage, which occurred at around age 19 years. First marriage for males was at about age 25 years.

These adolescents and young adults played productive social roles. Warriors defended existing territory and scouted for and annexed new lands. Maidens performed farm and domestic work; the value of their labor was a major rationale for the bride price demanded of prospective grooms. In addition, young people were given the freedom to lead quite active social lives, partly to maintain group solidarity, and partly to facilitate mate selection. There was a year-round cycle of dances, public demonstrations by warriors of physical and mental prowess (Cagnolo, 1933), and frequent group cross-sex socializing in young men's houses. Emphasis was placed on initiation cohort cohesiveness which would continue through adulthood for both sexes.

During the last 60 years, political and social change has obviated the role of warriors. Male circumcision is universal, but female circumcision was banned by the dominant Protestant churches in 1938 and is now discouraged by the state; although it is still practised, it is no longer universal. Initiation was also gradually deritualized, and the formation of age-sets or initiation cohorts has ceased. Instead, school is the major feature defining contemporary adolescent life. Education is valued equally for both sexes. Schooling is virtually universal, and most students remain enrolled through the first seven years to take the state comprehensive exam (CPE). Performance on this exam determines both whether one will be placed in a secondary school, and the quality of that school. Competition is intense since less than one-third of the students receive places in secondary school. The remainder must seek alternative job training or employment. Two further exams, after 4 and then 2 more years, also act as selective filters for continuation to higher education, which greatly increases employability. Enhancing employability is of great concern, since finding employment, especially initially, is becoming increasingly difficult.

Adolescents are expected to contribute labor or earnings to the family, the more so in return for parental investment in their schooling through foregone labor and school fees. Parents, usually the mother, assign them tasks for the family homestead, either in the compound, in the fields, or on errands, after school, on weekends or holidays, or during periods of unemployment.[3] Adolescent girls work primarily on the family compound, with their mother in the fields, or fetching water, fodder, and firewood. They are expected to perform numerous domestic and farm tasks independently, and their duties are far more extensive, home-bound, and supervised than are those of male adolescents. From childhood, males are assigned more unsupervised, compound-centripedal tasks such as herding and running errands, although they are also given farm and domestic duties on the homestead. Parents feel less able to command labor of their circumcised sons, which diminishes progressively as the sons become older. Young men rarely perform domestic duties, but often aid in compound maintenance or upgrading, and in heavier farm tasks.

Most adolescents spend regular, large blocks of time in school with peers. This time is heavily structured, however, and emphasis is placed on excelling individually vis-à-vis those peers. Individual allegiance is far less with the corporate peer group than it is with individual and family interests. Nevertheless, young men have the freedom and leisure to spend considerable time with male peers, thereby developing the social and verbal skills and the social network that will later be necessary for procuring employment and working the system in the traditional and modern sectors.

While it is now performed informally and not as a cohort ritual, circumcision still marks a turning point in puberty. This is particularly true of boys, for whom it is the unquestioned prerequisite for achieving manhood. Age-grade status terms are still employed and boys are promoted to *mwanake* status upon circumcision. Clear expectations and distinctions exist between what the circumcised and uncircumcised boy will think or do. After circumcision, he is expected to put away foolish and childish attitudes or behaviors, to behave responsibly and rationally, and is, furthermore, eligible to become sexually active. The median age at circumcision, for boys, now 15.9 years, has declined as male circumcision has come to be linked to a major scholastic rite of passage, sitting for the CPE (Herzog, 1973). Most boys are circumcised just subsequent to taking the exam. Thereafter, they will try to dress

---

[3] The importance of sex-differentiated task giving in patterns of socialization to different behavior styles, attitudes, and competencies is thoroughly discussed in Whiting, B. B. *The Company They Keep.* Book in preparation, 1984.

more stylishly, to seek the company of other young men, and to socialize with young women. Male adolescence ends with marriage, which occurs on average at age 23, whereupon age-grade status alters.

Because female circumcision is optional, and circumcision status is no longer made public, the structuring of female adolescence is not as clear as it is for males. One-half the young girls report that they expect to be circumcised, and approximately 40% are. These girls see circumcision as a way of taking control of their bodies and as a preparation for undergoing childbirth. Girls from families who do not have their daughters circumcised view it as unmodern, un-Christian, and unnecessary. If a girl is to be circumcised, it is still strongly preferred to do so prior to menarche, which occurs at a median age of 15.9 years. Median age of female circumcision for that group sanctioning circumcision is 14.5 years.

Conferring of the age-grade status of "initiated girls" is presently based on an informal estimate by the person addressing the girl of her physical maturity, not her circumcision status. Similarly, there are now no prescribed expectations of how the circumcised girl will behave; rather, as girls go through puberty they are expected and encouraged by their mothers to show more young ladylike behavior, emphasizing such characteristics as: demureness, modesty, neatness, and responsibility. Mothers of postmenarcheal girls make increased efforts to restrict and survey their daughters' activities to avoid unwanted pregnancy. Their daughters, on the other hand, may comply with most norms of demeanor, but may seek to increase their attractiveness to, and contact with, somewhat older members of the opposite sex.

The CPE exam is also perceived by girls as a major rite of passage, after which they feel they should have the equivalent of a postinitiate, fully adolescent status. Because most girls take the exam between age 15 and 16, at least one half are postmenarcheal. Adolescence ends for young women at marriage or first pregnancy, which occurs at a mean age of 20 years and brings a change in age-grade status.

Pubescent males move into individual boy's houses on the family compound. Traditionally, boys shifted residence to their father's separate house at about mid-to-late childhood. This separate man's house has vanished with the decline in polygyny and the rise of the nuclear family, but in its place the young man's home has become ubiquitous. Family size is large (7 ± 4, $\bar{x}\pm SD$, children in this sample) and a maturing male is problematic in the dense, intimate family context. Hence, the boy's house resolves potential psychological tension in the family while conceding to the adolescent male a tremendous increase in personal freedom and privacy. The median age at changing residence to a boy's house is 14.7 years.

BIOSOCIAL RELATIONSHIPS IN KIKUYU ADOLESCENCE

Although pubertal development is a continuous process, in the social management of that process, as well as in our study of it, it is usually divided into developmental stages (early, middle, late adolescence) or functional steps (pre-, postmenarcheal). An index variable or set of variables is required to track individual development and synchronize it with appropriate social inputs. An important limitation on such index variables is that they must be visible or readily measurable: hormone levels or Piagetian stage ratings are useless for this purpose. Hence, adolescence is widely characterized in societies by tests of skill acquisition and attention to attainment of hallmarks of physical maturation (e.g., facial hair).

Age has become so generally applied and ubiquitous an index variable in Western society that we find it difficult to conceptualize the human life cycle without it. It is well recognized, however, that due to the extent of individual variability in the timing of development, age is a poor index of physical maturation during puberty (Cheek et al., 1968; Tanner, 1962, 1975). Developmental dyssynchrony among adolescent peers also obtains among Kikuyu. Although the median age at entry into puberty for girls, for example, is 12.5 years,[4] girls were observed to have entered puberty by as early as 10.5 years, and to have not yet done so by as late as 16 years.

Traditionally, Kikuyu did not use age as a personal statistic. Currently, under pressure from bureaucratic requirements, they are increasing its use. Many of our adolescent subjects did not know their actual age, or were family records systematically kept; precise subject ages are known for research purposes from early records kept by the CDRU. There are many alternatives to age that societies use as indexes of individual development at puberty, including aspects of physical size, morphology, or the attainment of reproductive function, as well as indirect measures of mental or behavioral maturity and the acquisition of skills or capacities.

Kikuyu often use physical size as an index variable: they tend to start their children in school when they are "big" (not old) enough,[5] and they designate the tallest, usually just pre- and early pubescent children with the informal age-grade status of "bigboy" (kīhīī) or "small

[4] Because the number of observations of age at appearance of Breast Stage 2 is small, a more representative statistic may be derived from a probit analysis based on proportion by age of girls not in Breast Stage 1.

[5] Whiting, J. W. M. Personal communication, April, 1982, Variation in age at entry in nursery school was best explained by child size, rather than socioeconomic variables (e.g., mother's education, family modernity, income, sib order or number).

adolescent (initiated) girl" (kairītu). The goodness of fit of an index variable depends partly on the features for which it is to be used as an indicator. Height may be a reasonable index of emerging usefulness as a soccer player (a matter of concern for boys in this community), but it is a rather inadequate one of reproductive maturation in this population. Over the range of heights observed in very late childhood and adolescence (males: 119–173 cm; females: 120–167 cm), height is a poor predictor of sex character development, menarcheal status, and age.

To use the data for Kikuyu as an instance: first, although those girls who had reached menarche were all taller than 145 cm, the heights of premenarcheal girls extended across the entire range of heights observed. While all girls under 135 cm tall had no breast development (Breast Stage 1), there was a 20 cm range of heights (135–155 cm) including girls in Breast Stage 1 to those with more prominent breast development (Breast Stage 3). The taller girls (145–155 cm) showed all stages of breast development (Breast Stage 1–5), and only for those over 155 cm tall was breast development universal. The pattern of maturational diversity by height was similar for boys.

Overall, weight was better correlated than was height with pubertal development. It correlated with genital and pubic hair development in boys equally as well as it did with breast and pubic hair development in girls. However, when used as an index of maturation, it was as unsatisfactory as height.

Height and weight have been reported elsewhere to be unreliable maturational indexes (Marshall, 1978). The rating scales of secondary sex character development, however, have been repeatedly found to be well correlated with underlying endocrine function (Burr et al., 1970; Lee and Migeon, 1975; Lee et al., 1976; Sizonenko et al., 1970). These may be useful as index variables and, indeed, it appears that Kikuyu use breast development to time circumcision for girls. It will be recalled that girls must be circumcised before menarche, but it is also considered undesirable to circumcise them too early. Parents are faced with the problem of how to determine appropriate timing of their daughter's circumcision, despite the great population range in age at menarche (youngest postmenarcheal girl reported was 10.5 years, the oldest premenarcheal girls seen were 17 years). Although there are not sufficient cases to test the relationship on a prospective basis, it is most suggestive that the median age of female circumcision, 14.5 years, falls just after the mean age at first appearance of Breast Stage 3, at 14.2 years. It is then that breast development in a fully clothed individual first becomes readily visible to others. Appearance of Breast Stage 3 is probably the most proximate reliable indicator for increased probability of menarche:

in a sample of British girls, all but 1% reached menarche during or after Breast Stage 3 (Marshall and Tanner, 1969).

Timing for circumcision for males is usually set by the bureaucratic event of sitting for an exam, although the age at which it is taken may be determined by maturational variables, since the range of ages of exam takers is wide (13–18 years). School classes are, in general, multiaged, as students may enter school late, repeat classes, or take extended absences.

There is no prescribed parameter determining when boys take up residence in their own houses. The time at which they do so is dependent in large part on available family resources (e.g., space, building materials, extant boy's houses) in addition to the boy's maturational status. Most boys establish separate residence well before circumcision; three-quarters have done so by the time they are circumcised, but 10% never do have a boy's house, and are allocated their own space in the home instead. Hence, circumcision status was only weakly correlated to separate residency. Attainment of first emission, however, was rather better correlated, for nearly all boys who reported having had emissions lived separately. This suggests the inference that appearance of this maturational sign gives impetus to provision or acquisition of separate residency for those who did not already have it, perhaps confirming the presumed social-psychodynamic basis for existence of boy's houses as a solution for what to do with reproductively maturing males. However, the prospective data available are insufficient to validate this.

Kikuyu boys are, on average, quite as well into puberty at the median age for separate residency, 14.6 years, as are girls at median age for female circumcision, 14.5 years. In fact, boys show genital development (mean age, 12.5 years) at about the same average age as first appearance of breast development in girls. That adolescence is recognized later in males than in females—not only in Kikuyu culture, but also in Western and numerous other societies—is an excellent example of the potency of visible cues for shaping social conceptions of developmental process.

In populations reported to date, boys enter puberty later than girls on average, though how much later varies among studies (.5 to 2 years) and may reflect sample, methodological, or actual population differences (Marshall and Tanner, 1970; Thorner et al., 1977). These small or larger sex differences in age at entry are further magnified by sex differences in timing of growth and other changes in overall body appearance in the course of maturation. A most prominent distinction is in timing of maximum growth. Boys reach peak height velocity considerably later in puberty than do girls, reaching the growth spurt when genital development is well advanced (Genital Stage 4); girls attain peak growth rates a year after breast development has commenced (Marshall and Tanner, 1970). In Kikuyu adolescents, this resulted in a 2-year period (age 12.0–14.0 years) during which girls were on average appreciably taller (>4 cm) than boys.

Sex differences in pubertal growth schedules reflect differences in developmental patterns of gonadal steroid production. Gonadal steroids also influence overall somatotype by their effects on metabolism and body composition, specifically the amount and distribution of muscle and fat (Cheek, 1974; Malina, 1974). Elevation of estradiol levels coincides in girls with initiation of breast development (Lee *et al.*, 1976; Winter and Faiman, 1973a). Estradiol continues to rise until menarche and is involved in growth acceleration and redistribution of fat reserves, among other processes. In boys, on the other hand, the major increments in testosterone levels occur later in the maturational process, at Genital Stage 3 or 4 (Lee and Migeon, 1975; Winter and Faiman, 1972). Growth then accelerates and muscle mass increases, along with other signs of androgenization. Thus, sex differences in developmental schedule are exaggerated for the observer by the early appearance of height gains and altered body form in girls, and their late appearance in boys.

Both the pattern and degree of variability of pubertal development observed in the Kikuyu study population resembled that reported in other groups, with the exception that female maturation was especially late and prolonged. The median age at menarche, however, is consistent with the tendency to later menarcheal ages reported for other sub-Saharan Bantu populations (Eveleth and Tanner, 1975, p. 214). Although pubertal maturation may be characterized as a coherent physical process, the individual experience of that process can be obscured by interindividual variability from being generalizable to assessment of others, and prediction for oneself. The obscurity tends to be aggravated by the fact that many relevant physical variables are not discernable directly, and that intraindividual dyssynchronies may exist between the pubertal and other maturational processes, such as cognition or thought.

It was suggested at the outset of this chapter that anxiety, conflict, and cognitive dissonance could be drawn away from this period in the life cycle by offering a structure of meaningful, explicitly maturational experiences. The social structure of experience is thus of prime salience for modulating and focusing development at adolescence.

The social management of puberty and adolescence is in many ways distinctly different among Kikuyu from patterns prevalent in Western societies, although recent social change has greatly altered many aspects of adolescent experience. Emphasis on age is minimal, and the timing of rites of passage or major changes in status (circumcision, CPE exam, separate residence) is significantly influenced by individual maturation.

The practice of circumcision may play an especially important role, as indicated by its continued value even after it was deritualized, and the extent and persistence of its use for girls despite over 40 years' official disapproval. The meaning and function of circumcision rites have long been topics of interest and debate (e.g., Bettelheim, 1954; Mead, 1949; Van Gennep, 1909; Whiting et al., 1958). The more potent social rituals, such as circumcision, no doubt are so by virtue of their multiple levels of effect and significance. It is apparent that, besides its other functions, circumcision at puberty can be a powerful element in social modelling of adolescent experience: the operation is an excellent analog of pubertal maturation because it involves the transfiguration of primary sex characters, while offering the definite advantage of being a predictable event that can be endowed with universal elements. It can serve as a focal developmental funnel that explicitly merges physical with social maturation of the individual in a socially controlled way.[6] Important gains for the individual and for society can thereby be realized by synchronizing individual ontogenies within the social framework.

These effects of circumcision at puberty are possibly based on the incorporation of genital transformation with changes in social role and status. Hence, pubertal development is normalized and brought within the social sphere. The potential of developmental dyssynchronies within and among adolescents as a source of cognitive dissonance or conflict is reduced by placing emphasis on a biosocial event as a primary organizing maturational experience in puberty. The normative power of the event increases in proportion to the degree of actual conflict or potential dissonance it integrates.

Cultural beliefs which maintain that social interventions at puberty are fundamental to attaining physical maturity also advance rationalization of social structuring of development. Circumcision often functions in this manner. In the case of Kikuyu, true biological maturity for males entails circumcision, as the genital operation is seen as a necessary step in ontogeny. The dependence of physical processes on social factors can be emphasized in other ways. For example, some

---

[6] This is consistent with the theory of cognitive dissonance, which states that primary means of alleviating or avoiding dissonance are devaluation of dissonance-provoking elements and enhanced valuation of consonant ones (Zajonc, 1968, pp. 360–361).

groups such as Australian aboriginals[7] and !Kung San (Shostak, 1983) believe that intimacy with a male, by marriage or other arrangements, promotes maturation in pubescent females.

In summary, Kikuyu adolescents showed the same degree of variability in timing of pubertal development as has been observed in other populations, so that chronological age became a poor index of actual state of physical maturity in puberty. Logically, goodness of fit between adolescent social status and physical maturation may best be realized if the former is directly related to the latter. Index variables are crucial in this process. Kikuyu use a variety of index variables to track individual development and cue in social interventions.

SOCIAL STRUCTURE AND DEVELOPMENTAL PROCESS

It was reasoned in the previous sections that the continuous, complex, and variable nature of pubertal development necessitates the use of simplified social schemata to cue the social construction of adolescence to individual maturation. These points were illustrated with data on Kikuyu adolescence. In this section elements in the social construction of adolescent experience are outlined and the outcomes of different social schemata discussed.

The need for such schemata seems to arise from fundamental heuristics in human cognition (Lumsden and Wilson, 1981, pp. 86–90). Humans tend to fit present experience to a representative prototype on the lowest level of integration necessary to generate an efficient response pattern. Perceptions that are incongruent with the conceptual template are disregarded unless it is recognized that they threaten the utility of the functional schemata. Attention is also allocated in proportion to perceived relevance and variability. Human interest is thus directed differentially. Depending on the prototypes employed in these cognitive heuristics, a great deal of variance may be disregarded or subsumed. The array of schemata available in a society will therefore have considerable significance for individual experience and social management in puberty.

The cognitive-conceptual framework to be applied in a given situation is selected on the basis of fit between features of the immediate perception with those of a generalized framework, employing a minimum of variables necessary to achieve compatibility. A hierarchy of index variables that are heuristic devices for effecting fit of perception and prototype is evolved in the context of personal and cultural ex-

[7] Burbank, V. *Premarital sex norms: Cultural interpretations in an Australian Aboriginal Community.* Paper presented at the meeting of the American Anthropological Association, Chicago, November, 1983.

perience (Nisbett and Ross, 1980; Tversky and Kahneman, 1974). Decision making in determining behavior is similarly directed.

It has been emphasized that a necessary characteristic of an index variable is perceptibility. Thus, although in the study of adolescent development scientific progress had been made toward increasingly proximal measures of maturation, such as bone age (e.g., Tanner *et al.*, 1975), these are nearly inapplicable on the everyday cultural level because they are not readily seen. Index variables are usually selected that are indirect but representative reflections of the target state.

The cognitive heuristic power of a feature displayed by developing individuals may provoke its use as an index variable despite nonparallelism with the function it appears to track. A baby's first smiles are a good example (Konner, 1972). In puberty, menarche has been such a feature. Menarche, whether ritually marked or not, has been widely believed by societies to be a key event in female reproductive maturation (Brown, 1963, 1969). In fact, the social schemata based on assumptions of its importance may in a self-fulfilling way structure experience so that menarche does become a central occasion in organizing female development (Deutsch, 1944; Shainess, 1961; Koff *et al.*, 1978).

Nevertheless, recent findings in reproductive biology show that, far from being a definite physiological event indicating reproductive maturity, menarche is just an outcome in an ongoing physiological process to achieve fertile cyclicity (Lemarchand-Béraud *et al.*, 1982; Vihko and Apter, 1980: Winter and Faiman, 1973b). Perimenarcheal cycles are irregular and mainly anovulatory, generating a period of postmenarcheal infertility or subfecundity. Factors determining length of this period are little understood and interindividual variability is high, but on average, populations of young women have not reached mature ovulating frequency by five years after menarche. Menarche, then, is not a threshold event in reproductive maturation: it is only a rough indicator of approaching maturity.

Costs of maintaining a given social structure of adolescence are determined less by the actual congruence between the index variable and the maturational state it is supposed to represent than it is by the degree of congruence that is socially expected or sanctioned. For example, there is little cost for cultural maintenance of menarche as the index variable to reproductive maturity for females if it is not expected they commence childbearing immediately thereafter, but potential costs and conflicts increase if they are. Reciprocally, levels of cognitive dissonance generated by schemata determine whether they may be modified or discarded.

Index variables that track pubertal maturation may be intrinsic (size, age) or acquired (skills), and they may be treated in a continuous or

discontinuous manner. For example, degree of freedom or responsibility could be increased gradually as height increased, or conferred
in a single increment when a specific size is reached. Nature and application of indexes greatly influence the shaping of experience. If, as
a simplified instance, both height and age were tracked, dissonance
would of necessity occur if a privilege were given in puberty on the
basis of attainment in either.

Potential for cognitive dissonance generated by developmental variation at puberty may be modulated not only be social schemata, but
also by availability of peers among whom comparisons of maturational
progress may be made. Adolescence experienced in small, multi-age
groups would diverge in this and other respects from that experienced
primarily in larger, single-age groups. Peer groups can act as important
normative forces at puberty, but their influence depends on social modelling of their membership and roles.

Finally, a potent social means of transcending the vicissitudes of
developmental change consists of redirecting attention away from what
the adolescent *is* to what the adolescent is *becoming*. By this means
emphasis is transferred from uncertain process to valued outcome and
tolerance of intermediate circumstances is raised. The ethnographic
distribution of this device is wide. Under many guises, it sustains adolescents through socially decreed periods of often aversive conditions,
from the shorter periods of initiation and other rites of passage, to ap-
prenticeships (spiritual or technical), and prolonged phases of competitive tutelage.

To recapitulate briefly: With adolescents, society is confronted with
the task of fitting a continuous, variable process into social schemata
that serve as cognitive templates for integrating perceptions and di-
recting behavior. Index variables act as perceptual cues to fit appropriate schemata to experience. To be viable as indexes, variables must
be perceptible; hence, they must often be indirect measures of limited
validity. Obviously, selection of indexes included in schemata greatly
influences the structure of experience, as well as the potential for cognitive dissonance generated at puberty by developmental dyssynchrony.

In this final section, attention will be returned to Kikuyu adolescents
and the ways in which this model can characterize their experience.
In traditional Kikuyu society, adolescence was a particularly prominent,
prolonged phase of the life cycle with clearly defined roles and statuses.
Genital operations initiated both sexes into this phase. Age was not
tracked, but timing of circumcision was prescriptively linked to physical
maturation in females; for males, it came at the end of puberty, prior
to which they had moved into men's houses. Initiation year cohorts
were formed, within which cooperativeness, sociability, and mutual

support were strongly sanctioned. Males realized considerable freedom and autonomy—females less so. Leisure for varied recreation and peer sociability was granted.

Social supports (peer, ritual), disregard for age, positive valuation of roles, and lack of ambiguity in the structure of adolescence (boundaries, duration, content), definitely operated to fuse physical and social development in a normative framework. Today, some of these supportive features remain and mitigate the impact of social change on adolescent experience. In particular, schooling has induced intense competition among peers for access to opportunity and makes no concession to developmental differences while pressing for a fully age-tracked system. After school, there is usually an uncertain future for a rather undefined period in which the adolescent must somehow effect entry into the modernizing economy despite increasing competitive pressure. Peer supporters have become individual competitors, and the defining social structure of adolescence has become blurred.

Remaining supportive practices include continued use of age-grade terms, circumcision for boys and some girls, disregard for absolute age, and granting of personal freedom to boys. Data presented above demonstrated use of index variables (breast development, emissions, size) to gauge individual maturation and determine timing of social interventions (circumcision, separate residence, age-grade) that confer new statuses. Adolescence is nevertheless becoming an increasingly difficult, anxious period.

This Kikuyu community is only a specific example of the interplay of developmental process and social structuring in determining outcomes at adolescence. It has been argued here that some biosocial problems of adolescents in a particular cultural setting may not be strictly innate, but due to social modelling of experience. Other chapters in this volume (Vinovskis; Whiting et al.) document a tremendous range in the cultural management of adolescence, both across cultures and within societies over time.

This discussion has focused on physical parameters of adolescent maturation largely because there is much more comparative quantified data available. Further, physical processes of development are better understood than is cognitive, conceptual, behavioral, or psychological maturation in adolescence. Incorporation of these processes, however, will be vital to formulation of interactive models of culture and biosocial development.

ACKNOWLEDGMENT

This research was supported by an NIMH postdoctoral training grant, #MH14088-03, and by the Grant Foundation.

REFERENCES

Bettelheim, B. Symbolic wounds. Glencoe, Ill.: Free Press, 1954.

Brown, J. K. A cross-cultural study of female initiation rites. American Anthropologist, 1963, 65, 837–853.

Brown, J. K. Female initiation rites: A review of the current literature. In D. Rogers (Ed.), Issues in adolescent psychology. New York: Appleton-Century-Crofts, 1969, pp. 74–87.

Burr, I. M., Sizonenko, S.L., Kaplan, S. L., and Grumbach, M. M. Hormonal changes in puberty. I. Correlation of serum luteinizing hormone with stages of puberty, testicular size, and bone age in normal boys. Pediatric Research, 1970, 4, 25–35.

Burrell, R., Healy, J., and Tanner, J. M. Age at menarche in South African Bantu girls living in the Transkei Reserve. Human Biology, 1961, 33, 250–261.

Cagnolo, C. The Akikuyu: Their customs, traditions, and folklore. Nyeri, Kenya: Mission Printing School, 1933.

Cheek, D. B. Body composition, hormones, nutrition, and adolescent growth. In M. M. Grumbach, G.D. Grave, and F. E. Mayer (Eds.), Control of the onset of puberty. New York: Wiley, 1974, pp. 424–442.

Cheek, D. B., Migeon, C. J., and Mellitis, E. D. Concept of biologic age. In D. B. Cheek (Ed.), Human growth. Philadelphia: Lee & Febiger, 1968, pp. 541–567.

Deutsch, H. The psychology of women (Vol. I). New York: Grune & Stratton, 1944.

Eveleth, P. B. and Tanner, J. M. World-wide variation in human growth. New York: Cambridge University Press, 1975.

Harlan, W. R., Grillo, G. P., Cornoni-Huntley, J., and Leaverton, P. E. Secondary sex characteristics of boys 12 to 17 years of age: The U.S. health examination survey. Journal of Pediatrics, 1979, 95, 293–297.

Herzog, J. D. Initiation and high school in the development of Kikuyu youths' self-concept. Ethos, 1973, 1, 478–489.

Kenyatta, J. Facing Mount Kenya. London: Secker & Warberg, 1938.

Koff, E., Rierdan, J., and Silverstone, E. Changes in representation of body image as a function of menarcheal status. Developmental Psychology, 1978, 14, 635–642.

Konner, M. J. Aspects of the developmental ethology of a foraging pople. In N. G. Blurton Jones (Ed.), Ethological studies of child behaviour. Cambridge: Cambridge University Press, 1972, pp. 285–304.

Leakey, L. S. B. The Southern Kikuyu before 1903. London: Academic Press, 1977.

Lee, P. A., and Migeon, C. J. Puberty in boys: Correlation of plasma levels of gonadotropins (LH, FSH), androgens (testosterone, androstenedione, dehydroepiandrosterone and its sulfate), estrogens (estrone and estradiol) and progestins (progesterone and 17-hydroxyprogesterone). Journal of Clinical Endocrinology and Metabolism, 1975, 41, 556–562.

Lee, P. A., Xenakis, T., Winer, J., and Matsenbaugh, S. Puberty in girls: Correlation of serum levels of gonadotropins, prolactin, androgens, estrogens, and progestins with physical changes. Journal of Clinical Endocrinology and Metabolism, 1976, 43, 775–784.

Lemarchand-Béraud, T., Zufferey, M.-M., Reymond, M., and Rey, I. Maturation of the hypothalamo-pituitary-ovarian axis in adolescent girls. Journal of Clinical Endocrinology and Metabolism, 1982, 54, 241–246.

Lumsden, C. J., and Wilson, E. O. *Genes, mind, and culture.* Cambridge: Harvard University Press, 1981.

Malina, R. M. Adolescent changes in size, build, composition and performance. *Human Biology,* 1974, *46,* 117–132.

Marshall, W.A. The relationship of puberty to other maturity indicators and body composition in man. *Journal of Reproduction and Fertility,* 1978, *52,* 437–443.

Marshall, W. A., and Tanner, J. M. Variations in pattern of pubertal changes in girls. *Archives of Disease in Childhood,* 1969, *44,* 291–303.

Marshall, W. A., and Tanner, J. M. Variations in the pattern of pubertal changes in boys. *Archives of Disease in Childhood,* 1970, *45,* 13–23.

Mead, M. *Male and female.* New York: New American Library, 1949.

Murdock, G. P. *Africa: Its peoples and their cultural history.* New York: McGraw-Hill, 1959.

Nisbett, R., and Ross, L. *Human inference: Strategies and shortcomings of social judgment.* Englewood Cliffs, N.J.: Prentice-Hall, 1980.

Shainess, N. A re-evaluation of some aspects of femininity through a study of menstruation: A preliminary report. *Comprehensive Psychiatry,* 1961, 2, 20–26.

Shostak, M. *Nisa: The life and words of a !Kung San woman.* New York: Random House, 1983.

Sizonenko, P. C., Burr, I. M., Kaplan, S. F., and Grumbach, M. Hormonal changes in puberty. II. Correlations of serum luteinizing hormone and follicle-stimulating hormone with stages of puberty and bone age in normal girls. *Pediatric Research,* 1970, *4,* 36–45.

Tanner, J. M. *Growth at adolescence.* Oxford: Blackwell, 1962.

Tanner, J. M. Growth and endocrinology of the adolescent. *In* L. I. Gardner (Ed.), *Endocrine and genetic diseases of childhood and adolescence* (2nd ed.). Philadelphia: W. B. Saunders, 1975, pp. 14–64.

Tanner, J. M., Whitehouse, R. H., Marshall, W. A., Healy, M. J. R., and Goldstein, J. *Assessment of skeletal maturity and prediction of adult height.* New York: Academic Press, 1975.

Thorner, M. O., Round, J., Jones, A., Fahmy, D., Groom, G. V., Butcher, S., and Thompson, K. Serum prolactin and oestradiol levels at different stages of puberty. *Clinical Endocrinology,* 1977, *7,* 463–468.

Tversky, A., and Kahneman, D. Judgment and uncertainty: Heuristics and biases. *Science,* 1974, *185,* 1124–1131.

Van Gennep, A. *Les rites de passage.* Paris: Libraire Critique Emile Nourry, 1909.

Vihko, R., and Apter, D. The role of androgens in adolescent cycles. *Journal of Steroid Biochemistry,* 1980, *12,* 369–373.

Weiner, J. S., and Lourie, J. A. *Human biology: A guide to field methods.* Oxford: Blackwell, 1969.

Whiting, B. B., and Whiting, J. W. M. *Children of six cultures: A psycho-cultural analysis.* Cambridge, Harvard University Press, 1975.

Whiting, J. W. M., Kluckhohn, R. P., and Anthony, A. S. The function of male initiation ceremonies at puberty. *In* E. E. Maccoby, T. M. Newcomb, and E. L. Hartley (Eds.), *Readings in social psychology.* New York: Henry Holt, 1958.

Winter, J. S. D., and Faiman, C. Pituitary-gonadal relations in male children and adolescents. *Pediatric Research,* 1972, *6,* 126–135.

Winter, J. S. D., and Faiman, C. Pituitary-gonadal relations in female children and adolescents. *Pediatric Research,* 1973, *7,* 948–953.(a)

Winter, J. S. D., and Faiman, C. The development of cyclic pituitary function in adolescent females. *Journal of Clinical Endocrinology and Metabolism,* 1973, *37,* 714–718.(b)

Zajonc, R. B. Cognitive theories in social psychology. *In* G. Lindzey and A. Aronson (Eds.), *The handbook of social psychology, Vol. 1. Historical introduction, systematic positions* (2nd ed.). Reading, Mass.: Addison-Wesley, 1968, pp. 320–411.

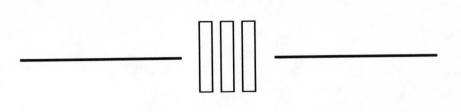

DEVELOPMENT: EMOTIONAL, COGNITIVE, AND SEXUAL

7

SUBSETS OF ADOLESCENT MOTHERS: DEVELOPMENTAL, BIOMEDICAL, AND PSYCHOSOCIAL ISSUES

Beatrix A. Hamburg

INTRODUCTION

The experience of being a mother represents a major developmental transition for all women, regardless of age. It is a time of new demands and challenges that lead to changes in values, attitudes, and behaviors that have an enduring impact on the future life course. The major trend among adult American women has been the evolving pattern to postpone childbearing until later in adult years after a stable period of time in the work force. At present, a large percentage of first births occur at 30 years or older. At the same time, among adolescents there is a countervailing trend toward earlier and earlier childbearing.

This discrepant timing of adolescent pregnancy inherently poses a stressful situation. It is a transition for which the individual has no prior preparation and societal supports are lacking. For these very young women, choices that are made in the process of resolution of the new developmental tasks and challenges offer possibilities for harmful foreclosure of growth and development with diminished life options for both mother and child. The pervasiveness of the highly adverse health, social, and economic consequences of adolescent parenthood and the continuing trend toward increasing numbers of very young adolescent mothers, particularly those 16 years of age and younger, are issues of continuing national concern. For a fortunate few adolescents, there is a mastery of the challenge and the achievement of significant gains in maturity and competence.

Progress in addressing the difficult and increasing problems of adolescent sexuality, pregnancy, and childbearing will depend on gaining insights into the complex interplay of biological, psychological, and developmental factors that interact in specific and differential ways to influence discrete subsets of the adolescent population.

In recent years, there have been major advances in behavioral and social sciences. There are now concepts and methods that suggest new approaches to clarifying the issues involved in differing life patterns of school-aged mothers. Systematic, interdisciplinary research is possible that adopts a developmental perspective in integrating the empirical knowledge and concepts from such diverse fields as epidemiology, psychology, pediatrics, obstetrics, psychiatry, public health, demography, and economics. A biopsychosocial perspective helps broaden our understanding of normal adolescent development and also serves to give new bases for comprehending the problem behaviors of contemporary youth in modern industrial society.

Three subsets of school-aged adolescents have been delineated, and their distinctive patterns of sexuality, pregnancy, and motherhood will be discussed in this chapter. The subsets of adolescents have been characterized as: (1) immaturity and problem-proneness; (2) alternate life course with competent coping; and (3) depressive disorder.

Although each of the three subsets of adolescent mothers will be discussed, there is a focus on early adolescence in relation to the subset of immaturity and problem-proneness. The reasons for delineating early adolescence as a distinct life stage are given. The developmental characteristics of this period are described in detail. The match of these characteristics and developmental tasks with pregnancy and motherhood is discussed. Typical medical, social, psychological, educational, and economic outcomes for the very young mother are presented. Some physical, cognitive, and psychosocial outcomes for the child are also given. These observations are placed in a life span context in which the implications of the asynchronous timing of events in the life cycle can help explain the altered maternal life course and the problems for the child, adolescent mother, and her family.

The range of negative medical, personal, and economic outcomes for adolescent pregnancy has been exceedingly well documented, but little attention has been given to understanding the good outcomes. The specific factors and mechanisms that mediate either good or bad outcomes among young mothers have been little studied. The fit between normative capabilities of adolescents at varying stages in their development in relation to the tasks of parenthood and outcomes has not been examined. There is little recognition that during adolescence there are chronological, biological, and social ages of an individual that may be markedly asynchronous. Yet, the known variability in the physical and psychosocial development of adolescents warrants the use of maturational status rather than chronological age in assessing biological and behavioral status during adolescence. For example, maternal adaptations to the needs of the infant may be intrinsically much more difficult for immature adolescents than for more mature mothers. Therefore, adolescent motherhood as a developmental challenge superimposed on the normative tasks of adolescents at differing developmental stages is an important, although neglected, line of inquiry. The developmental perspective should be broadly construed to include a life span perspective and developmental psychopathology.

Comparisons will be made with the subset of older, largely minority adolescents for whom their alternate life course results from sociocultural circumstances that predispose toward choosing a strategy of adolescent motherhood and represents competent coping. The typical medical, social, psychological, educational, and economic outcomes for these mothers and their children are discussed in detail by Furstenberg in Chapter 11.

Literature on adolescent sexuality, pregnancy, and motherhood will be reviewed from a developmental perspective. In doing so, there is an effort to identify gaps in knowledge and to highlight promising lines of inquiry for future research.

STAGES OF ADOLESCENCE

TERMINOLOGY AND DEFINITIONS

In the field of adolescent pregnancy, there is a notable lack of consensus within the ranks of medical professionals and social scientists on the meaning of most of the terms that are in common use. This semantic confusion has greatly complicated the tasks of trying to marshal relevant data, to sort out significant issues, and to determine their relationships to each other.

The lack of conceptual clarity derives in large part from the tendency to view adolescence, in general and "teenage pregnancy," in particular, as unitary phenomena. Without a clear understanding of the developmental and biopsychosocial bases for defining meaningful age groupings within adolescence, there are arbitrary and widely differing age-group choices. These arbitrary choices have often reflected targets of opportunity in sampling adolescent populations. Also, they derive from existing conventions of reporting national vital statistics. In this anachronistic tradition, national data concerning children and youth typically and grouped as 5–14 years and 15–24 years. Given these choices for defining adolescence, the prevalent practice has been to select the older age bracket and to compensate by adjusting downward and using 15–19 years as a "teenage" sample. This convention means that many meaningful data are washed out, and age categories that have developmental significance are unlikely to occur in studies that rely on such national data.

School-age pregnancy is a term that is preferable to "teenage" pregnancy. Across all subsets, the occurrence of pregnancy in a school-age girl poses high risk in the multiple ways that will be delineated in Chapter 18 by Klerman. The same issues do not apply to post-high school, 18- and 19-year-old mothers. In conventional usage, however, adolescent or teenage populations usually also include these persons who are, legally and in a functional sense, adult women. They do not belong in analyses of adolescent pregnancy and confound the findings.

The pervasive failure in studies of adolescent pregnancy and child-bearing to differentiate appropriately between early and late adolescence has obscured highly important differences in fertility rates and birth trends for the different teenage cohorts. Rates of childbearing for the oldest teenagers (aged 18–19) have shown a decline in recent years, whereas the rates for early adolescents (aged 11–15) are rising. However, much lumping of the data continues to occur, and some of this aggregated data can usefully be reported. In this chapter, *teenager* will be used to report such data and should signify that it is a unitary term that includes 18 and 19 year olds in addition to the younger age groups.

CONCEPTS OF AGE

Adolescence is a period during which it becomes important to recognize that there are actually three distinctive societal constructs and definitions of age. These constructs are chronological age, biological age, and social age.

Chronological Age. In industrial societies, the preponderant emphasis is on the calendar date of birth. The certificate of the date of birth is the earliest and one of the most crucial personal documents over the life span. Many significant societal milestones depend on this chronological age: the age of school entry, eligibility for military service, age of obtaining a driver's license, drinking age, voting age, etc. For most of the lifetime, the three kinds of ages are tightly yoked together. Their separability is not readily apparent, and there is a strong tendency to use chronological age as the single marker for all three. During the course of the lengthy modern adolescence, this is not appropriate. The salience of each of the age constructs will vary in accordance with the phase of adolescent development.

Biological Age. As will be discussed, there is a wide range in the normative chronological ages at which adolescents undergo the biological changes of puberty. There is also a gender difference. Females typically are 1–2 years ahead of males in normal pubertal change and, therefore, advanced in their biological age. Among early adolescents, both physical and psychological status is best understood by adopting a strong biological frame of reference. The concept of gynecological age has arisen to define the biological maturity of adolescent mothers. It is defined as the number of years following menarche at which a pregnancy occurs. For example, two young women may each have a gynecological age of 2 years if one had menarche at age 11 and became pregnant at age 13 and the other had menarche at age 16 and became pregnant at age 18 years.

Social Age. These are the ages at which cultural milestones are achieved for which there are social norms. This includes age at first marriage, age at birth of first child, age of adopting adult work roles, age of retirement, etc. When societal norms for these events are violated by being "off-time," too early or too late, there are social costs. A good example is teenage pregnancy.

For most individuals, these three age metrics are synchronized throughout the life span. However, during the lengthy period of modern adolescence there are many possibilities for asynchrony. When there is a lack of match between the three ages, usually some stress. At times, if the discrepancy is great enough, psychopathology may occur.

SUBSETS OF ADOLESCENT MOTHERS

PROBLEM-PRONENESS

The sexual and pregnancy behaviors of many adolescents of all ages have been shown to be highly intercorrelated with other adolescent problem behaviors such as alcohol, drug use, and drop in school achievement and motivation. Jessor and Jessor (1975) have suggested that engaging in problem behaviors serves important functions for the individuals that may include: (1) an instrumental effort to achieve otherwise unavailable goals; (2) a learned way of coping with personal frustrations and anticipated failure; (3) an expression of opposition to or rejection of conventional society; (4) a negotiation for developmental transition; (5) a badge of membership in peer subculture (or some combination of these alternatives). The survey and descriptive research has not generally addressed these broader psychosocial and personality implications and, in particular, does not account for the differential patterns of problem-proneness within adolescent cohorts.

The problem-proneness behavior theory of Jessor and Jessor (1977) holds that personality and social environment interact to set regulatory norms for individuals defining age appropriateness of their behaviors.

The likelihood of expression of problem behavior depends on the balance between instigations such as peer pressure and role models; the maturity of personal controls; and the psychosocial perceptions of the adolescent with respect to social supports, social constraint, expectations of others, particularly parents.

The Jessor's problem-prone behavior theory has lacked a developmental maturity component. The rising prevalence of problem behaviors among the youngest adolescents poses important questions about the relationship of problem-prone behaviors to processes of adolescent development. The developmental approach to the problem-prone behavior theory seems especially relevant to school-age pregnancy, since motherhood represents a major developmental transition. A major portion of this chapter will be devoted to a discussion of the likelihood that immaturity and problem-proneness are linked as a syndrome that represents a subset of adolescent pregnancy and motherhood in which there is double jeopardy. It is also proposed that this subgroup is at highest risk of biomedical casualty to both mother and child in terms of mortality and morbidity, and they are at very high risk of casualty in their caretaking as well.

ALTERNATE LIFE COURSE WITH COMPETENT COPING

As individuals move through the life span, their careers reflect a succession of culturally defined roles, which to a very great extent are age linked. As mentioned, rather explicit age norms exist for such major transitions as leaving home, getting married, having children, assuming adult work roles, and retiring. Neugarten (1979) has discussed the adverse consequences that can flow from pronounced deviations from the culturally approved time schedule—whether the "off-time" is too early or too late.

In the usual course of events, pregnancy is expected to occur in a mature adult who has completed schooling and has experienced a period of adjustment to the demands of marriage. Among mainstream adult women, there has been a trend toward early entry into the work force, later marriage, and quite late childbearing. The temporary, maternity-related retirement from the work force has been called the "M-dip," Masnick and Bane (1980). By these norms, adolescent pregnancy is markedly discrepant behavior. While it appears ill-timed and off-schedule according to the prevailing social norms, early fertility may not be ill-timed according to the developmental requisites of some adolescents (Cvetkovich et al., 1978; Zelnick et al., 1981; Hatcher, 1973), the requisites of teenaged male and female social relations (Furstenberg, 1976; Ladner, 1971), or the economic and social requisites of the subculture of which an individual adolescent is a member (Stack, 1974). In other words, prevailing societal norms may have little to say about the requirements—real and perceived—of survival and identity formation for a given adolescent whose own social context differs significantly from the mainstream societal norms. This might be true of individual adolescents of any socioeconomic status or of entire cohorts within disadvantaged subpopulations.

Established survey methodologies for studying rates of sexual and pregnancy phenomena (Zelnick and Kantner, 1980) are inappropriate to understand the social contexts of adolescence and the developmental issues peculiar to them. Instead, more naturalistic, ecologically valid, and in-depth interview techniques are needed. It will also be important to gather longitudinal data into the middle and late twenties of these young women in order to understand the chains of events and processes that connect social arrangements to the life situations and to the psychology of the individual. A charting of the long-term development of teenaged mothers would clarify the role of early pregnancy across the overall life course for distinctive groups of women. The importance of such research is suggested by Furstenberg's (1976) longitudinal study of teenaged mothers. By following the adolescent mothers into their early twenties, he discovered how erroneous some of our impressions of early parenthood have been. In particular, the notion that having an unplanned child in adolescence leads, inevitably, to lives of deprivation for both has been shown to be untrue.

Ethnographic studies provide descriptions of a normative, alternative life course within the black subculture (Ladner, 1971; Stack, 1974). In this subculture, the modal events for women of entry into the work force and childbearing are reversed. In adult life there is not a pattern of early entry into the labor force and time out from work or career to have children in late twenties or early thirties. An urban, poor, black woman who wishes to have children may find that her best option may be to commence childbearing in her teen years. This is her "time off" from the labor force (Hogan, 1978). Youth unemployment among blacks is high and has plateaued at about 50% in recent years. Furthermore, with adolescent pregnancy, her children will be old enough to manage substantial amounts of household responsibilities when the mother enters the work force. This may serve to relieve some of the stresses of being a working mother that a poor black mother could not afford to ease through other means.

Ethnographies also describe how early and out-of-wedlock fertility expands the kin networks on which poor, urban, black individuals depend for social and economic support. Full membership in this adult network can begin with childbearing, an incentive for early fertility.

These networks become especially significant when a young black woman enters the labor force. Network members can provide child care and other assistance unaffordable at a meager salary. Thus, it may be crucial for some black women that networks be well established by the time they enter the labor force. Black adolsecent mothers who initially reside with their families begin to establish their own households approximately 5 years after the birth of their first child. This observation lends plausibility to the thesis that black adolescent mothers use their first years of parenthood to consolidate their own growth and solidify their networks, in preparation for household headship once they are able to work. This suggests another adaptive feature of early fertility.

Consistent with this interpretation are analyses of the relationship between timing of the first birth and completed family size. While teenage fertility predicts continuing fertility and large completed family size for white women, it does not for blacks. Recent cohort analyses of these relationships reveal a decline in fertility rates for post-adolescent black women (Millman and Hendershot, 1980). Thus, as adults in their thirties, the completed family size and work status is roughly comparable for black and white females.

Converging lines of inquiry suggest that there is a subgroup of poor, urban, black young older adolescent women choosing to engage in early childbearing who are not immature, problem-prone, or emotionally symptomatic. They are hypothesized to have realistic perceptions of pregnancy and motherhood, capacity for sustained interpersonal relationships, mature and renegotiated relationships with their parents, and a realistic future orientation. For them, early childbearing is a strategy that promotes personal and social development and cultural survival, given their socioenvironmental contingencies. Further research is needed to describe in detail the social–psychological mechanisms by which this alternative strategy succeeds or fails.

DEPRESSION AND EARLY CHILDBEARING

The presence of clinical depression among school-age mothers is a prominent part of clinical experiences. Yet, there has been no systematic research attention to this phenomenon, despite the clear implications for likelihood of pregnancy and prediction of impairments in parenting. In general, adolescent depression has been a neglected area of inquiry. Recently, there has been an upsurge of interest in this area related to the sharp rises in adolescent suicide.

In 1980 there were 12.5 suicides per 100,000 persons aged 15–24 years. This is double the rate for 1970 (National Center for Health Statistics, 1980). Suicide is the second leading cause of death, after accidents, among adolescents. For every successful suicide attempt, it is estimated that there are at least 100 and perhaps as many as 200 suicide attempts. Male completed suicides still greatly outnumber females, but rates among males appear to be leveling off and those among females are continuing to rise. The data show that at all ages rates are highest among white males, followed by black males, white females, and black females in that order. Rates are lowest among all Hispanics, both male and female. The reasons for these differentials in risk of suicide are not known. However, there have been recent advances in methodology and measures that have given impetus to systematic studies of adolescent depression and suicide. It is now possible to carry out systematic assessment of depressive mood and depressive disorder in adolescent populations (Kandel and Davies, 1982).

The extent and level of depressive symptomatology in school-age mothers should be studied. It is also important to go beyond mere diagnosis of depression, to develop profiles of the attributes of these young women, and to characterize broad areas of their functioning or impairment. In addition to elucidating the role of loneliness and depression in the seeking of sexual intimacy, it is equally important to observe and characterize parenting behaviors and mother–infant interactions when the mother is depressed.

It has been a major finding that depressive mood is an important predictor of initiation into use of illicit drugs other than marijuana when the adolescent is at risk of such involvement by prior use of marijuana (Kandel, 1978). It has been suggested that this use of illicit drugs may represent a form of self-medication to relieve the depressed state (Kandel, 1978). The history of drug use in depressed pregnant young mothers is of high salience for the outcome of the baby. Smoking and alcohol use are known to have specific deleterious effects on a developing fetus. Illicit drug use can also result in damaged or addicted babies. The depressive status of the school-age mothers should be systematically related to the medical status, physical, and psychosocial development of her infant over time.

Clinical observations support the belief that when there is a healthy, easy to manage baby, the depressed mother may have a positive mothering experience. She may find the baby to be a gratifying extension of herself and enjoy a loving relationship. However, it has been observed that maternal depression, untreated, will tend to deepen as the infant reaches toddler status, makes more strident demands on the mother, and exhibits autonomous behaviors.

Some clinicians feel that when this occurs, such depressed mothers will try to recapture the sense of intimacy and love by becoming pregnant again. All of these issues have preventive implications and represent promising lines of inquiry.

DEVELOPMENTAL TASKS FOR EARLY ADOLESCENCE

BIOLOGICAL TASKS OF EARLY ADOLESCENCE

When completed, the biological changes of puberty endow individuals with the physical capability to perform adult functions. Among females, this chiefly refers to the constellation of anatomical and physiological changes that make childbearing and lactation possible. Among males, in addition to the development of secondary sex characteristics, the pubertal changes involve anatomical and physiological changes in respiratory, circulatory, and muscular systems that lead to remarkable increases in strength and endurance. There are also hormonal changes that enhance sexuality and aggressiveness. As the Western cultures have become more complex, the timing of adoption of adult roles has been increasingly delayed to later and later ages. Under circumstances in which postpubertal individuals with adult capacities are retained in child-like roles for lengthy periods of time, there are inherent opportunities for too early timing in the transition to adult roles such as pregnancy and motherhood.

The onset of menses is a dramatic biological event that is the marker of pubertal change in girls. Therefore, pre- and postmenarche are widely used as reference terms for females. No comparable referent exists for males. Tanner (1952) has detailed bodily changes of puberty for both males and females and specified five stages that encompass the full range of changes from Stage 1, prepuberty, where there is no observable change, to Stage 5, where there is complete acquisition of adult genital and secondary sex characteristics. On this Tanner scale, menarche is a relatively late event and occurs preponderantly in Stage 4. In the contemporary United States, the modal age of menarche is 12.8. In general, comparable Tanner stages for males lag 1–2 years behind those for females. The Tanner stages give a highly useful and practical way to ascertain the biological "age" or maturational status of a young person. Also, they can provide a stable reference point for differing terminologies of adolescence.

It is certainly true that the dominant themes of early adolescence are related to the endocrine changes of puberty. However, these changes transcend the changes in secondary sex characteristics or libido. There are biological changes in virtually every system of the body including, height, facial contours, fat distribution, muscular development, cardiovascular status, mood changes, and energy levels. These are of striking importance and function powerfully and independently in shaping the course of adolescent development. Also, the timing and rate of pubertal change has powerful impacts. The age of onset of puberty shows wide variation among normal children.

Some children have not yet begun any pubertal change at an age at which their peers have entirely completed all of the pubertal events. Mary Cover Jones (1965) has done long-term investigations of the differing impacts and varying outcomes of early versus late maturity in boys and girls. Others have shown significant interactional effects when diverse school contexts and social class were studied in relation to timing of puberty and maturational stage (Simmons *et al.*, 1973).

Classic studies of Jones and associates have made systematic comparisons between the behavior and personality characteristics of early- and late-maturing adolescents. Their results indicate that early maturity tends to carry distinct advantages for boys (Jones, 1957), but some disadvantages for girls (Jones and Mussen, 1958).

In early adolescence, early-maturing boys are given more leadership roles, are more popular, excel in athletic ability, were perceived as more attractive by adults and peers, and enjoyed considerably enhanced heterosexual status. When studied at 17 years of age (Jones, 1957, Clausen, 1975), the early-maturing boys showed more self-confidence, less dependency, and were more capable of playing an adult role in interpersonal relations.

With girls, a different and much more complex pattern emerges. When the relationships between the timing of puberty and perceptions of self are examined, those girls who perceive themselves to be "on time" in their physical maturation feel more attractive and more positive about their bodies than those who are either early or late. However, those girls who are late or perceive themselves as behind schedule have a body image more positive than those who mature early. The only individual component of pubertal development that is inconsistent with this pattern is breast development. Those girls with more breast development tend to feel more attractive regardless of timing (Tobin-Richards *et al.*, 1983). Body weight is an additional variable that contributes significantly to body image and self-esteem in girls. Average weight is most valued, and being thin is seen as next most desirable.

School context is also a critical variable. Experiencing grades 6 through 8 in elementary school is favorable for early-maturing girls. In junior high school settings, early-maturing girls experience specific stresses due to social pressures and their attractiveness to the older boys in upper grades (Simmons *et al.*, 1979).

All of the above factors are important variables that operate not only among peers but also in a family context. There is reason to believe that a positive view of pubertal changes, regardless of timing of puberty, is enhanced by greater acceptance of the reality of sexuality and physical maturation within the family (Brooks-Gunn and Ruble, 1983). This research also underscores the understudied but important role of the father as a determinant of the development of feminine identity in adolescent girls. Importance of the role of mother in the sex education of the daughter is discussed in Chapter 8 of this volume.

PSYCHOSOCIAL TASKS OF EARLY ADOLESCENCE

Early adolescence is a time of sharpest possible discontinuity with the past. There are two major psychosocial challenges that confront early adolescents: (1) the transition from elementary to junior high school and (2) the shift in role status from child to adolescent. The fact that these major life changes are superimposed on the profound biological changes of puberty amplifies the stressful impact. At this time of demand for totally new sets of behaviors and novel coping responses, we know little about the specifics of the development of social competence, cognitive styles, and information processing among early adolescents. Chapter 8 in this volume gives a review of the state of the field (Petersen).

JUNIOR HIGH OR MIDDLE SCHOOL

There is a cultural consensus that early adolescence be defined in terms of the social age of entry into junior high school (Hamburg, 1974). One of the striking aspects of a junior high school population is the wide diversity in the pubertal development of the students.

The drastic change in school format from the self-contained classroom of a small elementary school to the rotating classes of a very large junior high school represents one of the most abrupt and demanding transitions of the educational career. Elements that contribute to the high rate of distress are: (1) general sense of confusion about the bigness and complexity of the new school format; (2) insecurity about ability to cope with the interpersonal demand of having to relate to a different teacher and different group of students on an hourly basis; (3) concern about the ability to make and hold friends; (4) ignorance about role expectations now that they are considered to be adolescents; and (5) fear of academic failure.

A great many students have deep-seated fears of academic inadequacy and failure. An important issue for the early adolescent is the perception of sharp escalation in academic demands both in terms of expected output and complexity of tasks. Evidence tends to confirm that their fears may be well founded. Studies have demonstrated (Finger and Silverman, 1966) that there is a startling drop in school performance associated with junior high school. In a study by Armstrong in New York (1964), 45% of the boys and girls with good elementary school records performed at a fair or poor level in junior high school. The authors further noted that whereas grades in elementary school are highly related to intelligence, intelligence was largely unrelated to the change in performance at the junior high level.

COGNITIVE DEVELOPMENT IN EARLY ADOLESCENCE

Despite the fact that intelligence per se is not at issue in the school performance of early adolescents, it is worthwhile to re-examine their style of cognitive functioning. By and large, it has generally been assumed that these early adolescents have moved to logical operations and abstract thinking (Inhelder and Piaget, 1958). Several lines of evidence suggest that this is not generally true.

Cognitive abilities have great bearing on ways in which early adolescents respond to information and persuasion and how they make critical decisions in their lives. In making the transition into early adolescence, the young person confronts crucial, emotionally charged decisions about all spheres of functioning, that is, who to seek out and how to make friends in the larger social milieu of junior high school and what to do about pressures or temptations to experiment with smoking, alcohol, drugs, or sex. Reasoning is likely to still be mainly in terms of concrete operations. Even when formal reasoning has begun to develop, it may not be evident in the critical decisions. A useful distinction has been made between "hot" and "cold" cognitions. Hot cognitions are those that are highly charged with emotion and are involved in matters of perceived threat or in situations where cherished goals or values are in conflict or jeopardy. It has been shown that at all levels of intelligence and at the highest adult levels of formal reasoning, information processing and decision making are greatly impaired when dealing with hot cognitions (Janis and Mann, 1977). Early adolescents not only have immature cognitive levels but also confront a great many hot cognitions. They do show the typical impairments such as narrowing the range of perceived alternatives, overlooking long-term consequences, and distortion of expected outcomes. They also show, in exaggerated form, the heightened tendency to come to quick decision closures by an uncritical acceptance of peer advice, popular slogans for action, or submissive obedience to a "rule" of peers, family, or religion.

Recent research indicates that the junior high school student is deficient in ability to make valid generalizations, use symbols, and to process information with objectivity. Data indicate that although some formal operational abilities begin to emerge during the early adolescent period, abilities such as "controlling variables" (the strategy of holding other things constant in exploring the effect of one variable on an outcome) may be atypical among early adolescents. The results of Karplus et al. (1975) suggest that performance in these tasks may be benefited by instruction. However, further research is required to establish the degree of teachability of these skills for modal individuals at the early adolescent cognitive level. The National Science Foundation has reviewed cognitive development in early adolescents with emphasis on the implications for the teaching of science curricula to early adolescents (Hurd, 1978). Such research is also applicable to devising the appropriate junior high school curricula for the teaching of social skills, interpersonal relationships, and decision-making processes.

Investigations in other areas of reasoning are also relevant to early adolescents. Tversky and Kahneman (1971) have shown that some adults consistently tend to regard samples as overly representative of the populations from which they are drawn. The prevalence and significance of logical errors and biases of this kind in early adolescents should be investigated. Results from survey data show that early adolescents systematically overestimate the prevalence of certain peer behaviors. For example, when the actual baseline rate of smoking in a school was 15%, most students estimated the level of smokers to be over 80% (Fishbein, 1977). Similarly, Furstenberg (1976) reports that when asked about prevalence of sexual activity, early adolescents report with evident sincerity, "everybody is doing it." A consistent tendency to errors due to overgeneralization could help explain the exaggerated impact of peer pressure and media influences on early adolescents.

Elkind (1967) has described the egocentrism of adolescence as showing its peak in the ages that correspond to early adolescence (ages 12–15). As an aspect of the egocentrism, there can be a belief in personal uniqueness, called "personal fable" by Elkind. This cognitive stance may underlie a "here and now" time perspective in which long-term consequences and future happenings do not have salience. It may also explain ideas of invulnerability that allow early adolescents to persuade themselves that *they* can safely take a known risk. When this immediate time perspective and the sense of invulnerability are coupled with failure to comprehend laws of probability, young adolescents may be especially prone to engage in unprotected sexual encounters with a false sense of confidence. Also, disbelief and denial that she can actually be pregnant tends to lead any early adolescent girl to a pattern of delayed obstetrical attention. At time, this delay means that the pregnancy has progressed beyond the point when an abortion can be done with safety. Important prenatal care is deficient or absent for the same reason. Similar denials about the health and well-being of her infant could compromise the health care of the baby.

Just as there are wide normative variations in the timing of the biological changes of puberty, there is comparable variability in the timing and progression of cognitive skills among adolescents.

Middle and junior high school teachers are often unaware of the diversity in cognitive abilities that characterizes early adolescents (Martin, 1971). Further research is needed to establish the synchrony, if any, between timing of physical and cognitive maturity. In any case, it is known that even when more mature levels of cognitive functioning have been attained, there is a strong tendency for reversion to concrete information processing at times of stress and anxiety. It is important to realize that most early adolescents, regardless of level of cognitive functioning, are highly unlikely to be successful at improvising or making balanced, effective decisions when placed under the highly novel or disturbing situations that may arise in sexuality, pregnancy, and in parenting situations.

SELF-ESTEEM IN EARLY ADOLESCENTS

In large-scale studies in Baltimore and Milwaukee schools, Simmons (1973, 1979) has found that self-esteem typically drops when students are in junior high school. The young adolescent white girls (6th and 7th grade) showed the lowest self-esteem of the students tested. Further, it was found that early maturing girls with active dating behavior showed the lowest esteem of all students tested. When a matched group of early-maturing girls attending 6th and 7th grades in an elementary school was compared with 6th and 7th grade junior high school girls, the elementary school girls did not show the comparable fall in self-esteem. It was postulated that the early maturing girls in the elementary school situation was shielded from the added social and sexual pressures that characterized the junior high school experience. In prior studies of youth self-esteem, Rosenberg (1965) found that low self-esteem was correlated with characteristic attitudes and responses. The individual with low self-esteem is more vulnerable in interpersonal relations (deeply hurt by criticism); he is relatively awkward with others (finds it hard to make conversation, does not initiate contacts); he assumes that others think poorly of him or do not particularly like him; he tends to put up a "front" to people; and he feels relatively isolated and lonely. There is low faith in people. Rosenberg states: "Low self-esteem makes them relatively submissive or unassertive in their dealings with others" (p. 205). It is thus apparent that the individual's self-conception is not only associated with attitudes toward other people, it is also associated with his actions in social life and the position he comes to occupy in his high school peer groups. The attributes associated with low self-esteem represent attitudes and behaviors that would diminish coping potential, heighten stress, and accentuate any pre-existing tendencies to resort to maladaptive solutions.

ADOPTION OF ADOLESCENT ROLE

Entry into junior high school means leaving behind the familiar world of childhood and defines entry into the status of adolescence. For well-established major role transitions such as marriage or entering the work force, there are well-defined expectations for behaviors and, often, a prior period of preparation. Early adolescents are catapulted into their new role status with no preparation and very vague conceptions about the attitudes, behaviors, prescriptions, and prohibitions that are appropriate to the role. Unfortunately, there is a comparable ambiguity on the part of the adults who surround them. Adults feel frustrated and highly uncertain about the appropriate attitudes and behaviors on their part.

The newly labeled adolescent feels herself in immediate need of a new set of behaviors, values, and reference persons. She is aware that significant adults relating to her often have a reciprocal expectation that they will, in turn, now have different standards and new ways of relating to her. The uninitiated person, when aspiring to a new status, often tends to respond to the most conspicuous and stereotyped features of the new role. The early adolescent will often tend to assume postures of exaggerated independence with accompanying derisive and rebellious attitudes toward his parents, in particular, and perhaps adults, in general, in response to the stereotype of adolescent emancipation. He or she may also slavishly conform to styles of hair, clothing, and behaviors that are identified as characteristic of the youth culture. Sexual activity is a visible vehicle for testing new role behaviors.

The bulk of literature on adolescence actually derives from descriptions of the late adolescence phase. Unfortunately, these descriptions are generically applied to all adolescents. Parents, in seeking guidelines for their appropriate behavior in relation to their child's role transition, find an emphasis on the adolescent's need for independent decision-making and the development of autonomy. When taken literally, this can actually lead to a significant renunciation of parental participation and support. This type of response may, in turn, lead to heightened distress on the part of the early adolescent. The result is that in a time of major discontinuity, accustomed parental guidance is withdrawn, and the young person is thrust toward uncritical acceptance of the peer group as a model and as a major coping resource. While this uncritical allegiance to the peer group may be useful in allaying immediate anxieties, it has serious limitations. The peer group at this stage is usually too shallow in experience and limited in foresight to provide the necessary resources for growth and development. Loevinger and Wessler (1970) find that typical junior high school students are at Stage 2 of ego development which is characterized by impulsiveness

siveness and exploitativeness. When the peer group is organized around alcohol, drugs and/or acting-out behaviors, there is potential for considerable damage.

Before the invention of junior high school, when the child had continued into eighth grade in an elementary school setting, premature issues of autonomy had little emphasis. The early adolescent, the junior high school student, is typically between 12 and 14 years of age. Thus, there is a 4- to 6-year period before the actual separation from the home and parents will occur. A strong posture of independence at this early stage is not linked with a valid developmental transition. Therefore, it is inappropriate to convey to early adolescents and their parents an emphasis on the achievement of independence. Instead, emphasis should be placed on parental stability and guidance at the time of major superimposed biological, school, and social discontinuity. The early adolescent cannot possess the competence and mastery needed for full independence. However, the early and middle-adolescent phases are the necessary training grounds and biological preparation for the achievement of autonomy by the end of late adolescence. The success with which each of these earlier phases are negotiated will, of course, affect the final outcome of adolescent development.

ADOLESCENT SEXUALITY

A review of adolescent sexuality and pregnancy is presented in Chapter 10 of this volume. This brief review analyzes the existing research from a developmental perspective with particular attention to early adolescence. Unfortunately, the lack of developmental perspective is very striking in the literature on adolescent sexuality. In particular, very little is known about the sexual behavior, knowledge or attitudes of the youngest group. Although it was sometimes acknowledged that special issues might arise for the early adolescent, very few articles discussed this group independently or even reported the data with age difference as a separate variable (Elster and McAnarney, 1980; Jaffe and Dryfoos, 1976; Phipps and Yonas, 1980). Methodological limitations occur in many studies of adolescent sexuality. These should be noted.

First, most data is reported by age groupings rather than by single age years, precluding further analysis of age as a factor. It is difficult to make comparisons among studies or even to know if the general conclusions of the research are equally applicable to all of the ages represented in the study.

Second, there is no uniformity of approach on the issue of age reporting. Adolescence is often treated as a unitary stage in development, encompassing the entire period between ages 12 and 20. Although the bulk of the research comprises studies of adolescents 16 and older, the findings from this older group have been ascribed to adolescents as a whole. Young adolescents aged 12–15, if they are included at all, usually represent a small percentage of subjects in a study that includes adolescents through age 19. A mean age of 16 to 17 years is typical. Because the proportion of younger pregnant teenagers is small when compared to the proportion of older pregnant teenagers in the total study population, a highly significant low frequency behavior which has its highest prevalence among the younger teenagers may be overlooked. Other studies use arbitrary age groupings, e.g., 15–19, 10–14, or 16–18, with no explanation or discussion of the theoretical basis for the choice.

Third, only a few authors utilize the distinct developmental periods within adolescence (Hatcher, 1973; Hamburg, 1980). The biological, cognitive, psychological, and social differences between the 13- and the 19-year-old adolescent are so substantial that these kinds of differences clearly need to be taken into account in attempts to understand adolescent sexuality.

SEXUAL KNOWLEDGE

No systematic study has been done on the extent of sexual knowledge in early adolescence or on its relation to sexual behavior. As might be expected, adolescent exposure to information about reproductive physiology, contraceptive methods, abortion, and venereal disease increases steadily from ages 13–18 (Reichelt and Werley, 1975; Zelnick and Kantner, 1979). By age 15, 62% of female adolescents have had a sex education course, generally in a school setting. However, completion of a sex education course does not guarantee adequate knowledge of sexuality. In one survey, only 33% of the 15–19 year olds who had taken sex education knew the time of greatest risk of pregnancy within a menstrual cycle (Zelnick and Kantner, 1979). Thus far, the effectiveness of the schools is limited (Hamburg, 1980). One reason for this limitation is that the educational techniques may not be properly designed in terms of the cognitive maturity levels of subgroups of adolescents and may not address content or motivations that are developmentally relevant. When material has been offered in schools, it was often highly anatomical, overly didactic, and of little practical use. Many schools continue to avoid sex education because of parental and political pressures based on the conviction that presenting the issues would lead to promiscuity.

Accumulated evidence shows that there is very little communication about sex in the home (Bloch, 1972; Fox, 1979; Rothenberg, 1978). These studies indicate that parents are never cited by adolescents as their first or major source of sex instruction. It was typical to find that for 7th grade girls, 20% of mothers had never told daughters about menstruation, 50% had not discussed the male role in reproduction, and 68% had not discussed any aspect of birth control. When any reading matter or sexual discussion was offered in the family, the mother was the usual agent. However, it was also noted that impact of parental communication about sex is significant. (Chapter 8 in this volume discusses these issues in detail.) Research shows that even minimal sex education from the family (mother) is associated with postponement of age of initiation of sex activity. Also, when daughters are sexually active, parental discussions about sex seem to be related to more effective use of contraception (Fox, 1979; Furstenberg, 1976). Unfortunately, methods to enhance parental involvement in sex instructions for their children have not been seen as an important ingredient of family planning services for teenagers. On the contrary, there is a pervasive belief that adolescents benefit from disengagement from parents, particularly in sexual discussions and decisions.

Early adolescents have been dependent, for the most part, on haphazard and often distorted information largely derived from peers and media. Physicians are viewed by adolescents as a potentially good source of information (Yankelovich et al., 1979) but adolescents seldom visit a physician.

The biology of pregnancy, medical aspects of childbirth, and facts of child development have, if possible, received even less attention in the education of early adolescents. Again, this ignorance has serious consequences for both parent and child. Even at the high school level, most adolescents are unaware of the early pregnancy risks for mother and child. Often they do not know about the hazards to the fetus of smoking or alcohol consumption. This ignorance may contribute to their failure to seek early or regular prenatal care.

SEXUAL BEHAVIOR

The work of Vener et al. (1972; Vener and Stewart, 1974) provides the best available information on stages of sexual activity of the young teenagers. In 1969, they studied the entire population of white adolescents ($N = 4220$), ages 13 to 17, in three Michigan communities of middle-level economic status. One community was resurveyed in 1973. A significant contribution of the research is the use of an eight-level scale of sexual activity to measure the degree of experience of the adolescents ranging from simple petting to coitus with several partners. Such a scale is far more descriptive of sexual activity than is merely determining whether or not intercourse has occurred, which most investigators have done.

From the study conducted in 1969, Vener et al. (1972) concluded that the sexual climate for middle American adolescents had changed little in the 20 years since World War II. In contrast, their resurvey 4 years later (in 1973) demonstrated a significant increase in coital activity at all ages. In particular, 33% of the males and 17% of the females aged 13–15 had experienced coitus, compared to 19% and 9% in the initial study in 1969. The greatest increase in sexual activity was recorded for ages 14 and 15. Also, they were significantly more deeply involved in advanced sexual behaviors.

The recent significant rise in level of sexual activity among adolescents and the trend toward increasingly younger ages of initiation is well documented. It seems unlikely that these trends can be largely attributable to earlier maturation. Since about 1850, the secular trend toward earlier menarche has averaged 3 months per decade resulting in an average currently of 12.8 years in affluent and healthy nations. In the United States, these secular declines appear to have leveled off halfway through this century. In any event, the sharp rises in sexual activity of adolescents have far outstripped the rates of biological changes and there has been an explosive rise in rates of sexual activity starting in the 1970's. This is exemplified in the data on sexual activity in 15-year-old girls in the United States. Kinsey (1953) reported their rate as 3%; in 1966 the rate was 6% (Lake, 1967); for 1971 and 1976, Zelnick and Kanter (1977) reported rates of 13.8 and 18%, respectively. The continuing increase in sexual activity at younger ages was corroborated in their report of a national sample of black and white women ages 15–19 between 1971 and 1979 (Zelnick and Kantner, 1980). *Age 15 was, unfortunately, the youngest age surveyed.* For the entire sample, the proportion who had experienced intercourse rose from 30% in 1971 to 50% in 1979. In their 1971 survey the investigators found that the level of sexual activity was higher for adolescent black women than for adolescent white women. However, for whites between 1971 and 1979, the level of sexual activity has increased continuously, while for blacks, there was virtually no change between 1976 and 1979. These studies show that in 1980 for 19 year olds, 65% of white females and 89% of black females were sexually experienced.

In the 15-year-old subgroup, the proportion of sexually active females increased from 13.8 to 23%. In 1979 15-year-olds blacks were still over twice as likely as whites to have had intercourse (41 vs. 18%) and blacks were found to initiate intercourse about 1 year before whites.

EARLY ADOLESCENT PREGNANCY

Birth control and contraceptive behaviors are inadequate among teenagers. Increasingly higher percentages of sexually active young women are becoming pregnant. Pregnancy rates of sexually active adolescents 15–19 years old were 28% in 1981, 30% in 1976, and 33% in 1979. The major findings from an on-going statistically reliable sample survey on adolescent sexuality and pregnancy document that the rate of pregnancy among 15–19 year olds almost doubled between 1971 and 1979. The rates increased from 9.0 in 1971 to 16.2 in 1979 (Zelnick and Kantner, 1980).

The changing trends are even more evident for the youngest age group of early adolescents. Data from the National Center for Health Statistics document a 50% increase in births to adolescents 15 years old and younger from 26,380 in 1960 to 39,635 in 1978 (National Center for Health Statistics, 1980). Almost one in ten early adolescents becomes pregnant the first month after initiating intercourse, and this increases to one in five after only 6 months (Zabin et al., 1979; Zelnick and Kantner, 1979). One-half of all teenage pregnancies which occur in the first 2 years after initiating intercourse will begin in the first 6 months (Zabin et al., 1981).

Contraceptive usage by early adolescents has been especially poor. In 1976, almost 40% of 15-year-old women had never used contraception, and only 30% always used some method of birth control (Zelnick and Kantner, 1977). By contrast 25% of 18- or 19-year-old sexually active women have never used any contraception (Zabin et al., 1979; Zelnick and Kantner, 1979). Even among those who were sufficiently motivated to seek the services of a family planning clinic, only one half of the 14 year olds and two-thirds of the 15 year olds regularly used contraception (Akom et al., 1976). A recent study suggests that participation by the mother in the clinic visit to obtain birth control can improve compliance by the daughter (Scher et al., 1982).

Lindemann's model of three stages of contraceptive usage is particularly appropriate to a developmental analysis of adolescent sexuality (Lindemann, 1974). The first or "natural" stage is characterized by unpredictability of coitus, a belief in the spontaneity and naturalness of sex, infrequency of coitus, recent establishment of heterosexual interests, and little awareness of the possibility of pregnancy and the need for contraception.

The second or "peer prescription" stage is characterized by discussing pregnancy prevention with friends and by experimenting with nonprescription methods of birth control, which may be used either spontaneously or with planning, depending on the nature of the relationship. A major problem is misinformation.

The third or "expert" stage involves willingness to contact a professional to obtain a prescribed method of birth control. Adolescents at this stage have intercourse more frequently (usually in a steady relationship), are developmentally mature, and are committed to sexual behavior. An adolescent usually passes through these stages in sequence, although retrogression or skipping is also possible. Regrettably, Lindemann does not attempt to correlate these stages with age or maturity. One might expect to find that the majority of early adolescents are at the "natural" stage of contraceptive usage.

An additional explanation of the inadequate contraceptive behavior postulates that some adolescents adopt a personal cost–benefit perspective in which both the cost of using contraception and the benefits of physical intimacy and of becoming pregnant are considered to be high (Luker, 1975; Rogel et al., 1980; Miller, 1973a, b).

In survey studies of young women who were seen because of suspected pregnancy, a variety of explanations were given for the lack of adequate contraception. These include unexpected intercourse, disbelief of reproductive capability, and desire for pregnancy (Zelnick and Kantner, 1979).

The obvious result of unprotected intercourse in a large percentage of teenagers is pregnancy. Dating from the landmark Supreme Court decision in 1973, the proportion of young adolescent pregnancies ending in abortion has risen. In 1977, five out of ten pregnant 15 year olds and seven out of ten aged 14 or younger chose to abort (Baldwin, 1980). Even though abortion is frequently used to terminate the pregnancy there are still significant numbers who elect to maintain the pregnancy. Of the 500,000 births to teenaged mothers each year, approximately 10% are born to adolescents aged 15 or less. Most pregnant teenagers who decide to continue the pregnancy also choose to keep their baby. The consequence of this decision is multifactorial with medical, psychological, sociological, and economic ramifications.

BIOMEDICAL OUTCOMES

OBSTETRICAL AND NEONATAL OUTCOMES

Teenage pregnancy is associated with a constellation of negative medical outcomes for both mother and child. Some well-designed studies find that negative outcomes for the teenage mother range in severity from excessive weight gain in pregnancy to maternal mortality and include anemia (Jorgensen, 1972), nutritional deficiencies (Naeye, 1981), mild and severe toxemia of pregnancy (Graham, 1981; Duenholter, 1975), prolonged or abrupt labors (Naeye et al., 1977), cephalopelvic disproportion (Battaglia et al., 1963; Bochner, 1962), and caesarean section (Jorgensen, 1972; Finkelstein, 1983). In addition, a variety of negative outcomes have been documented in infants born to teenage mothers (Grant and Heald, 1972; Merrit et al., 1980) and include prematurity (Hulka and Schaaf, 1964), low birth weight for gestational age

(Israel *et al.*, 1964), congenital malformations, neurological defects, perinatal mortality and childhood growth failure (Bailey, 1981; Oppel and Royston, 1971). It has been postulated that these increased medical risks may be preferentially associated with adolescents less than 15 or 16 years of age (Hulka and Schaaf, 1964; Horon *et al.*, 1983), with those teenage mothers of low gynecological age, age at conception minus age at menarche (Zlatnick and Burnmeister, 1977; Hollingsworth, 1981; Elkan *et al.*, 1971).

It has been suggested that for all mothers poor medical outcome is strongly associated with inadequate prenatal and perinatal care (Jorgensen, 1972; McArnarney, 1978; Briggs *et al.*, 1962). The corollary to this latter hypothesis is that many adverse medical outcomes of teenage pregnancy are not age-specific phenomena but can be avoided by appropriate medical care. This further underscores the seriousness of the tendency of the early adolescent to neglect prenatal care.

A variety of these investigations have looked at the medical complications of teenage pregnancy for mothers and their babies in comparison to adult mothers and their babies. Some investigators classified all teenagers under the age of 20 in one group, whereas others subdivided the study population into age-stratified groups in which the groups span only 2 or 3 years. Because the proportion of the youngest pregnant teenagers is small when compared to the proportion of older pregnant teenagers in the total study population, the investigations which do not differentiate between these groups may overlook a low frequency morbid event which has a high prevalence among the youngest teenagers.

Furthermore, the racial compositions of the populations must be considered as there is a documented increase in negative obstetrical outcomes among non-white women and among those of low socioeconomic status (Horon, 1983). In addition the selection of the control population must also be scrutinized. For controls, some studies look at the morbidity and mortality associated with all pregnancies, thus including the known high-risk pregnancies to women over the age of 35. In the absence of appropriate controls, studies may minimize the relative risks for morbidity and mortality from teenage pregnancy as compared to pregnancy in women in their 20's and early 30's.

Physiological immaturity has been postulated as a risk factor for a negative outcome of teenage pregnancy. One convenient way of assessing this possibility is to examine outcomes for teenagers of the same chronological age and socioeconomic status but who differ with respect to gynecological age.

There is some controversy about the validity of gynecological age as a variable. Gynecological age is defined as the number of years following menarche at which a pregnancy occurs. Adolescents of the same chronologic age can have different gynecological ages depending on their age at menarche. Hollingsworth and Kreutner (1980) point out that menarche may not be accurately remembered, that it does not imply maturity, and that skeletal maturation may be a more valid marker. However, it is impossible to use retrospective data in determining time of skeletal maturation. However, most investigators agree that for early adolescents menarche is such a recent and salient event that recall is likely to be accurate.

Elkan *et al.* (1971) studied 261 pregnancies of 12 to 15 year olds in low socioeconomic status blacks in Baltimore during the years 1957–1967. Low birth weight babies (2500 gm) were born to 23.4% and of that number 14.4% experienced toxemia of pregnancy. When the same data was examined according to gynecological age, 31.4% of those less than 2 years gynecological age had a low birth weight baby. In contrast, only 16.0% of those greater than 2 years had a low birth weight baby (p 0.01). A similar association was noted between low gynecological age and toxemia of pregnancy. Thus this study clearly indicates a high risk associated with low gynecological age irrespective of chronological age.

A separate study of 1005 predominantly white teenagers was done by Zlatnick and Burnmeister (1977) at the University of Iowa in 1970–1975. In general agreement with Elkan *et al.*, (1971), they found that increased numbers of low birth weight babies was associated with a gynecological age of less than 2 years, 17% as opposed to 9% for those greater than 2 years (p 0.05). In contrast to Elkan, there was no influence of young gynecological age on the prevalence of toxemia in their studies. The reason for this discrepancy is unclear but may reflect the improvements in obstetrical care since the early 1970's.

In addition, *irrespective of gynecological age* they found that there is a significant increase in numbers of low birth weight infants in young teenagers, 15 years of age or less, when compared to older teenagers. However, there was approximately the same risk for a low birth weight infant in older teenagers of less than 2 years gynecological age when compared to young teenagers of greater than 2 years gynecological age.

NUTRITION AND PREGNANCY OUTCOME

One possible association with low gynecological age is nutritional status and requirements of the adolescent. The most rapid rate of growth and nutritional requirement for adolescent girls is prior to menarche. By 2 to 3 years postmenarche, the rate of growth declines to adult levels (Garn and Petzold, 1983). It has been documented that pregnant teenagers often have nutritional deficiences in iron, vitamin A, and calcium.

In addition, the young teenagers had a twofold risk of developing acetonuria, a possible indication of metabolic acidosis, a condition which is associated with a high incidence of perinatal death (Naeye, 1981).

Naeye (1981) examined the relationship between prepregnancy weight and growth retarded fetuses for young teenagers, ages 11–15. There was transient, early childhood growth retardation in the children of both normal and underweight mothers whereas this was not observed in overweight mothers. This has suggested potential competition for nutrients between the growing fetus and the growing adolescent mother. Further investigation is warranted to confirm the possibility of nutritional deficiencies interacting with physiological immaturity as risk factors for negative pregnancy outcome.

Several authors including Dwyer (1974) and Zuckerman et al. (1983) feel that the adverse medical outcomes in early adolescence can be avoided to large extent by aggressive, early, and ongoing prenatal care. The problem with this approach is that over 50% of pregnant adolescents receive no prenatal care in the first trimester and 16% have not received health care by the end the second trimester.

In summary, most investigators agree that very early teenage pregnancy is associated with maternal toxemia and low birth weight of the infant. Studies have identified several variables associated with negative outcomes. The aggregated data show that women at highest risk are very young, black, have a low gynecological age, are thin, are from a low socioeconomic status, and do not seek prenatal care. At all ages, adolescent women with a gynecological age of less than 2 years experience higher risks in pregnancy than do women in their twenties.

Data from a recent study done in Rochester, New York (McAnarney, 1978) show that between 1967 and 1978 there has been a trend of an increasing proportion of low birth weight babies born to adolescents below 15 years of age. This has been more pronounced in the white than the nonwhite population. The rates for the white adolescents have dramatically increased from 9.1% in 1967 to 19.2% in 1978. The authors speculate that one reason for this drastic increase is that those teenagers who are at low risk for pregnancy-associated morbidity may more frequently choose abortion and high-risk mothers elect to continue their pregnancy. However, those authors indicate that they find no conclusive evidence regarding identifiable overall risk factors for low birth weight in adolescent pregnancy. It would seem urgent to identify those subgroups at high risk as well as to understand the specific factors that are determinants in this condition that appears to have an increasing morbidity.

Personal factors such as eating behaviors, smoking alcohol or illegal drug use have been reported for aggregated populations of adolescents (Zuckerman et al., 1983). These results have been inconclusive. There is a need to analyze these factors in differentiated groups of adolescents to ascertain whether or not there are subsets for whom these factors do pose high risk. Psychosocial factors such as quality of social networks and social support have been neglected in research on biomedical outcomes. When studied, these factors appear to have significant effects (Dott and Fort, 1976; Zuckerman et al., 1979). They seem to provide clues to understanding the understudied phenomenon of favorable outcomes among high-risk adolescent mothers.

CONCLUSION

After a decade of national concern and substantial public and private efforts there continue to be highly prevalent problems of adolescent pregnancy and childbearing. There is a challenge to develop research designs that represent fresh approaches to these seemingly intractable problems.

An interdisciplinary approach that integrates data from a range of biological and behavioral fields suggests several lines of inquiry. On the basis of current knowledge, it seems possible to delineate distinctive subgroups among adolescents who are at high risk for pregnancy and parenthood. For each subgroup, and for quite different reasons, there is a selective imperviousness to current sex education efforts or attempts to increase use of contraceptives. These subgroups also pose differing risks for specific medical and psychosocial outcomes for mother and child. Much more needs to be learned about the major determinants, correlates, and consequences for each subgroup. In general, too little attention has been given to the careful study of the personal and psychosocial factors that have fostered good outcomes among certain of these high risk young mothers.

Special emphasis has been placed on the youngest adolescents who represent a small but rising percentage of school-age mothers. One group of these early adolescents appear to be both immature and problem-prone. As such, they pose exceedingly high risk to themselves and the child for biomedical casualty as well as problems in parenting behaviors. A greater understanding of the patterns of determinants, motivations and behaviors for each subgroup will make it possible to design more targeted and effective preventive and remedial interventions.

ACKNOWLEDGMENT

This work was supported in part by grants from the Robert Wood Johnson Foundation and the John D. and Catherine T. MacArthur Foundation.

REFERENCES

Akpom, C.A., Akpom, D., and Davis, M. Prior sexual behavior of teenagers attending rap sessions for the first time. *Family Planning Perspectives*, 1976, *8*, 203–208.

Armstrong, C. *Patterns of achievement in selected New York State schools.* Mimeo 1964. Albany: New York State Educational Department.

Anzar, R., and Bennett, A.E. Pregnancy in the adolescent girl. *American Journal of Obstetrics and Gynecology*, 1961, *81*, 934–940.

Baldwin, W. The fertility of young adolescents. *Journal of Adolescent Health Care*, 1980, *1*, 54–59.

Bailey, L.B., Mahan, C.S. and Dimperio, M.S. Folacin and iron status in low-income pregnant adolescent and mature women. *American Journal of Clinical Nutrition*, 1980, *33*, 1997–2001.

Battaglia, F., Frazier, T., and Hellegers, A. Obstetric and pediatric complications of juvenile pregnancy. *Pediatrics*, 1963, *32*, 902–910.

Bloch, D. Attitudes of mothers toward sex education. *American Journal of Public Health*, 1979, *69*, 911–915.

Bloch, D. Sex education practices of mothers. *Journal of Sex Education and Therapy*, 1972, *7*, 1–18.

Brooks-Gunn, J., and Ruble, D.N. The experience of menarche from a developmental perspective. In J. Brooks-Gunn and A.C. Petersen (Eds.), *Girls at puberty: Biological and psychosocial perspectives.* New York: Plenum, 1983, pp. 155–178.

Bochner, K. Pregnancies in juveniles. *American Journal of Obstetrics and Gynecology*, 1962, *83*, 269–271.

Briggs, R.M., Herren, R.R. and Thompson, W.B. Pregnancy in the young adolescent. *American Journal of Obstetrics and Gynecology*, 1962, *84*, 436–441.

Bureau of the Census. Fertility of American Women: June, 1979. *Current Population Reports* Series P-23, No. 358, 1980, Washington, D.C., U.S. Department of Commerce.

Clausen, J. The social meaning of differential physical and sexual maturation. In S. Dragastin and G.H. Elder, Jr. (Eds.), *Adolescence and the life cycle.* New York: Wiley, 1975.

Coates, J. Obstetrics in the very young adolescent. *American Journal of Obstetrics and Gynecology*, 1970, *108*, 68–72.

Cvetkovich, G., Grote, B., Lieberman, G.J., and Miller, W.B. Sex role development and teenage fertility behavior. *Adolescence*, 1978, *13*, 231–236.

Dott, A.B., and Fort, A.T. Medical and social factors affecting early teenage pregnancy. *American Journal of Obstetrics and Gynecology*, 1976, *125*, 532–536.

Duenholter, J.H., Facoq, J.M.J., and Bauman, G. Pregnancy performance of patients under 15 years of age. *Obstetrics and Gynecology*, 1975, *46*, 49–52.

Dwyer, J.G. Teenage pregnancy. *American Journal of Obstetrics and Gynecology*, 1974, *118*, 373–376.

Elkan, K.A., Rimer, B.A., and Stine, D.C. Juvenile pregnancy role of physiologic maturity. *Maryland State Medical Journal*, 1971, *20*, 50–52.

Elkind, D. Egocentrism adolescence. *Child Development*, 1967, *4*, 1025–1034.

Elster, A.B. and McAnarney, E.R. Medical and psychosocial risks of pregnancy and childbearing during adolescence. *Pediatric Annals*, 1980, *9*, 89–94.

Finger, J., and Silverman, M. Changes in academic performance in junior high school. *Personnel and Guidance Journal*, 1966, *45*, 157–164.

Fishbein, M. Consumer beliefs and behavior with respect to cigarette smoking: A critical analysis of the public literature. In Federal Trade Commission. Report to Congress: Pursuant to the Public Health Cigarette Smoking Act. For the Year 1976, May (1977). U.S. Government Printing Office: Washington D.C.

Fox, G.L. The family's influence on adolescent sexual behavior. *Children's Today*, May–June, 1979, 21–36.

Furstenberg, F. *Unplanned parenthood: The social consequences of teenage childbearing.* 1976, New York: The Free Press, 1976.

Garn, S.M., and Petzold, A.S. Characteristics of the mother and child in teenage pregnancy. *American Journal of Diseases of Children*, 1983, *137*, 365–368.

Graham, D. The obstetric and neonatal consequences of adolescent pregnancy. *Birth Defects*, 1981, *17*, 49–67.

Grant, J.A., and Heald, F.P. Complications of adolescent pregnancy survey of the literature on fetal outcome in adolescence. *Clinical Pediatrics*, 1972, *11*, 567–570.

Guttmacher Institute. *Teenage pregnancy: The problem that won't go away.* Alan Guttmacher Institute, Planned Parenthood Federation of America, 1981.

Hamburg, B.A. Early adolescence: A specific and stressful stage of the life cycle. *In* G. Coelho, D.A. Hamburg, and J.E. Adams (Eds.), *Coping and adaptation.* New York: Basic Books, 1974, pp. 102–124.

Hamburg, B. Teenagers as parents: Developmental issues in school-age pregnancy. *In* E. Purcell (Ed.), *Psychopathology of children and youth: A cross-cultural perspective*, New York: Josiah Macy, Jr. Foundation, 1980, pp. 299–321.

Hassan, H.M., and Falls, F.H. The young primipara. *American Journal of Obstetrics and Gynecology*, 1964, *88*, 256–269.

Hatcher, S.L.M. The adolescent experience of pregnancy and abortion: A developmental analysis. *Journal of Youth and Adolescence*, 1973, *2*, 53–102.

Hogan, D.P. The effects of demographic factors, family background and early job achievement or age at marriage. *Demography*, 1978, *15*, 161–165.

Hollingsworth, D.R. and Kreutner, A.K.K. Teenage pregnancy: Solutions are evolving. *New England Journal of Medicine*, 1980, *303*, 516–518.

Hollingsworth, D.R. and Kotchen, J.M. Gynecologic age and its relation to neonatal outcome. *Birth Defects*, 1981, *17*, 91–105.

Horon, I.L., Strobino, D. M., and Mc Donald, H.M. Birth weights among infants born to adolescent and young adult women. *American Journal of Obstetrics and Gynecology*, 1983, *146*, 444–449.

Hulka, J.F. and Schaaf, J.H. Obstetrics in adolescents. A controlled study of deliveries by mothers 15 years of age and under. *Obstetrics and Gynecology*, 1964, *23*, 444–449.

Hurd, P.D. *Early adolescence:perspectives and recommendations to the National Science Foundation.* U.S. Superintendent of Documents Stock No. 038-000-00390-9, 1978.

Hutchins, F.L., Kendall, N., and Rubino, J. Experience with teenage pregnancy. *Obstetrics and Gynecology*, 1979, *54*, 1–5.

Inhelder, B. and Piaget, J. *The growth of logical thinking from childhood to adolescence: An essay on the construction of formal operational structures.* New York:Basic Books, 1958.

Israel, S.L., and Duetschberger, J. Relation of the mother's age to obstetric performance. *Obstetrics and Gynecology*, 1964, *24*, 411–417.

Jaffe, F., and Dryfoos, J. Fertility control services for adolescents: Access and utilization. *Family Planning Perspectives*, 1976, *8*, 167–175.

Janis, I.L. and Mann, L. *Decision making: A psychological analysis of conflict, choice and commitment.* New York: Free Press, 1977.

Jessor, R., and Jessor, S.L. *Problem behavior and psychosocial development.* New York: Academic Press, 1977.

Jessor, S., and Jessor, R. Transition from virginity to nonvirginity among youth: A social-psychological study over time. *Developmental Psychology,* 1975, *11,* 473–484.

Jessor, R., Graves, T.D., Hanson, R.C., and Jessor, S.L. *Society personality and deviant behavior.* New York: Holt, Rinehardt and Winston, 1968.

Jones, M.C. The later careers of boys who were early or late maturing. *Child Development,* 1957, *28,* 113–128.

Jones, M.C. Psychological correlates of somatic development. *Child Development,* 1965, *36,* 899–911.

Jones, M.C. and Mussen, P.H. Self-conceptions, motivations and interpersonal attitudes of early and late maturing girls. *Child Development,* 1958, *29,* 491–501.

Jorgensen, V. Clinical report on Pennsylvania Hospital's adolescent obstetrics clinic. *American Journal of Obstetrics and Gynecology,* 1972, *112,* 816–818.

Kaltreider, D.F., and Kohl, S. Epidemiology of pre-term delivery. *Clinical Obstetrics and Gynecology,* 1980, *23,* 17–31.

Kandel, D.B. *Longitudinal research in drug use.* New York: Halstead Press, 1978.

Kandel, D., and Davies, M. Epidemiology of adolescent depressive mood: an empirical study. *Archives of General Psychiatry,* 1982, *39,* 1209–1212.

Karplus, R., Karplus, F., Formisano, M., and Paulson, A. Proportional reasoning and control of variables in seven countries:Advancing education through science oriented programs, Report 10-25. Lawrence Hall of Science: Berkeley, California, 1975.

Kinsey, A., Pomeroy W. and Gebhard, P.H. *Sexual behavior in the human female.* Philadelphia: W.B. Saunders, 1953.

Klein, L. Early teenage pregnancy, contraception and repeat pregnancy. *American Journal of Obstetrics and Gynecology,* 120, 249–256.

Ladner, J. *Tomorrow's tomorrow: The black woman.* New York:Doubleday, 1971.

Lake, A. Teenagers and sex: A student report. *Seventeen,* 1967, *26,* 88–131.

Lindemann, C. *Birth control and unmarried young women.* New York: Springer, 1974.

Loevinger, J., and Wessler, R. *Measuring ego development.* San Francisco: Jossey-Bass, 1970.

Luker, K. *Taking chances: Abortion and the decision not to contracept.* Berkley, California: University of California Press, 1975.

McArnarney, E., Roghman, K.J., Adams, B.N. Obstetric, neonatal psychosocial outcomes of pregnant adolescents, *Pediatrics,* 1978, *61,* 199–205.

Marchetti, A.A., and Menaker, J.J. Pregnancy and the adolescent. *American Journal of Obstetrics and Gynecology,* 1950, *59,* 1013–1020.

Martin, E.C. Reflections on the early adolescent in school. *Daedalus,* Fall, 1971, 1087–1103.

Masnick, G., and Bane, M.J. *The nation's families: 1960–1990,* Cambridge, Mass.: Joint Center for Urban Studies of MIT and Harvard, 1980.

Mednick, B.R., Baker, R.L., and Sutton-Smith, B. Teenage pregnancy and perinatal mortality. *Journal of Youth and Adolescence,* 1979, *8,* 343–357.

Miller, W. Psychological vulnerability to unwed pregnancy. *Family Planning Perspectives,* 1973, *5,* 199–201. (a)

Miller, W. Sexuality, contraception and pregnancy in a high school population. *California Medicine*, 1973, 2, 14–21. (b)

Millman, S.R., and Hendershot, G.E. Early fertility and lifetime fertility. *Family Planning Perspectives*, 1980, 12, 139–149.

Morrison, J.H. Primipara under age fourteen. *American Journal of Obstetrics and Gynecology*, 1962, 84, 442–444.

Naeye, R.L. Teenaged and pre-teenaged pregnancies. Consequences of the fetal-maternal competition for nutrients. *Pediatrics*, 1981, 67, 146–150.

National Center for Health Statistics. Final Natality Statistics, Advance Report. *Monthly Vital Statistics*, Report 29, 1, Suppl., April 28, 1980.

Nelson, J.D., Patterson, K.A., and Mercer, R.T. Pregnancy outcomes for adolescents receiving prenatal care by nurse practitioners in extended roles. *Journal of Adolescent Health Care*, 1983, 4, 215–221.

Neugarten, B. Time, age and the life cycle. *The American Journal of Psychiatry*, 1979, 135, 887–894.

Phipps-Yonas, S. Teenage pregnancy and motherhood: A review of the literature. *American Journal of Orthopsychiatry*. 1980, 50, 403–431.

Presser, H. Age at menarche, socio-sexual behavior and fertility. *Social Biology*, 1978, 25, 94–101.

Reichelt, P. and Werley, H. Contraception, abortion, and venereal disease— Teenagers' knowledge and the effect of education. *Family Planning Perspectives*, 1975, 7, 83–88.

Rogel, M.J., Zuehlke, M.E., Petersen, A.C., Tobin-Richards, M., and Shelton, M. Conceptive behavior in adolescence. A decision-making perspective. *Journal of Youth and Adolescence*, 1980, 9, 491–506.

Rosenberg, M. *Society and the adolescent self-image.* Princeton, N.J.: Princeton University Press, 1965.

Rothenberg, P.B. Mother-child communication about sex and birth control. Presentation at Population Association of America. Atlanta, Georgia, 1978.

Rothenberg, P.B. Communication about sex and birth control between mothers and their adolescent children. *Population and Environment*, 1980, 3, 35–50.

Ryan, G., and Schneider, J. Teenage obstetric complications. *Clinical Obstetrics and Gynecology*, 1978, 21, 1191.

Sarrel, P.M., and Klerman, G.V. The young unwed mother. *American Journal of Obstetrics and Gynecology*, 1969, 105, 575–578.

Scher, P.W., Emans, S.J., and Grace, E.M. Factors associated with compliance to oral contraceptive use in an adolescent population. *Journal of Adolescent Health Care*, 1982, 3, 120–123.

Semmens, J.P., and McGlamory, J.C. Teenage pregnancies. *Obstetrics and Gynecology*, 1960, 16, 31–43.

Simmons, R. Rosenberg, F., and Rosenberg, M. Disturbance in the self-image at adolescence. *American Sociological Review*, 1973, 38, 553–568.

Simmons, R.G., Blyth, D.A., Van Cleave, E.F., and Bush, D.M. Entry into early adolescence: The impact of school structure, puberty, and early dating on self-esteem. *American Sociological Review*, 1979, 44, 948–967.

Stack, C. *All our kin.* New York: Harper and Row, 1974.

Stine, O.L., Rider, R.V., and Sweeney, E. School leaving due to pregnancy in an urban adolescent population. *American Journal of Public Health*, 1964, 54, 1.

Tanner, J.M. Physical development. *In* P.H. Mussen (Ed.), *Carmichael's manual of child psychology (Vol. I).* New York: Wiley, 1970, pp. 77–156.

Tobin-Richards, M.H., Boxer, A.M., and Petersen, A.C. The psychological significance of pubertal change: Sex differences in perceptions of self during early adolescence. *In* J. Brooks-Gunn and A.C. Petersen (Eds.), *Girls at puberty: Biological and psychosocial perspectives.* New York: Plenum, 1983, pp. 127–154.

Tversky, A. and Kahneman, D. Belief in the law of small numbers. *Psychological Bulletin,* 1971, *76,* 105–110.

Tyrer, G.B. Complications of teenage pregnancy *Clinical Obstetrics and Gynecology,* 1978, *21,* 1135.

United Nations Department of International Economic and Social Affairs, Table II, *Demographic Yearbook,* 1978, United Nations, New York, 1979.

Vener, A.M. and Stewart, C.S Adolescent sexual behavior in Middle America revisited: 1970–1973. *Journal of Marriage and the Family,* 1974, *36,* 728–735.

Vener, A.M., Stewart, C.S., and Hager, D.L. The sexual behavior of adolescents in middle America: Generational and American-British comparisons. *Journal of Marriage and the Family,* 1972, *34,* 696–705.

Wallace, H.M. Teen-aged pregnancy. *American Journal of Obstetrics and Gynecology,* 1965, *92,* 1125–1131.

Weiner, G. and Milton, T. Demographic correlates of low birthweight. *American Journal of Epidemiology,* 1970, *91,* 260–270.

Yankelovich, Skelly and White, Inc. The General Mills American Family Report, 1978–1979: Family health in an era of stress. General Mills, Inc., Minneapolis, 1979.

Zabin, L.S., Kantner, J.F., and Zelnick, M. The risk of adolescent pregnancy in the first months of intercourse. *Family Planning Perspectives,* 1979, *11,* 215–222.

Zabin, L.S., Kantner, J.F., and Zelnick, M. The risk of pregnancy in the first months of intercourse. *In* F. Furstenberg, R. Lincoln, and J. Menken (Eds.),*Teenage sexuality, pregnancy and childbearing.* Philadelphia: University of Pennsylvania Press, 1981.

Zelnick, M. and Kantner, J.F. Sexual and contraceptive experience of young unmarried women in the United States, 1976 and 1971. *Family Planning Perspectives,* 9 (2), March/April, 1977, 55–71.

Zelnick, M., and Kantner, J. Sex education and knowledge of pregnancy risk among U.S. teenage women. *Family Planning Perspectives,* 1979, *11,* 355–357.

Zelnick, M., and Kantner, J.F. Sexual activity, contraceptive use and pregnancy among metropolitan area teenagers: 1971–1979. *Family Planning Perspectives,* 1980, *12,* 230–237.

Zelnick, M., Kantner, J.F., and Ford, K. *Sex and pregnancy in adolescence (Vol. 133).* Beverly Hills: Sage Library of Social Research, 1981.

Zlatnick, F.J. and Burnmeister, G.F. Low "Gynecologic age" : An obstetric risk factor, *American Journal of Obstetrics and Gynecology,* 1977, *128,* 183–186.

Zuckerman, B., Winsmore, G., and Alpert, J.J. A study of the attitudes and support systems of inner city adolescent mothers. *Journal of Pediatrics,* 1979, *95,* 122–125.

Zuckerman, B., Alpert, J.J., Dooling, E., Hingson, R., Kayne H., Moorelock, S., and Oppenheimer, E. Neonatal outcome: Is adolescent pregnancy a risk factor? *Pediatrics,* 1983, *71,* 489–495.

PUBERTAL DEVELOPMENT AND ITS RELATION TO COGNITIVE AND PSYCHOSOCIAL DEVELOPMENT IN ADOLESCENT GIRLS: IMPLICATIONS FOR PARENTING

Anne C. Petersen
Lisa Crockett

INTRODUCTION

The rise in adolescent pregnancies and childbearing has led to increased interest in the factors potentially affecting child rearing competence in teenage mothers. Clearly, competent child rearing requires that a parent have mature judgment, the ability to anticipate the child's needs, and the resources to meet the child's needs, as well as those of the parent. From the start, then, it would seem that adolescent mothers are at a disadvantage developmentally, because they have typically not reached adult levels of cognitive, psychological, and social functioning. Lacking the necessary cognitive abilities and psychosocial maturity, they would be less able to meet the challenges of child rearing.

Although it seems relatively clear that young adolescents are developmentally disadvantaged with respect to child rearing, there appears to be some question regarding the factors responsible for their relative immaturity. Age would seem an important factor, since older girls are more likely to have developed the cognitive capacity and psychosocial skills important for competent mothering. It has often been assumed, however, that reproductive maturity (sometimes termed "gynecological age") is also a key variable. Proponents of this view believe that child rearing competence is linked to reproductive competence. From a developmental perspective, this would mean that cognitive and psychosocial functioning are related to the pubertal changes involved in the maturation of the reproductive system. Gyne-cological age (or the more easily assessed menarcheal age), rather than chronological age is held to be the primary factor.

One way to test the hypothesis relating reproductive maturity to child rearing competence would be to determine whether greater menar-cheal age is in fact associated with higher levels of functioning in the cognitive and psychosocial domains that may figure importantly in child rearing. Studies utilizing menarcheal age in the investigation of ad-olescent developmental patterns are rare, and, consequently, almost no data relevant to the question are currently available. Therefore, we will review some of the important changes in cognitive and psycho-social development associated with adolescence and describe our own findings concerning the relationship of these developments to men-archeal age.*

THEORETICAL MODELS

Two theoretical models provide particularly useful conceptualizations of the link between pubertal maturation and cognitive and psychosocial development, although others could be proposed as well. One is a *generalized maturation model*, in which cognitive and psychosocial maturity are assumed to be a function of physiological or reproductive maturity. For example, it is possible that pubertal development is re-lated to brain maturation and that pubertal brain growth permits the emergence of abstract reasoning. Similarly, the mature biological status of postmenarcheal girls, because it marks the completion of the bio-logical transition, could lead to a more integrated self-image as well as to greater social status. If the generalized maturation model were correct, we would see positive linear relationships between increasing menarcheal age and cognitive and psychosocial maturity. Girls reaching puberty early would be no more at risk than later maturers in terms of their degree of cognitive and psychosocial maturity since cognitive and psychosocial competence would develop at the same time as reproductive competence.

Alternatively, it is possible that there is a period of disruption in the lives of young girls as they become biologically mature. We know that

---

*Since this chapter is primarily a review, we will describe our own sample and measures here rather than disrupt the flow of the text to do so. The data are taken from a longitudinal study of biopsychosocial development in early adolescence. Samples selected at the beginning of sixth grade were followed in a cohort-sequential longitudinal design, with the second cohort serving to replicate the first. Two primarily white, suburban middle to upper-middle class school districts were randomly sampled. The total sample size is 335. Data on girls in Cohort I will be presented here ($n = 78$), although we refer to other results from this study from time to time.

the development of a mature menstrual cycle is a lengthy process in which menarche is but a single event (Petersen, 1979; Petersen, 1983a; Petersen and Taylor, 1980). The endocrine changes associated with this process could directly disrupt cognition and psychological functioning, and consequently affect cognitive performance and social relationships. If this *pubertal disruption model* were correct, we would see curvilinear relationships between menarcheal age and cognitive or psychosocial measures such that performance would be lowest for girls currently in the midst of pubertal change. Therefore, girls who have recently begun menstruation would be at particular risk as childrearers.

Tentative support for both models can be obtained from the literature on development in adolescence. However, it should be noted that the research findings are often contradictory. Even when findings appear to be largely consistent with one model, they must be interpreted with caution, since the link between reproductive maturation and cognitive or psychosocial functioning has rarely been directly examined; rather, it has been assumed (perhaps erroneously) on the basis of age comparisons.

Interestingly, models making the opposite predictions from those described above could be proposed on logical or empirical grounds. We could argue that puberty brings with it a general deterioration, rather than a generalized maturation effect. For example, some of the data on the development of sex differences (e.g., Maccoby and Jacklin, 1974; Petersen, 1980) would suggest that, beginning in early adolescence, girls begin to decrease their rate of growth in achievement, decline in self-esteem, and come to be at increased risk for depression. Such phenomena could be part of an underlying process of *maturationally based decline*.

The opposite of the pubertal disruption model would be a period of *pubertal enhancement*. Although there is little theoretical or empirical support for such a model, we could entertain the possibility that increased pubertal hormones temporarily enhance some behavioral processes. Belief in hypersexuality during adolescence might be consistent with this model.

DEVELOPMENTAL CHANGE IN ADOLESCENCE

PUBERTAL DEVELOPMENT

The dramatic changes accompanying puberty are described elsewhere in this volume (Lancaster, Chapter 2; Reiter, Chapter 4). Although we have learned a great deal in the past decade or so about the typical pattern of pubertal changes, the nature of variations in patterns—for example, variations associated with social class (Clausen, 1975) or race (Worthman, this volume, Chapter 6)—have been only superficially examined.

Of the few studies examining pubertal status in relation to other aspects of development, most have used a measure of relative timing of maturation. Typically, these studies examine those who are early or late in their timing relative to most adolescents, using age at menarche or the adolescent growth spurt as the marker (e.g., Jones and Bayley, 1950; Jones and Mussen, 1958; Mussen and Jones, 1957). Only recently have more direct biological measures been used (Duke *et al.*, 1982; Gross and Duke, 1980). Even so, we do not know, except in a general way, what the association is between biological indicators of pubertal status and reproductive status. For example, we know that ovulation (and, consequently, reproductive capability) may begin shortly after menarche in a few girls while, in most, ovulation occurs a year or so after the initial menstrual period.

In addition to asynchronies within individuals in the initiation of the various events and processes involved in reproductive maturation, measurement of pubertal status is further impeded by inaccurate reporting of pubertal events. There can be real confusion about the identification of menarche since the first instance of bleeding may not be followed by another for months. Young adolescents often asked us if by menarche we meant the first time of *regular* bleeding or the first bleeding per se. In these instances of ambiguity we used the first bleeding since we felt that this was likely to be the psychologically meaningful event. First bleeding may not, however, be the most meaningful event in a general biological sense, or in terms of reproductive potential. More research is needed before we will be able to gauge the appropriateness of this measure.

Apart from confusion about the "real" first menstruation, some girls—particularly early maturers—may misreport menarche. We found that

TABLE 8.1. Menarcheal Age at Six Assessment Times[a]

	Grade 6		Grade 7		Grade 8	
Menarcheal status	Fall (%)	Spring (%)	Fall (%)	Spring (%)	Fall (%)	Spring (%)
More than 1 year before	81	42	31	28 ⎱		
7–12 months before	10	32	24	13 ⎰	[b]28 ⎱	[b]28
1–6 months before	8	13	20	13	9 ⎰	
0–6 months after	1	8	15	27	19	17
7–12 months after	0	5	8	8	23	17
More than 1 year after	0	0	3	13	21	38

[a] $n = 78$ girls; numbers may total more than 100% due to rounding error.
[b] At these times it is not possible to determine when a girl not yet menarcheal will begin to menstruate.

many early maturers denied menarche when it had occurred (based upon vivid reports from the mothers as well as their own later accounts) (Petersen, 1983a). In our data, the actual date can be ascertained because we have multiple reporters and multiple assessments over time.

Table 8.1 gives some idea of the distribution of menarcheal age with data from one cohort of girls in our study. At each time of assessment, each girl is classified into one of six categories relative to menarche: more than 1 year before, between 6 and 12 months before, 6 or fewer months before, 6 or fewer months after, between 6 and 12 months after, and more than 12 months after.

COGNITIVE DEVELOPMENT

Adolescence is thought to be a time of major cognitive advances which profoundly alter children's conceptions of themselves and the world, and which bring their intellectual capacities up to those of adults. Typically between the ages of 12 and 15 years, the child enters the stage of formal operations—and final stage of cognitive development (Inhelder and Piaget, 1958; Piaget, 1972). Formal operations permit hypothetical thinking, in which the child reasons on the basis of verbally stated hypotheses and logical deduction. The child with formal operations can determine what is logically implied by a proposition regardless of whether or not that proposition is true. Essentially, then, formal operations free the child from reliance on the actual and concrete. Adolescents do not have to reason by manipulating concrete objects but can imagine hypothetical circumstances and anticipate possible outcomes given those circumstances. In short, the adolescent can reason abstractly. No longer intellectually constrained by the contingencies that actually obtain in the here and now, he or she can generate alternatives.

Linked to the development of abstract reasoning are cognitive advances that affect the adolescent's conceptualization of self and others and which permit the development of greater insight and more accurate judgment (Damon and Hart, 1982). First, adolescents who can imagine circumstances other than those currently affecting them are better able to take the perspective of another and to understand the wants of the other. At the same time, such people have the capacity for self-reflection and can attempt to view themselves as others might. Second, adolescents can conceptualize a past and a future as well as the present; their expanded time frame allows them to consider plans for the future and the long-term consequences of current action. Such intellectual advances are potentially important for child rearing, since a mother must frequently anticipate the needs of a child who may be wholly dependent on her, and must weigh alternative courses of action in light of their long-term consequences for herself and the child. Of course, the development of an extended time perspective and the capacity for self-reflection do not guarantee either insight or mature judgment. Particularly among young adolescents, sensitivity and good judgment often seem the exception rather than the rule. The cognitive advances of adolescence mean only that young people have the intellectual underpinnings necessary for the development of these capacities; the expression of these capacities, however, is likely to require motivation and the right kinds of practical and interpersonal experience as well.

Almost without exception, studies utilizing the tasks developed to measure formal reasoning (Inhelder and Piaget, 1958) report that performance on these tasks (and presumably formal reasoning) improves throughout adolescence (Keating, 1980; Petersen; 1983b). Several cross-sectional studies have demonstrated a steady increase in the proportion of children exhibiting formal operations, as one moves from grade school to junior high to high school groups (e.g., Keating and Clark, 1980; Martorano, 1977; Roberge, 1976; Ronning, 1977; reviewed in Neimark, 1975a, 1982). Similarly, the sole large-scale longitudinal study of formal reasoning showed that many children advance to the level of formal operations in junior high or high school (Neimark, 1975b).

Contrary to Piaget's conclusion, however, not all individuals studied demonstrate formal reasoning capability by age 15; in fact, many adults fail to show formal operations on Inhelder tasks (e.g., Dulit, 1972; Elkind, 1975; Tomlinson-Keasey, 1972; reviewed in Neimark, 1975a). For instance, Tomlinson-Keasey (1972) observed formal reasoning in only about one-half of the middle-aged women in her study and in two-thirds of the college women. Similarly, in a study by Dulit (1972), less than one-third of the adolescents and adults performed at a fully formal level. Overall, only 40–60% of college students and adults in Western cultures seem to attain formal operations (Keating, 1980), and the percentage of individuals reaching formal operations in non-Western cultures is even lower (Ashton, 1975; Bart and Lane, 1982; Neimark, 1975a). Differential familiarity with the test situation and materials as well as different cultural demands regarding the development of formal reasoning skills may account for the cross-cultural variation, but the fact remains that formal operations (as measured by Inhelder tasks) are not universally attained. Furthermore, some people who show formal reasoning on one task may not show it on others, or may show it to a lesser degree (Neimark, 1975a). This lack of consistency could indicate that the tasks tap somewhat different skills (which develop at different rates or to different degrees in the same person), that they tap a skill which individuals are more likely to apply to some task situations than to others, or that they tap the same skill with differential accuracy. The inconsistency could also reflect differential task difficulty.

Thus, it seems that formal reasoning is not as pervasive a phenomenon as Piaget originally anticipated, in terms of its prevalence in the adult population and in terms of its consistent use by individuals across all situations. The development of (or at least the manifestation of) formal reasoning may be confined to areas of individual talent, interest, and specialization (Piaget, 1972). If this last possibility proves true, the Inhelder tasks may not be the most efficient way to tap formal operational capability, since the tasks and materials may be unfamiliar or uninteresting to many people.

In addition, many recent studies have failed to substantiate Piaget's assertion that the emergence of formal operations constitutes a discrete, pervasive shift in cognitive functioning (i.e., a new cognitive stage). Instead, adolescent cognitive development may be more accurately characterized as a "continuous quantitative and multidimensional growth in abilities" (Keating, 1980, p. 231). Although the controversy regarding continuous versus discontinuous development may never be resolved, investigators on both sides of the issue agree that formal abstract reasoning capacity increases in adolescence. At least, we can say that older adolescents have a greater probability than younger adolescents of consistently manifesting formal operations and abstract thought. Older adolescents thus have a greater likelihood of exhibiting cognitive maturity.

Although the steady improvement in formal reasoning ability would seem consistent with the general maturation model described above, it should be kept in mind that the findings mentioned are based on age effects only; the hypothesized link between reproductive maturation and formal reasoning ability was not tested or examined. A relationship between pubertal status and cognition has been hypothesized, however, with respect to spatial ability, an ability to visualize the rearrangement of objects or features of objects. Spatial ability has been found to correlate strongly with formal reasoning ability as measured by a paper-and-pencil version of a Piagetian proportional reasoning task; in a factor analysis, formal reasoning factors with spatial rather than verbal measures (Petersen and Gitelson, in preparation). Thus, evidence of an association between pubertal status and spatial ability could indicate a parallel link between pubertal processes and formal reasoning capabilities.

In an attempt to establish a link between puberty and spatial ability, Waber (1976, 1977) suggested that pubertal hormones initially promote brain development but ultimately curtail it in a manner analogous to their effect on skeletal growth. If this hypothesis were true, early maturers (whose brain development is presumably curtailed at a younger age) should perform more poorly than late maturers on test of spatial ability. Consistent with this argument, Waber (1976) found that later maturers outperformed early maturers on some spatial tests, a finding that has been replicated in several more recent studies (Carey and Diamond, 1980; Newcombe et al., 1983; Petersen and Gitelson, in preparation). Other studies, however, have failed to find a relationship between timing of maturation and spatial performance (Herbst and Petersen, 1979; Petersen, 1976; 1983b). It should also be noted that if such a relationship does exist, it is directly contrary to the generalized maturation model, since instead of being more advanced cognitively, girls reaching puberty at a young age are disadvantaged relative to their later maturing peers, at least in the spatial processing domain.

The fact that performance on formal reasoning tasks may be related to spatial ability raises a further interesting point. Sex differences are frequently found when adolescents and adults are tested on the Piaget and Inhelder tasks (e.g., Dulit, 1972), and on this basis it has often been assumed that females are less capable of abstract reasoning than are males. A strong correlation between formal reasoning performance and spatial ability would cast doubt on this conclusion, since the sex differences on Piaget and Inhelder tasks might be attributable to the well-documented sex difference in spatial ability, rather than to a gender-related difference in the capacity for abstract thought. Tasks drawing heavily on spatial ability may simply be inappropriate for the measurement of abstract reasoning. Even Piaget (1972) has observed that formal operations are most likely to be observed in those domains in which an individual's talents, interests, and experience are focused; since spatial ability is considered a male, rather than a female, domain, tasks utilizing spatial skills would be unlikely to tap abstract reasoning capability in many girls and women.

Another set of findings on cognitive performance has been interpreted as evidence favoring the pubertal disruption model. Adolescents exhibit a performance dip in the encoding and recognition of unfamiliar faces (Carey, 1981; Carey and Diamond, 1980; Carey et al., 1980; Flin, 1983). Performance on this task increases until the age of 10 years, then drops temporarily between ages 12 and 14, returning to former high levels by age 16. Carey and her associates attribute the dip in performance to physiological events associated with the onset of puberty, since girls in the midst of pubertal change do more poorly on face recognition tasks than do like-aged girls who are prepubertal or late pubertal (as measured by secondary sex characteristics) (Diamond et al., 1983). However, not all of the data on face recognition is consistent with the pubertal disruption hypothesis. The main incongruency is that no studies have found a sex difference in the timing of the dip in performance (Carey et al., 1980; Diamond et al., 1983; Flin, 1980, 1983). Since boys tend to mature later than girls, we would expect any disruption caused by pubertal events to occur later in boys than in girls. Yet studies conducted thus far suggest that boys and girls decline in performance at approximately the same age. Thus, evidence for pubertal disruption is found only with girls; a general pubertal disruption model has not been supported.

In our own data, we have found that cognitive test performance—including tests of spatial ability, field independence, and fluent production, as well as one component of Piagetian cognitive development—increases steadily in both boys (unpublished data) and girls (Petersen, 1983b) over the early adolescent years (see Fig. 8.1). There was no sex difference in the pattern of change, although the predictable sex differences in *level* of performance on each variable emerged (i.e., girls scored higher on fluent production, boys higher on the other tasks). This pattern of change would fit the *generalized maturation model* except that it is grade-related and not related to menarcheal age (see Table 8.2).

Studies examining the relationship between achievement test scores and pubertal status have found no association between the two in girls (Duke *et al.*, 1982; Gross and Duke, 1980; Simmons *et al.*, 1982). In our

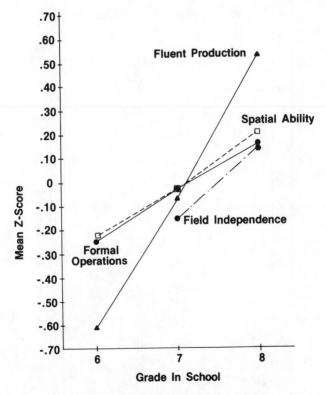

FIGURE 8.1. Longitudinal trends in girls' performance on cognitive tests. (Field independence was not assessed in sixth grade.)

TABLE 8.2. Analyses of Variance of Menarcheal Age on Cognitive Tests with and without IQ Controlled[a]

Cognitive tests	Sixth grade					Seventh grade					Eighth grade				
	F	p	η	β	R^2	F	p	η	β	R^2	F	p	η	β	R^2
Abstract reasoning															
Physical	0.61		.22	.23	26	1.74		.32	.33	30	1.05		.20	.18	23
Verbal	1.55		.38	.37	30	1.19		.31	.31	11	0.54		.12	.15	5
Spatial ability															
Visualization	1.10		.34	.31	32	1.15		.25	.31	26	0.76		.22	.22	22
Horizontality	0.43		.22	.22	16	[b]					[b]				
Embeddedness	[b]					0.26		.15	.14	16	0.74		.10	.15	30
Fluent production	0.23		.14	.16	8	1.55		.36	.37	18	0.15		.12	.11	2
Achievement tests															
Reading	0.48		.20	.12	50	[b]					1.86		.09	.18	59
Mathematics	1.30		.24	.18	57	[b]					3.07	.03	.13	.24	56
Total	0.93		.22	.14	58	[b]					2.96	.04	.11	.21	64

[a] F is the statistic measuring the effect of menarcheal age when IQ is controlled, p is the significance level if .05 or less, η is the effect size, β is the effect size controlling for IQ, R^2 is the percentage of variance accounted for by menarcheal age and IQ.
[b] Not given at these ages.

data, we see no effects of menarcheal age on IQ. But when IQ is controlled we do see significant effects of menarcheal age on two eighth grade achievement test scores: mathematics and an overall score (based on mathematics and reading achievement as well as other aspects of achievement) (see Table 8.2). In both cases, performance increased dramatically (looking like an exponential curve) with increasing menarcheal age. Before we conclude, however, that the *generalized maturation model* is correct, we must note that no effects were seen with these tests in sixth grade. Although only a few girls were postmenarcheal in sixth grade, some effect of menarcheal age would be expected. When linear and quadratic polynomials were fit to the sixth and eighth grade data, to directly test the proposed generalized maturation and pubertal disruption models, respectively, neither described the achievement test data to the extent necessary for statistical significance.

Course grades for science, mathematics, social studies, literature, and language arts were also fit to polynomials representing the proposed models. Table 8.3 shows that no effects of menarcheal age were seen. When effects of IQ were controlled, there were no effects at seventh and eighth grade, and only one effect at sixth grade—a *positive* linear effect on math grades. Therefore, more mature girls tend to get higher grades in one academic domain. These results are consistent with the generalized maturation model, although a single significant finding could easily appear on the basis of chance alone.

These results should be considered in the context of the effects of grade level in school. For both boys and girls, course grades *declined* significantly over the early adolescent years (Kavrell and Petersen, 1984) (see Fig. 8.2). The same decline has been found in another study (Simmons et al., 1982). This result appears to reflect increasingly difficult grading practices on the part of teachers. There were no sex differences in the pattern of decline although girls, overall, had higher grades than boys.

Taken together, our data indicate that school performance, as measured by course grades, shows *maturational decline*, across grades, although there may be a circumscribed positive effect of menarcheal age within grades. Recall, however, that a quite different pattern appears with cognitive test scores, in that they increase steadily and show no association with pubertal status. These combined results would suggest that the underlying cognitive processes are not disrupted by reproductive maturation. Only school performance appears to be affected, and in this case, the observed decline in grades could well be due to more stringent grading practices on the part of teachers. Therefore, social processes, such as the social responses given to individuals with more mature bodies, appear to be implicated.

TABLE 8.3. Linear and Quadratic Trends in the Effect of Menarcheal Age on Course Grades[a]

| | Grade 6 | | | | Grade 7 | | | | Grade 8 | | | |
| | Linear | | Quadratic | | Linear | | Quadratic | | Linear | | Quadratic | |
Grades	T	p	T	p	T	p	T	p	T	p	T	p
Language arts	.86		− .89		.12		− .50		− .22		− .10	
Literature	.20		− .18		−1.04		.58		−1.13		.98	
Mathematics	1.69		−1.45		− .40		− .38		− .71		.08	
Science	− .38		.35		−1.02		.14		−1.46		1.26	
Social studies	1.27		−1.18		−1.19		.79		− .92		1.08	
Grades (controlling for IQ)												
Language arts	1.36		−1.36		.24		− .32		− .52		.23	
Literature	.66		.60		−1.23		1.13		−1.73		1.64	
Mathematics	2.18	.03	−1.88		− .37		− .24		− .91		.30	
Science	− .07		.08		−1.07		.39		−1.90		1.74	
Social studies	1.81		−1.67		−1.27		1.13		−1.62		1.93	

[a] T is the statistic measuring the effect of menarcheal age; p is the significance level at .05 or less.

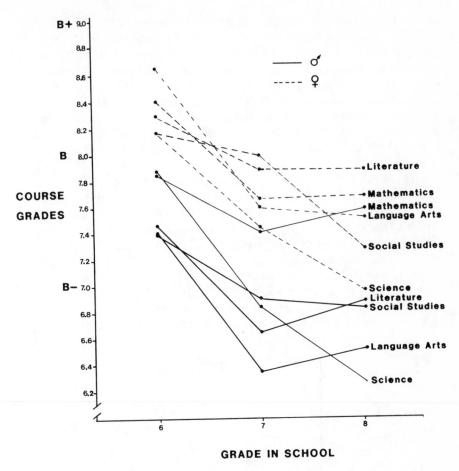

FIGURE 8.2. Longitudinal trends in course grades.

PSYCHOSOCIAL DEVELOPMENT

Psychosocial maturation is also in evidence during the pubertal years and would be important for child rearing. Although psychosocial functioning often appears to involve a strong cognitive component, especially in the cases of moral reasoning and ego development (Rowe and Marcia, 1980; Walker and Richards, 1979), cognitive factors alone cannot account for behavior in this domain (Youniss, 1981). Similarly, psychosocial maturation in adolescence may be in part a function of cognitive maturation occurring during the same period, but cannot be wholly explained by this single factor.

Ego Development. One psychosocial construct of potential importance to child rearing competence is ego development. Loevinger (1966,

1976) has theorized that ego or character development proceeds through
a series of stages or milestones, each of which involves a characteristic
mode of ego functioning. "Mode of ego functioning" refers to a loosely
organized composite of impulse control and depth of character, orientation toward self and others, interpersonal style, and degree of cognitive complexity (Loevinger, 1979). Thus, a girl's level of ego functioning
has profound consequences for her conceptualization of self and others
and for her mode of interpersonal interaction. It could, therefore, importantly affect her capacity and motivation to care for and nurture a
young child.

   Early studies of ego development employing a cross-sectional design
found significant increases in level of ego functioning across the adolescent years (Loevinger, 1979; Loevinger and Wessler, 1970), a finding
that has been substantiated in a recent series of longitudinal studies
(Redmore and Loevinger, 1979) (see Fig. 8.3). The longitudinal studies
were based on several samples covering a broad range of socioeconomic levels. All samples, retested at intervals of 1½ to 6 years, showed
an increase in average ego level, although at the higher grade levels
(e.g., eleventh to twelfth grade), the increase was not statistically significant, perhaps indicating that ego development tapers off at this time.

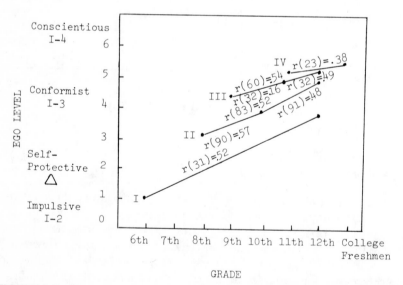

FIGURE 8.3. Average ego level by grade and correlations over 1.5, 2, 3, and
            6 years for longitudinal samples. Note: SES (0=high) for Group
            I=6, for Group II=3, and for Groups III and IV=2. I: inner city
            school (black); II: inner city, suburban (black and white), prep
            school (white); III: suburban (white), prep school; IV: prep school.
            Reproduced with permission from Redmore and Loevinger, 1979.

The findings also suggest that changes in ego functioning proceed relatively slowly, since a 2-year interval often yields a gain of only one-half a stage or less. Thus a change would probably not be detected using a test–retest interval of only a year. Indeed, in our data we found no significant change in level of ego development over the three years of the study, a result similar to those summarized by Redmore and Loevinger over the same age range.

Overall, the studies present strong evidence that ego functioning develops over the course of adolescence. These findings are based, however, only on age increases, or increases in grade level. When we examined ego level in relation to menarcheal age among girls in our sample, we found no such association.

Self-Esteem. We are not aware of any studies demonstrating a link between self-esteem and mothering competence in adolescent girls, but it seems likely that high self-esteem would promote a psychologically healthier mother–infant relationship, since the young mother would rely less on her child to bolster her feelings of personal worth. Less dependent on the child's positive responses to her, she would be less threatened by occasional negative transactions and more able to take them in stride. Less likely to overidentify with the child, she would be more likely to differentiate the child's needs from her own and attend to them appropriately.

Although most of the studies assessing self-image (reviewed by Wylie, 1979) have failed to demonstrate increments during adolescence, it has been noted (McCarthy and Hoge, 1982) that the great majority of the studies (75%) employed cross-sectional designs; in contrast, of the longitudinal studies reviewed, six out of seven found that self-esteem increases with age. More recent longitudinal studies have also reported that self-esteem increases over the course of adolescence (McCarthy and Hoge, 1982; O'Malley and Bachman, 1983). Since longitudinal studies are able to detect subtle intraindividual changes often missed by cross-sectional studies, it seems likely that self-esteem does increase during adolescence, although the changes may not be large or dramatic. In our own data, we do not find significant increases over the early adolescent period.

Self-esteem may not, however, increase steadily and linearly during adolescence. Simmons and her colleagues (Simmons *et al.*, 1979; Simmons *et al.*, 1973) reported a drop in self-esteem among seventh graders. Among boys, the decline was linked to environmental changes such as the transition from elementary to junior high school, while in girls pubertal variables as well as environmental ones were important (Simmons *et al.*, 1979). Specifically, girls who had recently changed schools, experienced menarche, and begun to date exhibited particularly low self-esteem. Thus, in addition to the support for the general

TABLE 8.4. Analyses of Variance of Menarcheal Age on
Psychological Tests[a]

	Grade 6		Grade 7		Grade 8	
	F	p	F	p	F	p
Self-image						
Impulse control	2.16	.05	0.22		2.20	.05
Emotional tone	2.13	.05	0.77		0.46	
Body image	0.13		0.94		0.44	
Social relationships	0.56		1.75		0.74	
Family relationships	2.86	.04	1.64		1.57	
Mastery and coping	1.44		0.43		0.75	
Vocation/education	0.45		1.55		0.17	
Psychopathology	0.69		0.39		0.89	
Superior adjustment	0.20		1.19		0.92	
Total	1.75		0.80		0.88	
Ego development	0.55		0.74		0.41	

[a] F is the statistic measuring the effect of menarcheal age; p is the significance level if .05 or less.

maturation model suggested by the overall increase in self-esteem over the adolescent years, there may also be a perimenarcheal effect of pubertal changes or of psychological responses to pubertal change. The perimenarcheal effect would be consistent with the pubertal disruption hypothesis.

In our own data, we do not find evidence of pubertal disruption in self-image. Table 8.4 reveals only one significant association with menarcheal age. When linear and quadratic polynomials are fit to the data to test systematic increases, decreases, dips, or humps over time, effects are seen with only a few aspects of self-image. In sixth and eighth grades there are significant effects with Impulse Control. In sixth grade, the best impulse control is seen in girls just postmenarcheal while the worst impulse control is seen in girls 6 to 12 months before menarche. In eighth grade, there is a similar pattern except that girls 12 months or more postmenarcheal have the lowest impulse control. Taken together, these results suggest that the perimenarcheal girls show the best impulse control; this is opposite from what a pubertal disruption hypothesis would predict.

Two other effects are seen on self-image scales. In sixth grade, positive Emotional Tone appears to decline with girls closer to menarche. In eighth grade, family relations are most positive for girls in a perimenarcheal status. These results may be meaningful but need to be considered in relation to the general lack of replication over time and the few results obtained.

Although menarcheal age seems unrelated to self-image, we have

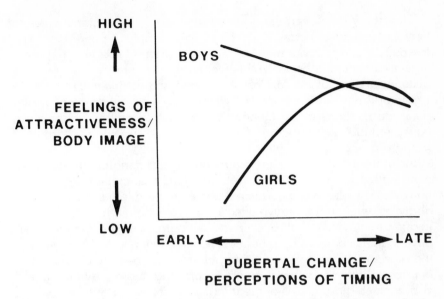

FIGURE 8.4. The model describing the relationship of pubertal change to body image and feelings of attractiveness.

found that pubertal status as indexed by several other characteristics is related to body-image and feelings of attractiveness, but with distinctly different patterns for boys and girls (Tobin-Richards et al., 1983). The general pattern observed with most characteristics is shown in Fig. 8.4. Note that whereas increased development is a positive factor for boys, it is negative for girls, with "on-time" girls reporting the most positive attitudes about their bodies. Other studies, focusing only on early and late maturation, have found similarly that early maturers report a more negative psychological picture (Jones and Mussen, 1958; Peskin, 1973; Simmons et al., 1973).

The experience of menarche may also affect girls' images of their bodies. Studies of girls within the same school grade show that post-menarcheal girls draw pictures of mature women while premenarcheal girls draw children (Koff et al., 1978). Assuming that this measure provides information about body image, these results suggest that girls dramatically change their views of themselves once they have menstruated. We are conducting similar studies but have focused on the broader spectrum of pubertal changes (e.g., Petersen, 1983a), in order to understand the psychological meaning of puberty to girls. Personal attitudes are difficult to study because feelings about pubertal change are not often expressed in our society. Nevertheless, there is accumulating evidence that personal meaning mediates the impact of pubertal change on behavior and affect.

One study, however, suggests caution in ascribing significance to personal attitudes (Rogel et al., 1981). In a sample of poor black adolescents, feelings about menarche were uniformly negative but there was no association between this feeling and any measures of sexual attitudes and behavior. This lack of results could be due to the restricted range of the feelings measured, which would attenuate any correlations. But feelings about menarche may not be embedded within a consistent meaning structure. Or, there may be subcultural variations in these processes.

In summary, we find some evidence for perimenarcheal enhancement (rather than pubertal disruption) on impulse control. In general, however, few effects of menarcheal age were seen in our data. In other analyses, we found *negative* effects of increasing maturation on body image and feelings of attractiveness, with girls who are "on-time" relative to their peers having the most positive feelings. We believe that the personal meaning attached to puberty may be a potent mediator of pubertal effects, although we recognize that there may be cultural variations in the patterns of meanings that are important.

Conformity and Other Aspects of Social Development. An integrated picture of social development in adolescence has not been presented in the literature, but several processes pertaining to this aspect of development have potential relevance for teenage pregnancy and/or child rearing competence. We know, for instance, that the importance of the peer group increases in adolescence; girls especially turn more and more to their friends for standards of behavior and emotional support (Conger and Petersen, 1984). One important aspect of these friendships is the development of emotional intimacy and of reciprocal relationships based on mutual support, appreciation, and consideration. Unfortunately, the teenager whose first concern is with peer acceptance and reciprocity in social relationships is unlikely to be psychologically prepared to care for a wholly dependent infant in what is an intrinsically unilateral relationship.

At the same time, the need for acceptance and support from peers during this period of transition from childhood to adulthood may cause adolescents to follow the crowd, rather than making responsible decisions for themselves. The tendency to follow the crowd, combined with increased libido and a need for emotional intimacy, may lead some girls to become involved in early sexual relationships, increasing the likelihood of early pregnancy.

The tendency to conform to group opinion and pressure seems to follow a clear developmental course (Costanzo and Shaw, 1966). Most studies comparing degree of conformity across age groups have found a striking increase in this tendency in early adolescence as compared to preadolescence and late- to postadolescence; in most cases conformity peaks at about age 13 (Coleman, 1980; Conger and Petersen, 1984). Although conformity is usually measured experimentally by determining whether an individual changes his or her judgments so that they are in accord with the judgments of the group, the principle is clearly applicable to the way in which adolescents behave outside the laboratory as well. Peer group conformity has long been a stereotypic attribute of adolescence within this culture, although it does not describe the behavior of all adolescents, nor all of the behavior of any one adolescent. Rather, conformity to peers occurs primarily in behavioral domains (such as taste in dress and in music) where modeling the parent will not necessarily prove useful; in other areas such as values, adolescents often internalize parental guidelines (Conger and Petersen, 1984).

Conformity is likely to peak in adolescence because the pubertal years bring changes in role expectations as well as in physical and cognitive changes. Adolescents attempting to behave in an adultlike fashion, but finding many of the changes confusing or difficult to apprehend, turn to peers as models for behavior and as support groups. In light of the importance of peers as sources of deep friendship and support, and most of all, acceptance (Conger and Petersen, 1984), it is not surprising that conformity to peers is especially high in early adolescence when the child is first confronted with simultaneous physical, psychological, and social changes. As the adolescent becomes more comfortable and secure with his or her developing self, the need to conform to peers wanes.

Since puberty includes the development of adultlike secondary sex characteristics, pubertal status is likely to affect one's status within the adolescent group and within the broader social context. In particular, deviant rates of maturation (e.g., too early or too late) may be disturbing to adolescents, given their strong need for conformity.

Studies report contradictory findings regarding the social implications of pubertal maturation. Some studies find social advantages of early maturation (e.g., Faust, 1960) while others find that early maturers are disadvantaged socially (e.g., Jones and Mussen, 1958). There are class differences that may explain these discrepancies; Clausen (1975) found that early maturing working-class girls had lower self-confidence than later maturers, while the reverse effect was seen among middle-class girls. Among boys, the social effects of early maturation seem to be uniformly positive.

In the study of black adolescent girls mentioned earlier (Rogel et al., 1981), timing of menarche was related to sexual attitudes and behavior such that girls with earlier menarche expressed more positive feelings about sex. Interestingly, the interval between menarche and first intercourse as well as first pregnancy was longer for the early maturing girls, so that the average ages of the latter two events were similar to those of "on-time" girls. Later maturing girls were later in both first intercourse and first pregnancy. This result is somewhat similar to that of Presser (1980) who found that among black, but not white girls, there was an association between age at menarche and first intercourse.

More research is needed on the relationship between menarcheal age and social development. The limited results currently available are contradictory. Studies of primates and of boys showing associations between pubertal status and social dominance (Freedman, 1979; Savin-Williams, 1979; Steinberg and Hill, 1978) would suggest that we might also expect associations between these two areas for girls. Nevertheless, the lack of similarity between boys and girls in other important areas, e.g., aggression (Maccoby and Jacklin, 1974, 1980), would suggest great caution in generalizing from primates and boys to girls. Furthermore, we believe that a better understanding of preadolescent social relationships is essential for understanding those that occur during adolescence.

Moral Development. Over the course of adolescence, boys and girls also develop a greater understanding of, and concern with, moral issues. Their progress has been documented by two complementary lines of theory and research which focus on what might be referred to as the cognitive and affective aspects of moral development. Research on the cognitive aspect, the development of moral reasoning, has a longer history since it dates back at least as far as Piaget (1932), who noted two levels of moral judgment in children. Younger children, in the stage of moral realism, base their judgments entirely on the concrete or objective aspects of the situation and ignore such subjective aspects as the transgressor's intentions. For them, naughtiness is wholly a function of how much physical damage has been done (i.e., how many cups were broken accidentally). For children aged 11 or older, subjective contingencies are likely to outweigh the assessments of physical damage. Thus, a boy who breaks one cup while attempting to steal jam is naughtier than a boy who breaks 15 cups but who was not engaged in intentional wrong doing. Piaget believed that the older child's greater sensitivity to the subjective context was due partly to a more advanced stage of cognitive functioning and partly to more extensive social experience.

Piaget's conceptualization considered only two levels of moral reasoning, with little development occurring after the shift to the second in early adolescence. Kohlberg (1964, 1976), however, expanded Piaget's formulation of moral development to encompass six stages of moral reasoning. With this more detailed formulation, Kohlberg has been able to detect changes in moral reasoning level during adolescence. The changes occur slowly, but from age 10 or 11 years to young adulthood, there is a gradual shift away from primitive (preconventional) modes of moral reasoning to more sophisticated modes (Hoffman, 1980; Rest, 1975, 1979). Both cross-sectional and longitudinal studies have demonstrated that the incidence of preconventional reasoning decreases markedly while that of conventional reasoning increases. There is also an increase in the number of individuals showing principled reasoning, although the incidence remains low.

It has been conceptualized by Piaget and Kohlberg, moral reasoning depends heavily on cognitive processes. Despite the relationship between the formulations of cognitive and moral development, and despite the role that cognitive processes undoubtedly play in moral reasoning, the two concepts are not identical. Chronologically, not all moral transitions follow cognitive reorganizations; thus, these transitions must have a different source of impetus. Empirically, it has been demonstrated that a given level of cognitive development may be a necessary, but not sufficient, condition for the corresponding level of moral development (Walker, 1980; Walker and Richards, 1979. Thus, in addition to cognitive development, moral development appears to depend on other factors, in particular, on social and educational experiences that force the individual to confront moral issues.

Gilligan (1977) has delineated a second dimension of moral development that may characterize the moral reasoning of girls and women better than does the Kohlbergian formulation. The interpersonal orientation of many females leads them to be assigned to the conformist stage of moral reasoning. However, if an interpersonal orientation is viewed as reflecting a different moral orientation rather than a single stage of moral thought, levels along this new moral dimension can be discerned. Gilligan has outlined five stages in moral development with respect to interpersonal relations which describe a progression from selfishness to conformity with cultural norms to nonviolence (not hurting others) as moral principles. Future studies with adolescent girls may be able to validate the hypothesized progression and document changes in moral level over the pubertal years. Although we expect that there are gradual changes in moral development, we doubt that they would be linked to pubertal status. Such changes would, however, be relevant to the teenage girl's interpersonal relations, and with respect to the focus of this chapter, to a teenage mother's behavior toward her child.

Although much attention and research has been devoted to cognitive aspects of moral development, some investigators have offered alternative conceptualizations of moral behavior. Hoffmann (1980) has delineated a model in which morality is based on the experience of empathy. According to this model, empathy involves an affective arousal component deriving from a vicarious response to another's pain or distress. High levels of empathy require a capacity for understanding distress cues and a conception of the other as a person who exists in time and therefore may experience difficulties or pain not just momentarily but chronically. The person concept that plays a role in more sophisticated empathic responses, allows vicarious distress to be combined with the less immediate sense of compassion (sympathetic distress) for the other as a separate person who is suffering. It is compassion that allows a person to help the suffering individual despite the helper's vicariously experienced discomfort. Compassion may also allow the individual to experience guilt when he or she is the cause of another's distress or fails to relieve it. Empathic distress, compassion, and guilt, then, provide the motivational bases for moral action.

Although research has shown that people do respond empathetically to another's distress and that empathic or sympathetic distress and guilt contribute to helping behavior, the developmental picture of the relationship between empathy and moral action is not yet clear. It does seem, however, that the differentiated concept of another person required for responses of compassion and guilt would be unlikely to develop without the expanded time frame and self-awareness that emerges with the development of abstract reasoning in adolescence. It also seems likely that empathic responding and mature compassion would be important aspects of competent parenting.

Moral development was not measured in our study and to our knowledge has not been related to pubertal development in other research. Based on the work reviewed here, we would be surprised if there were an association. Moral development is strongly related to cognitive development and to a lesser extent, ego development and neither of these constructs has shown associations with menarcheal age.

SUMMARY

From the above discussion, it can be seen that advances in cognitive capacity and in psychosocial functioning occur over the course of adolescence. The development of formal operations opens up new intellectual abilities to adolescents which may also contribute to psychosocial maturation. In this regard, many of the psychosocial variables we have discussed (e.g., moral reasoning, empathy, social cognition) clearly draw on cognitive skills and others (e.g., self-concept) are made possible by the concomitants of formal operations (in this case, self-reflection). Thus, although having the cognitive underpinning does not ensure psychosocial advances, it makes such advance possible.

The question remains whether the important cognitive and psychosocial advances of adolescence are linked to reproductive maturation,

TABLE 8.5. Summary of Menarcheal Age Effects

| | Developmental hypotheses | | |
Kind of test	Generalized maturation	Pubertal disruption	Perimenarcheal enhancement
Cognitive	Verbal abstract reasoning Mathematics achievement Total achievement Math grades		Verbal abstract reasoning
Psychological		Emotional tone	Impulse control Family relationships

and, more precisely, to pubertal status and development. Unfortunately, the relationship between *pubertal* maturation and cognitive or psychosocial functioning has rarely been tested. Despite this gap in the empirical evidence, many researchers strongly believe that competence in mothering is somehow tied to reproductive maturation and, specifically, to menarcheal age.

Table 8.5 summarizes the effects that were found in our own data. Improved performance with increasing gynecological age was found with verbal abstract reasoning as well as mathematics and total achievement test scores and math grades. Evidence for pubertal disruption was found with emotional tone. Perimenarcheal enhancement was seen with verbal abstract reasoning, impulse control, and family relationships. Given the number of effects examined, these could all be chance results.

DISCUSSION

While we believe that puberty, in general, and menarcheal age, in particular, are important influences on *some* aspects of cognitive, psychological, and social functioning for *some* girls, we are coming to believe that a global hypothesis—such as the generalized maturation model or the pubertal disruption model—is not appropriate for understanding development at this age. We are finding psychological factors that mediate the direct effects of puberty, factors that operate differently for subgroups of individuals. One of the goals in our current research is to identify these subgroups in order to better understand the processes of development during the pubertal years. It is quite clear that boys and girls constitute two important subgroups in terms of pubertal effects. In addition, very early maturing girls have been identified as an important subgroup (Petersen, 1983a). Another dimension that we think will be an important mediator of social effects is size—height, weight, and bulk. This would seem to have an obvious influence on various aspects of interpersonal relationships and other psychosocial behaviors, yet it has been virtually ignored in studies of human adolescents.

On the basis of our experiences with the young adolescents in our study, as well as our analyses of the data on pubertal effects, we have come to appreciate the complexity of the processes that we are examining. Pubertal change and the development of reproductive potential involve several interrelated processes. More importantly, we must attend to the meaning of these changes to girls. Because in our society we have no puberty rites or clear transitional rituals based on maturational status, this change becomes more individually integrated. It should not be surprising to find few correlates of pubertal status when the salient influences on young adolescents are social and, for many, transmitted through the social structure of grade in school. Indeed, except for early maturing girls, all young adolescents seem to behave as though they were "pubertal" once some "critical mass" has made the transition to biological pubertal status. We believe that young adolescents learn vicariously about the various changes involved and prepare themselves for their own pubertal transition. Our results support this interpretation of social structure effects (i.e., grade in school) rather than maturationally driven developmental changes in adolescence.

IMPLICATIONS FOR CHILD REARING

The findings reviewed here have important implications for the child rearing capacities of adolescent girls. We see clearly that most aspects of cognitive and psychosocial development increase steadily over the adolescent years. Therefore, a sixth-grade girl is much less mature, both cognitively and psychosocially, than a twelfth-grade girl. When the increase in experience gained over these years is also considered, the case is even stronger for greater maturity in older adolescents.

But have we simply confounded age with biological maturation status? Are girls who mature earlier biologically the ones who also mature earlier in other respects? From the limited research addressing this question, the answer appears to be "NO." There are few consistent patterns of relationships that would suggest a strong link between biological maturation and psychosocial or cognitive development. If there are any relationships between menarcheal age and other aspects of development, they appear to depend on the aspect of development, and perhaps the subgroup of individuals such as ones determined by social class.

Furthermore, since the changes across adolescence are greater than those during the early adolescent years when pubertal change is occurring, postpubertal developmental changes would give an advantage to older girls even if there were some changes linked to menarcheal status during the pubertal years. Therefore, chronological age is likely to be a more potent factor than pubertal status even if some effects of puberty are found in future research.

Together with the possibility of greater biological risk associated with pregnancy among young adolescents (i.e., those under 15 years of age), the present conclusions would suggest that strong efforts be made to postpone pregnancy in this age group. Young adolescent girls would, in general, appear likely to be poor mothers, given their significantly less mature developmental status. Although the passage of a few more years cannot guarantee adequate mothering competence, most girls do acquire increased psychosocial and cognitive maturity over the course of adolescence, as well as increased experience with the demands of adult status. If childbearing is postponed, these few years of experience and psychological growth are likely to permit the development of personal resources important to the welfare of the adolescent and her future children.

SUMMARY

The increase in adolescent pregnancy and childbearing has caused concern about the capacities of young adolescent girls to function adequately as parents. This chapter reviewed current knowledge about cognitive and psychosocial development in adolescence, particularly in relation to biological development. We concluded that among girls who are able to bear children (and who are therefore postmenarcheal), the key factor related to parenting capacity is not menarcheal age but chronological age. Older girls are more likely than younger girls to have sufficient cognitive and psychosocial maturity as well as the appropriate knowledge and experience to function as an adequate parent. Younger adolescents, even if they are postpubertal and at no risk biologically as a parent, are at risk because of their relative immaturity in terms of cognitive and psychosocial development.

ACKNOWLEDGMENT

Harry Jarcho's work with the data analyses presented here is gratefully acknowledged. This work is supported by grant MH30252/38142 to Anne Petersen.

REFERENCES

Ashton, P. Cross-cultural Piagetian research: An experimental perspective. *Educational Review*, 1975, *45*, 475–506.

Bart, W. M., and Lane, J. F. *Cross-cultural patterns of formal operations development.* Paper presented at the meeting of the American Educational Research Association, Montreal, 1983.

Carey, S. E. *Maturation and the development of spatial ability in children.* Paper presented at a conference "Gender-Role Development: Conceptual and Methodological Issues," National Institutes of Health, Bethesda, MD, 1981.

Carey, S. E., and Diamond, R. Maturational determination of the developmental course of face encoding. *In* D. Caplan (Ed.), *Biological studies of mental processes.* Cambridge, MA: The MIT Press, 1980.

Carey, S. E., Diamond, R., and Woods, B. Development of face recognition—A maturational component? *Developmental Psychology*, 1980, *16*, 257–269.

Clausen, J. A. The social meaning of differential physical and sexual maturation. *In* S. E. Dragastin and G. H. Elder, Jr. (Eds.), *Adolescence in the life cycle: Psychological change and social context.* Washington, D. C.: Hemisphere, 1975.

Coleman, J. C. Friendship and the peer group in adolescence. *In* J. Adelson (Ed.), *Handbook of adolescent psychology.* New York: John Wiley, 1980.

Conger, J. J., and Petersen, A. C. *Adolescence and youth* (3rd ed.). New York: Harper & Row, 1984.

Costanzo, P. R., and Shaw, M. E. Conformity as a function of age level. *Child Development*, 1966, *37*, 967–975.

Damon, W., and Hart, D. (1982). The development of self-understanding from infancy through adolescence. *Child Development*, 1982, *53*, 841–864.

Diamond, R., Carey, S., and Back, K. J. Genetic influences on the development of spatial skills during early adolescence. *Cognition*, 1983, *13*, 167–185.

Duke, P. M., Carlsmith, J. M., Jennings, D., Martin, J. A., Dornbusch, S. M., Gross, R. T., and Siegel-Gorelick. B. Educational correlations of early and late sexual maturation in adolescence. *Journal of Pediatrics*, 1982, *100*, 633–637.

Dulit, E. Adolescent thinking *a la* Piaget: The formal stage. *Journal of Youth and Adolescence*, 1972, *1*, 281–301.

Elkind, D. Recent research on cognitive development in adolescence. *In* S. E. Dragastin and G. H. Elder (Eds.), *Adolescence in the life cycle.* Washington, D.C.: Hemisphere, 1975.

Faust, M. S. Developmental maturity as a determinant of prestige in adolescent girls. *Child Development*, 1960, *31*, 173–184.

Flin, R. H. Age effects in children's memory for unfamiliar faces. *Developmental Psychology*, 1980, *16*, 373–374.

Flin, R. H. *The ups and downs of face recognition: A unique developmental trend?* Paper presented at the Society for Research in Child Development meeting in Detroit, 1983.

Freedman, D. G. *Human sociobiology: A holistic approach.* New York: The Free Press, 1979.

Gilligan, C. In a difference voice: Women's conceptions of the self and of morality. *Harvard Educational Review*, 1977, *47*, 481–517.

Gross, R. T., and Duke, P. M. The effect of early versus late physical maturation on adolescent behavior. *Pediatric Clinics of North America*, 1980, *27*, 71–77.

Herbst, L., and Petersen, A. C. *Timing of maturation, brain lateralization, and cognitive performance in adolescent females.* Paper presented at the Fifth Annual Conference on Research on Women and Education, Cleveland, 1979.

Hoffman, M. L. Moral development in adolescence. In J. Adelson (Ed.), *Handbook of adolescent psychology*. New York: John Wiley, 1980.

Inhelder, B., and Piaget, J. *The growth of logical thinking from childhood to adolescence*. New York: Basic Books, 1958.

Jones, M. C., and Bayley, N. Physical maturing among boys as related to behavior. *Journal of Educational Psychology*, 1950, *41*, 129–148.

Jones, M. C., and Mussen, P. H. Self-conceptions, motivations, and interpersonal attitudes of early- and late-maturing girls. *Child Development*, 1958, *29*, 491–501.

Kavrell, S. M., and Petersen, A. C. Patterns of achievement in early adolescence. *In* M. L. Maehr and M. W. Steinkamp (Eds.), *Women and science*. Greenwich, CT: JAI Press., 1984.

Keating, D. P. Thinking processes in adolescence. *In* J. Adelson (Ed.), *Handbook of adolescent psychology*. New York: John Wiley, 1980.

Keating, D. P., and Clark, V. Development of physical and social reasoning in adolescence. *Developmental Psychology*, 1980, *16*, 23–30.

Koff, E., Rierdan, J., and Silverstone, E. Changes in representation of body image as a function of menarcheal status. *Developmental Psychology*, 1978, *14*, 635–642.

Kohlberg, L. Development of moral character and moral ideology. *In* M. L. Hoffman and L. W. Hoffman (Eds.), *Review of child development research* (Vol. 1). New York: Russell Sage Foundation, 1964.

Kohlberg, L. Moral stages and moralization: The cognitive-developmental approach. *In* T. Likona (Ed.), *Moral development and behavior*. New York: Holt, 1976.

Loevinger, J. The meaning and measurement of ego development. *American Psychologist*, 1966, *21*, 195–206.

Loevinger, J. *Ego development: Conceptions and theories*. San Francisco: Jossey-Bass, 1976.

Loevinger, J. Construct validity of the Sentence Completion Test of ego development. *Applied Psychological Measurement*, 1979, *3*, 281–311.

Loevinger, J., and Wessler, R. *Measuring ego development 1. Construction and use of a sentence completion test*. San Francisco: Jossey-Bass, 1970.

McCarthy, J. D., and Hoge, D. R. Analysis of age effects in longitudinal studies of adolescent self-esteem. *Developmental Psychology*, 1982, *18*, 372–379.

Maccoby, E. E., and Jacklin, C. N. *The psychology of sex differences*. Stanford, CA: Stanford University Press, 1974.

Maccoby, E. E., and Jacklin, C. N. Sex differences in aggression: A rejoinder and reprise. *Child development*, 1980, *51*, 964–980.

Martorano, S. C. A developmental analysis of performance on Piaget's formal operations task. *Developmental Psychology*, 1977, *13*, 666–672.

Mussen, P. H., and Jones, M. C. Self-conceptions, motivations, and interpersonal attitudes of late and early maturing boys. *Child Development*, 1957, *28*, 243–256.

Neimark, E. D. Intellectual development during adolescence. *In* F. D. Horowitz (Ed.), *Review of child development research* (Vol. 4). Chicago: University of Chicago Press, 1975. (a)

Neimark, E. D. Longitudinal development of formal operations thought. *Genetic Psychology Monographs*, 1975, *91*, 191–225. (b)

Neimark, E. D. Adolescent thought: Transition for formal operations. *In* B. B. Wolman (Ed.) *Handbook of developmental psychology*. Englewood Cliffs, NJ: Prentice-Hall, 1982.

Newcombe, N., Bandura, N. M., and Taylor, D. G. Sex differences in spatial ability and spatial activities. *Sex Roles*, 1983, *9*, 377–386.

O'Malley, P. M., and Bachman, J. G. Self-esteem: Change and stability between ages 13 and 23. *Developmental Psychology*, 1983, *19*, 257–268.

Peskin, H. Influence of the developmental schedule of puberty on learning and ego development. *Journal of Youth and Adolescence*, 1973, *2*, 273–290.

Petersen, A. C. Physical androgyny and cognitive functioning in adolescence. *Developmental Psychology*, 1976, *12*, 524–533.

Petersen, A. C. Female pubertal development. *In* M. Sugar (Ed.), *Female adolescent development*. New York: Brunner/Mazel, 1979.

Petersen, A. C. Biopsychosocial processes in the development of sex-related differences. *In* J. E. Parsons (Ed.), *The psychobiology of sex differences and sex roles*. Washington, D.C.: Hemisphere, 1980.

Petersen, A. C. Menarche: Meaning of measures and measuring meaning. *In* S. Golub (Ed.), *Menarche*. New York: D.C. Heath, 1983. (a)

Petersen, A. C. Pubertal change and cognition. *In* J. Brooks-Gunn and A. C. Petersen (Eds.), *Girls at puberty: Biological and psychosocial perspectives*. New York: Plenum Press, 1983. (b)

Petersen, A. C., and Gitelson, I. B. *Toward understanding sex-related differences in cognitive performance*. New York: Academic Press, in preparation.

Petersen, A. C., and Taylor, B. The biological approach to adolescence: Biological change and psychological adaptation. *In* J. Adelson (Ed.), *Handbook of adolescent psychology*. New York: John Wiley, 1980.

Piaget, J. *The moral judgment of the child*. New York: The Free Press, 1932.

Piaget, J. Intellectual evolution from adolescence to adulthood. *Human Development*, 1972, *15*, 1–12.

Presser, H. Sally's Corner: Coping with unlearned motherhood. *Journal of Social Issues*, 1980, *36*, 107–129.

Redmore, C. D., and Loevinger, J. Ego development in adolescence: Longitudinal studies. *Journal of Youth and Adolescence*, 1979, *8*, 1–20.

Rest, J. R. Longitudinal study of the Defining Issues Test of moral judgment: A strategy for analyzing developmental change. *Developmental Psychology*, 1975, *11*, 738–748.

Rest, J. R. *Development of judging moral issues*. Minneapolis: University of Minnesota Press, 1979.

Roberge, J. J. Developmental analyses of two formal operational structures: Combinatorial thinking and conditional reasoning. *Developmental Psychology*, 1976, *12*, 563–564.

Rogel, M. J., Fleming, J. P., and Zuehlke, M. E. *Responses to menarche as indicators of sexual attitudes and behaviors*. Paper presented at the annual meeting of the American Psychological Association, Los Angeles, 1981.

Ronning, R. R. Modeling effects and developmental changes in dealing with a formal operations task. *American Educational Research*, 1977, *14*, 213–223.

Rowe, I., and Marcia, J. E. Age identity status, formal operations, and moral development. *Journal of Youth and Adolescence*, 1980, *9*, 87–99.

Savin-Williams, R. C. Dominance hierarchies in groups of early adolescents. *Child Development*, 1979, *50*, '23–935.

Simmons, R. G., Blyth, D. A., Van Cleave, E. F., and Bush, D. M. Entry into early adolescence: The impac. of school structure, puberty, and early dating on self-esteem. *American Sociological Review*, 1979, *44*, 948–967.

Simmons, R. G., Blyth, D. A., Carlton-Ford, S., and Bulcroft, R. *The adjustment of early adolescents to school and pubertal transitions*. Paper presented at a meeting of the Life Span Development Committee of the Social Science Research Council, Tucson, Arizona, 1982.

Simmons, R. G., Rosenberg, F., and Rosenberg, M. Disturbance in the self-image at adolescence. *American Sociological Review*, 1973, *38*, 553–568.

Steinberg, L. D., and Hill, J. P. Patterns of family interaction as a function of age, onset of puberty, and formal thinking. *Developmental Psychology*, 1978, *14*, 683–684.

Tobin-Richards, H. M., Boxer, A. M., and Petersen, A. C. The psychological significance of pubertal change: Sex differences in perceptions of self during early adolescence. *In* J. Brooks-Gunn and A. C. Petersen (Eds.), *Girls at puberty: Biological and psychosocial perspectives.* New York: Plenum Press, 1983.

Tomlinson-Keasey, C. Formal operations in females from eleven to fifty-four years of age. *Developmental Psychology*, 1972, *6*, 364.

Waber, D. P. Sex differences in cognition: A function of maturation rate? *Science*, 1976, *192*, 572–574.

Waber, D. P. Sex differences in mental abilities, hemispheric lateralization, and rate of physical growth at adolescence. *Developmental Psychology*, 1977, *13*, 29–38.

Walker, L. J. Cognitive and perspective-talking prerequisites for moral development. *Child Development*, 1980, *51*, 131–139.

Walker, L. J., and Richards, B. S. Stimulating transitions in moral reasoning as a function of stage of cognitive development. *Developmental Psychology*, 1979, *15*, 95–103.

Wylie, R. C. *The self-concept* (rev. ed., Vol. I and II). Lincoln: University of Nebraska Press, 1979.

Youniss, J. Moral development through a theory of social construction: An analysis. *Merrill-Palmer Quarterly*, 1981, *27*, 385–403.

9

ADOLESCENT FATHERS: THE UNDER STUDIED SIDE OF ADOLESCENT PREGNANCY

Arthur B. Elster
Michael E. Lamb

Researchers have traditionally been concerned with the parental behavior of middle-class adult mothers, and have only recently begun to systematically study paternal influences and adolescent parents. The interest in father–child relationships probably resulted from a renewed concern for the welfare of children and from a reassessment of traditional sex-role expectations brought about by the Women's Movement. Previously, mothers were believed to have a disproportionate impact on child development because biological factors ensured that they spent more time with their children than did fathers. Societal mores, which enforced traditional work-role segregation patterns, also served to maximize maternal and minimize paternal involvement with children. It is now thought, however, that cultural rather than hormonal factors affect the degree of parental involvement and that the influence exerted on child development by each parent may be imperfectly related to the amount of involvement (Lamb and Goldberg, 1982; Nash and Feldman, 1981). Most developmentalists now agree that fathers, like mothers, can have a significant influence on child development (Lamb, 1981; Parke, 1981).

As more has been learned about the factors affecting the adequacy of parental behavior, researchers have begun studying "high-risk" parents. Young parents are often considered at high risk for parenting failure because they are assumed to be psychologically and physically immature, poorly prepared for parenthood, to have unstable relationships with their sexual partners and parents, and to experience added emotional stress resulting from the negative circumstances which surround "premature" pregnancies. Consequently, research on adolescent parents has burgeoned in response to the emergent concern with parents and children who are "at risk." The convergent and simultaneous interest in paternal behavior and in adolescent parents has lead researchers and clinicians to seek an understanding of the special circumstances and needs of adolescent fathers and their children, but because that is a recent trend, our knowledge is still very limited. This chapter reviews the available evidence and makes suggestions regarding the services needed by adolescent fathers.

EPIDEMIOLOGY

Approximately 4% of all births in the United States are fathered by men under 20 years of age (National Center for Health Statistics, 1981). Although fewer than 40% of teen mothers have partners who are adolescents, 97% of teen fathers have adolescent partners. Overall, about 36% of babies are born into families where both parents are under age 20. Unfortunately, it is impossible to determine how many school-aged fathers there are because the National Center for Health Statistics (NCHS) does not analyze by paternal age in as much detail as maternal age. Thus, paternal age is categorized as "less than age 15" and then successively by 5-year intervals (i.e., 15–19, 20–24). Because of this, it is not possible to distinguish the number of school-age fathers (those 18 and under) who presumably would be most adversely affected by parenthood, from those who are 19. Based on our clinical experience, we estimate that probably 30–50% of pregnant adolescents have school-age partners. Unfortunately, the NCHS does not provide statistics on the relationship between paternal age and potentially important factors such as parity, birth weight, birth order, or prenatal care.

Comparisons between the absolute number of children fathered by teens and the number fathered by older men are less informative than are live birth rates, which represent the number of births per 1000 in specific age groups. In 1979, the live birth rate for 15- to 19-year-old males was 18.9, which was a 26% decline from 1970 (NCHS, 1981). By contrast, the birth rate for 15- to 19-year-old females declined by 22% to 53.4 between 1970 and 1979.

Evidently, although there are fewer adolescent fathers than adolescent mothers, the former still constitute a sizable group. Because of the sheer number of young people who become parents each year, it is important to ask about the quality of parental behavior that can be expected of these young mothers and fathers.

DIMENSIONS OF PARENTAL BEHAVIOR

Over the last few decades, many theorists have come to believe that a pattern of parental behavior involving warm, sensitive responsiveness to children's needs or signals coupled with a rational, inductive disciplinary style in later years facilitates secure, trustful infant–parent attachments, a self-confident and assertive style of interaction with peers, an internalized conscience, cognitive competence, and an enthusiastically resourceful approach to challenging tasks (Ainsworth et al., 1978; Arend et al., 1979; Baumrind, 1976; Clarke-Stewart, 1973; Hoffman, 1970; Lamb and Easterbrooks, 1981; Pastor, 1981; Lamb et al., 1984). Although researchers have generally studied the effects of "sensitive," "optimal," or "authoritative" maternal behavior, the few studies of fathers that have been completed confirm that a similar pattern of effects is also obtained with them (Clarke-Stewart, 1978; Belsky, 1979; Radin, 1981). To our knowledge, however, no one has yet investigated the parental behavior of adolescent fathers.

Originally, theorists assumed that the ability to provide sensitive parental care was an intrinsic characteristic of the parent, with individual differences in sensitivity constituting an enduring characteristic or trait. It has become increasingly clear, however, that although some enduring personality characteristics may be correlated with sensitivity, parental competence may vary substantially depending on the parent's circumstances and the child's characteristics (Lamb and Easterbrooks, 1981; Belsky, Robins, and Gamble, 1984). Most relevant, in the present context, are findings showing that both adult and teenage mothers behave less sensitively and have less securely attached infants when they are subject to substantial social stress (Crockenberg, 1981; Crnic et al., 1981) and/or lack reliable social support networks (Colletta and Gregg, 1981; Crockenberg, 1981; Crnic et al., 1981). Likewise, mothers who resent the infants' intrusion into their lives are more likely to behave insensitively and have infants whose attachments to them are less secure (Owen et al., 1982). It seems reasonable to assume that stressful circumstances experienced by teenage fathers would have similar effects on their parental behavior, and, consequently, on their children's development. Furthermore, as indicated in the next section, there are good reasons to believe that many adolescent fathers are subject to substantial psychological stress.

PSYCHOSOCIAL PROBLEMS OF TEENAGE FATHERS

Parenthood and marriage are considered normal developmental "crises" (Dyer, 1965; Miller and Sollie, 1980; Parad and Caplan, 1965). One reason for concern about adolescent fathers is that these crises coincide with the "crisis" of normal adolescent development. The combination of stresses associated with each of these "crises" may adversely affect young males, especially those who are psychologically immature and who have weak or inconsistent social support networks. Two clinical studies suggest that pregnancy and parenthood indeed subject young fathers to a considerable amount of stress (Elster and Panzarine, 1980, 1983).

Our first study, performed in Rochester, New York, was designed to investigate the emotional reaction of prospective fathers involved with the teenagers attending the Rochester Adolescent Maternity Project (Elster and Panzarine, 1980). Sixteen young men, 19 years of age or younger (average age 17.4 years), were studied during a 5-month period. All were single at the time of their interview. The mean gestational age when interviewed was 18 weeks. The subjects were predominantly from lower-middle to lower socioeconomic backgrounds; ten were black, five were white, and one was hispanic. The subjects were self-selected in that information about the study was delivered through the female partner. While the fathers who were studied were demographically representative of the RAMP population, they may have felt more stress, or more of a need to discuss their situation, than the youths who chose not to participate.

The research interview focused on perceptions of changes that had occurred since the pregnancy. The teens' response upon learning of the pregnancy was categorized as positive (proud, happy, pleased), intermediate (ambivalent), or negative (angry). The manner in which the fathers were coping with pregnancy and prospective parenthood was categorized as adequate, moderately good, or poor. This rating was assigned from review of the audiotaped interviews. Adequate coping was defined as the acceptance of responsibilities associated with being a father, and the resolution of ambivalent, guilty, or confused feelings regarding pregnancy; poor coping was defined as a lack of acceptance of responsibilities associated with being a father, and incomplete resolution of ambivalent, guilty, or confused feelings regarding the pregnancy; moderately good coping was defined by responses between the two extremes.

Eight subjects reported initially positive feelings, two stated that they had been ambivalent, and one reported anger upon learning of the pregnancy. Two teens reported both positive and ambivalent feelings, and three reported a combination of ambivalent and angry feelings. Nine of the teens appeared to be coping adequately, four moderately well, and three poorly. Six subjects were referred for counseling because of apparent depression. Correlations between the subjects' initial reactions to the pregnancy and the adequacy of their coping showed that the teens' initial reactions seemed to be good predictors of the way in which they coped with the stresses of pregnancy and prospective parenthood.

These results suggested that at least some young fathers needed and wanted help adjusting to the stresses of pregnancy and prospective parenthood. Before making recommendations about effective counseling, however, we clearly needed to learn more about the nature of these stresses.

The second study, which was conducted in Salt Lake City, Utah, was designed to identify the types of problems experienced by prospective young fathers and the ways in which these problems changed over time (Elster and Panzarine, 1983). Subjects were again recruited through information delivered by the pregnant teen. We interviewed twenty fathers who were 18 years of age or younger, at various times during the prenatal period as well as 4–6 weeks after delivery. Semistructured interviews were used to elicit comments about the type and severity of the stresses perceived by the subjects.

The subjects we studied were predominantly from middle and lower-middle socioeconomic backgrounds and were, in general, representative of the total group of prospective fathers in our teenage pregnancy program: eighteen were white and two were hispanic. All pregnancies were conceived premaritally; by delivery, however, 15 of the 18 couples were married. There were a total of 44 interviews: 4 during the first trimester (at an average of 12 weeks gestation), 12 during the second trimester (at an average of 22.2 weeks gestation), 17 during the third trimester (at an average of 32.7 weeks gestation), and 11 postpartum (at an average of 4.5 weeks). Five subjects were interviewed once, seven were interviewed twice, seven were interviewed three times, and one was interviewed four times. The reported stresses were graded by degree of severity from one (low) to three (high). Four major groups of stresses were identified: vocational-educational concerns, concerns about the health of mother and infant, concerns about parenthood, and problems with relationships. An average score per trimester for each perceived stress was calculated by multiplying the frequency with which the stress was reported by the corresponding degree of severity and then dividing the sum of the number of subjects interviewed. Changes over time in the severity of each group of stresses were then plotted.

Vocational-educational concerns were of greatest severity during the first trimester, but remained at a relatively high level throughout the pregnancy and into the neonatal period. Health concerns peaked during the third trimester and declined following delivery. Parenting concerns arose during the second trimester, dropped slightly during the third trimester, and increased postpartum. Concerns about problems with relationships were greatest during the first trimester and declined thereafter. Viewed differently, it appeared that relationship issues caused the most concern during the first and second trimesters, health concerns were greatest during the third trimester, and vocational-educational worries were strongest during the neonatal period.

We then wondered if circumstances other than marital status could have affected the level of stress reported by these teen fathers. From our clinical experience, we knew that some young couples were not surprised by conception although most did not plan to get pregnant. We had the impression that when pregnancies were "expected," teen fathers had less difficulty with the "crises" of pregnancy and prospective parenthood. The data from our second study allowed us to investigate this hypothesis.

Each subject was asked in the first interview whether or not he had expected the pregnancy to occur. Eleven (58%) responded "YES," eight (42%) responded "NO," and the information was not obtained from one person. There were no substantial differences between the two groups with respect to age of subject, age of female partner, or likelihood of marriage by the time of delivery. However, compared to fathers who had not expected the pregnancy to occur, the fathers who expected the pregnancy had dated the mother for a longer time (18 as compared to 14 months) and learned of the pregnancy earlier (7 as compared to 9 weeks postconception). To determine whether the teens in these groups differed in their response to pregnancy, we compared the average total stress scores obtained in the third trimester interview ($n = 9$ for the expected group and $n = 7$ for the not-expected group). The teens who had anticipated the pregnancy had an average stress score of seven whereas the others had an average score of nine. For both groups combined, there was only a slight negative correlation between the length of time that the pregnancy had been known and the third trimester stress score.

In summary, the results of this second study confirmed that the crises of pregnancy and prospective parenthood indeed affect young prospective fathers. Fathers who are more committed to their mates are apparently less surprised by the pregnancy and are able to cope better with the stresses involved. The strength of the couples' relationships may also affect decisions regarding outcome of the pregnancy and future contraceptive practices. Thus, pregnant teens who choose to deliver instead of aborting have longer, more stable relationships (Fischman, 1977; Gispert and Falk, 1976). Following delivery unmarried couples with stronger relationships have higher rates of continuing contraceptive use than those who are less committed (Ewer and Gibbs, 1975).

Studies conducted by Hendricks (1981) have further elucidated the problems experienced by young fathers. Twenty black unmarried fathers in Tulsa, Oklahoma, and 27 black unmarried fathers in Chicago, Illinois, were interviewed after delivery. The average age of the fathers at the time of delivery was 17.8 years (range: 15–20 years) for the Tulsa group and 17.2 years (range: 14–20 years) for the Chicago group. When asked to identify some of the problems faced by young fathers, men in both groups listed such items as financial responsibilities, parenting skills, education, employment, transportation, relationship with girl-friend, and "facing life in general."

Overall, the results of these three studies suggest that the immediate events surrounding pregnancy and parenthood can be stressful for teenage fathers. Pregnancy and parenthood, however, not only have an immediate effect on young fathers, but also affect educational achievement and future vocational attainment. Age at birth of first child is directly related to the amount of schooling completed — the younger the age at parenthood, the less formal education a father achieves (Card and Wise, 1978; Kerckhoff and Parrow, 1979). The long-term consequence of this is that young fathers are at a vocational disadvantage when compared with men who postpone parenthood until a later age.

Pregnancy is also a major precipitant of teenage marriage. The results of a nationwide study by Zelnik and Kantner (1978) suggested that although 70% of first births to white adolescents and 95% of first births to black teens in 1976 were *conceived* premaritally, only 25% of white infants and 85% of black infants were *born* out-of-wedlock. Thus, 45% of white teen mothers and 10% of black teen mothers married followed conception, but before delivery. The younger the adolescent, the greater the likelihood of a "legitimated" birth. In 1973, 40% of births to women aged 14–17 occurred within seven months of marriage, compared with 26% of births to teens aged 18–19, and 20% of births to women older than 19 years of age (McCarthy and Menken, 1979).

Age at the time of marriage also appears related to the likelihood of marital discord and divorce. The results of a study by Burchinal (1965) suggested that males who married before 16 years of age were more likely to divorce than were males who married at a later age. This may be explained partially by the fact that young parents tend to have larger families than do couples who begin family formation later in life (Moore and Hofferth, 1978), and the combination of large family size and lower educational attainment probably ensure that these families suffer greater financial stress than families formed by older couples.

PROBLEMS ASSOCIATED WITH MALADAPTATIONS TO PREGNANCY AND PARENTHOOD

The psychological problems associated with teenage fatherhood should be of concern to us for at least two reasons. First, if stress and maladjustment are as widespread as these few studies suggest, then the mental anguish experienced by young fathers merits attention from clinicians and counselors in its own right. Second, it is likely that when young fathers so remain involved their psychological status affects their children's development, whether mediated directly via effects on the father–child relationship, or indirectly via effects on the mother–child relationship (Belsky, 1981; Parke et al., 1979). Thus, a concern for the welfare of these children demands that attention be directed to the psychological problems of their fathers.

The lack of appreciation by health providers, social service workers, and the girls' parents for the problems experienced by teen fathers often results in their total exclusion from prenatal care and, in some cases, the denial of opportunities to see their female partners or children. Some teenage fathers may thus have little opportunity to develop relationships with their children. Although adverse effects are apparently quite rare, children with single parents are more likely than those from two-parent families to have behavior problems and difficulty interacting with members of the opposite sex, exhibit less sex-stereotyped behavior, and perform more poorly in school (Biller, 1981; Shinn, 1978). In the case of teenage parents, the likelihood of effects such as these surely depends on the living arrangements of mother and child, since "father absence" may mean very different things when the child lives with its mother and grandparents rather than alone with an impoverished and socially isolated mother. However, Furstenberg and Crawford's (1978) longitudinal study of adolescent mothers indicated that parenthood frequently led teens, regardless of marital status to establish their own households, thus separating them from potentially useful social supports. Five years after delivery, 26% of the teen mothers (11% never married and 15% previously married) were living alone.

This is not to imply that the children of teenaged parents are necessarily better off when their parents marry. As stated previously, couples who marry during adolescence are more likely to experience marital discord than are couples who marry later (Burchinal, 1965; Moore, et al., 1978). This is a source of concern since poor relationships between parents seem to have a more predictably negative effect on child development than any other family event, including divorce and single parenthood (e.g., Rutter, 1973; Rutter et al., 1975).

Researchers have not yet explored the relationship (if any) between child abuse and paternal age. However, several studies (Bolton, 1980; Kinard, 1980; Leventhal, 1981) have found a relationship between child abuse and *maternal* age. Specifically, women who began childbearing as teenagers appear more likely to abuse or neglect their children than mothers who began childbearing in their twenties, although the actual abusive incidents often do not occur while the mothers are in their teens. In fact, the victims of the abuse may often be children who were themselves born when their mothers were older. These facts suggest that maternal age, per se, is not the critical factor. Rather, factors associated with maternal age — such as social isolation, single parenthood, economic stress, poor wage-earning abilities, large family size — may interact to place "teen mothers" at risk for abuse.

When teenage fathers remain with their partners and children, some of the stresses experienced by young mothers are alleviated, particularly if the fathers have stable employment. Thus, under favorable circumstances, the fathers' presence may indirectly improve the quality of their children's lives by facilitating better maternal care. Overall, however, the problems experienced by teenage couples, in general, and teenage fathers, in particular, may increase the likelihood that they will behave abusively or neglectfully (e.g., Belsky, 1980).

In summary, there are several reasons for concern that the psychosocial circumstances of teenage fathers may adversely affect the quality of their parental behavior. Psychological immaturity, lack of parenting skills, economic stress, and stresses implicit in premature role transitions are problems that psychological and vocational counselors have to address. It is important to remember, however, that some teenage fathers cope effectively and responsibly, and that many children develop perfectly well despite stressful family circumstances. Further research is necessary to determine more clearly what factors distinguish these individuals and families from those whose adaptations are not so favorable.

CLINICAL INTERVENTION WITH ADOLESCENT FATHERS

The medical and psychosocial problems associated with teenage pregnancy started receiving attention during the 1960's and over the next 20 years many special programs were developed to provide care for this group of high-risk mothers. Few programs, however, actively attempted to involve the male partners (Goldstein and Wallace, 1978). It was apparently assumed that since unwed fathers often did not remain involved with their partners, special efforts should not be made to include them in clinical services (Lorenzi et al., 1977). We believe that this conclusion may well have been incorrect, in that many fathers do remain involved with their children even if the couple does not marry (Furstenberg, 1978; Rivara, Sweeney, and Henderson, 1985).

In our teenage pregnancy program at the University of Utah we have adopted a systems approach to adolescent pregnancy. Each person involved with the teenager (such as her parents, the father of the baby, and her friends) affects the pregnancy and, the pregnancy affects each of these individuals. Intervention can thus be directed in various ways to ensure better professional outcomes. Providing services to young fathers serves to assist him, and also to influence young mothers and their children.

WHY INVOLVE ADOLESCENT FATHERS IN CLINICAL SERVICES?

In our opinion, there are several reasons why young fathers *should* receive psychosocial services. First, participation in prenatal services may promote the fathers' involvement with their infants. It seems reasonable to assume that fathers who (1) come to prenatal visits, (2) are included in discussions with the clinical staff about the pregnancy, and (3) whose role in assisting the pregnant teen through gestation, labor, and delivery is promoted, will begin preparing themselves for parenthood earlier than fathers who do not participate. Such fathers may later be more involved than those who are alienated or confused about their roles. Such fathers contribute to child development directly (through sensitive interaction, play, and role modeling), and indirectly, by providing material and emotional support to mothers which, in turn, enhances the quality of their parental behavior (Parke et al., 1979).

Second, by helping teens to communicate more effectively with each other, prenatal programs may assist these couples in making more thoughtful and realistic decisions regarding their pregnancy and future. Unfortunately, young pregnant couples frequently make passive decisions regarding their future, such as concluding "we're pregnant and have no choice except to get married." The high divorce rate among these couples is at least partially attributable to these precipitous decisions. Better communication would help teens resolve their angry or guilt-laden feelings toward each other and thus allow them to make more rational, rather than emotional, decisions.

Third, young fathers often need instruction about childbirth, child rearing, and contraception. Adolescent males, whether or not they are prospective fathers, are frequently ignorant about reproductive physiology and contraception (Elster and Panzarine, 1980; Finkle and Finkle, 1975; Hendricks et al., 1981), and at least some young fathers are interested in learning more about childbirth and child rearing (Elster and Panzarine, 1980).

Fourth, service programs may provide direct assistance to young fathers. As mentioned earlier, prospective and new teen fathers frequently need individual psychosocial counseling (Elster and Panzarine, 1980). Such counseling may help them manage the stresses they are experiencing and assist them in locating job-training programs or actual employment. Informal support groups and peer counseling may also be helpful.

In summary, there are multiple reasons why adolescent fathers should be provided with clinical services. These services would, in many cases, benefit not only the men themselves, but also their partners, future partners, and children.

WHAT FACTORS LIMIT THE PARTICIPATION OF ADOLESCENT FATHERS?

The involvement of young fathers in adolescent pregnancy programs is limited primarily by the attitudes of the clinical staff. Clinicians who work with pregnant teens generally strive to improve the mothers' welfare and often view prospective fathers as the cause of the couples' problems. They seldom pursue the "other side of the story" told them by the pregnant teens, or attempt to identify the problems and needs of the male partners. Unless the staff take a broad, comprehensive view of teen pregnancy and its implications, they cannot appreciate the roles played by teen fathers (or, for that matter, grandparents!). This lack of appreciation may lead the staff to provide subtle, negative messages to the males, less-than-thorough psychosocial assessments of the mothers and their situation, and weak outreach efforts directed at teen couples. Contrary to popular stereotype, many teen fathers are willing to accept some responsibility for their actions if service providers can be understanding rather than accusatory.

WHAT PROGRAM COMPONENTS ARE NECESSARY IF ADOLESCENT FATHERS ARE TO BE INVOLVED?

Two components are essential if programs for adolescent fathers are to be successful. First, programs must establish and maintain links with community facilities providing financial, educational, vocational, and psychosocial counseling services to young fathers. It is futile to assess the problems of teens unless one can help them obtain the services they need. Thus, both knowledge of available service agencies and a system for ensuring successful referrals are necessary. Second, the clinical staff must be empathetic toward teen fathers and knowledgeable regarding the unique aspects of adolescent psychological development. Work with adolescent fathers is uniquely demanding in that health providers need to understand relevant devlopmental issues *in addition* to issues surrounding pregnancy.

CONCLUSION

In sum, there is much that we do not know about adolescent fathers as parents, but we have every reason to believe that a focus on their unique circumstances will yield information of both practical and theoretical significance. Like teen mothers, young fathers must negotiate the stressful crises of adolescence and parenthood simultaneously rather than sequentially. As fathers, they often feel special concern about their ability to provide for their partners and children — a concern that is realistic, given their educational attainments and vocational potential. As males, they are often blamed for the pregnancy. Unfortunately, while a more sympathetic service-oriented attitude has developed toward teen mothers, the needs of teen fathers have often been ignored. Closer attention to their needs is likely to be beneficial not only to themselves — as recipients of psychosocial, financial, and vocational counseling — but to their partners and children as well. Teenaged couples need help in dealing with issues surrounding their relationship, so they do not feel pressured into marriage. Whichever way these issues are resolved, both parents will be relieved of some of the stress which may be inimical to sensitive interaction with the baby. If the couple choose not to maintain their relationship, they may agree on ways to permit the father–child relationship to grow: if they choose to continue their relationship, the emotional support for one another may again enhance the quality of parent–child interaction. Now that we as a society have come to understand the medical needs of teenaged parents, we need to recognize that relief of this group's high-risk status depends on our adoption of a broad family-centered multidisciplinary approach to the provision of care.

REFERENCES

Ainsworth, M. D. S., Blehar, M. C., Waters, E., and Wall, S. *Patterns of attachment*. Hillsdale, N.J.: Erlbaum Assoc., 1978.

Arend, R., Gove, F. L., and Sroufe, L. A. Continuity of individual adaptation from infancy to kindergarten: A predictive study of ego-resiliency and curiosity in preschoolers. *Child Development*, 1979, *50*, 950–959.

Baumrind, D. *Early socialization and the discipline controversy*. Morristown, N.J.: General Learning Press, 1975.

Belsky, J. A family analysis of parental influence on infant exploratory competence. *In* F.A. Pedersen (Ed.), *The Father-infant relationship: Observational studies in a family context*. New York: Praeger, 1980.

Belsky, J. Mother–father–infant interaction: A naturalistic observational study. *Developmental Psychology*, 1979, *15*, 601–607.

Belsky, J. Early human experience: A family perspective. *Developmental Psychology*, 1981, *17*, 3–23.

Belsky, J., Robins, E., and Gamble, W. Characteristics, consequences and determinants of parental competence: Toward a contextual theory. *In* M. Lewis and L. Rosenblum (Eds.), *Beyond the dyad*. New York: Plenum, 1984.

Biller, H. B. Father absence, divorce, and personality development. *In* M. E. Lamb (Ed.), *The role of the father in child development* (Rev. ed.). New York: Wiley, 1981.

Bolton, F. G., Laner, R. H., and Kane, S. P. Child maltreatment risk among adolescent mothers: A study of reported cases. *American Journal of Orthopsychiatry*, 1980, *50*, 489–504.

Burchinal, L. G. Trends and prospects for young marriages in the United States. *Journal of Marriage and the Family*, 1965, *27*, 243–254.

Card, J. J., and Wise, L. L. Teenage mothers and teenage fathers: The impact of early childbearing on the parents' personal and professional lives. *Family Planning Perspectives*, 1978, *10*, 199–205.

Clarke-Stewart, K. A. Interactions between mothers and their young children: Characteristics and consequences. *Monographs of the Society for Research in Child Development*, 1973, *38* (Serial number 153).

Clarke-Stewart, K. A. And daddy makes three: The father's impact on mother and young child. *Child Development*, 1978, *49*, 466–478.

Colletta, N. D., and Gregg, C. H. Adolescent mothers' vulnerability to stress. *Journal of Nervous and Mental Disease*, 1981, *169*, 50–54.

Crnic, K. A., Greenberg, M. T., and Ragozin, A. S. *The effects of stress and social support on maternal attitudes and on the mother–infant relationship.* Paper presented at the Biennial Meeting of the Society for Research in Child Development, Boston, 1981.

Crockenberg, S. B. Infant irritability, mother responsiveness, and social support influences on the security of infant–mother attachment. *Child Development*, 1981, *52*, 857–865.

Dyer, E. D. Parenthood as crises: A re-study. *In* H. J. Parad (Ed.), *Crises intervention: Selected readings.* New York: Family Service Association of America, 1965.

Elster, A., and Panzarine, S. Unwed teenage fathers: Emotional and health educational needs. *Journal of Adolescent Health Care*, 1980, *1*, 116–120.

Elster, A., and Panzanine, R. Teenage fathers: Stresses during gestation and early parenthood. *Clinical Pediatrics*, 1983, *10*, 700–703.

Ewer, P., and Gibbs, J. O. Relationships with putative father and use of contraceptions in a population of black ghetto adolescent mothers. *Public Health Reports*, 1975, *90*, 417–423.

Finkle, M. L. and Finkle, D. J. Sexual and contraceptive knowledge, attitudes, and behavior of male adolescents. *Family Planning Perspectives*, 1975, *7*, 256–260.

Fischman, S. H. Delivery or abortion in inner-city adolescents. *American Journal of Orthopsychiatry*, 1977, *47*, 127–133.

Furstenberg, F. F., and Crawford, A. G. Family support: Helping teenage mothers to cope. *Family Planning Perspectives*, 1978, *10*, 322–333.

Gispert, M., and Falk, R. Sexual experimentation and pregnancy in young black adolescents. *American Journal of Obstetrics and Gynecology*, 1976, *126*, 459–466.

Goldstein, H., and Wallace, H. M. Services for and needs of pregnant teenagers in large cities of the United States. *Public Health Reports*, 1978, *93*, 46–54.

Hendricks, L. E., Howard, C. S., and Caesar, P. P. Help-seeking behavior among selected populations of black unmarried adolescent fathers. *American Journal of Public Health*, 1981, *71*, 733–735.

Hoffman, M. L. Moral develpment. *In* P. H. Mussen (Ed.), *Carmichael's manual of child psychology.* New York: Wiley, 1970.

Kerckhoff, A. C., and Parrow, A. A. The effect of early marriage on the educational attainment of young men. *Journal of Marriage and the Family*, 1979, *41*, 97–107.

Kinard, E. M., and Klerman, L. V. Teenage parenting and child abuse: Are they related? *American Journal of Orthopsychiatry*, 1980, *50*, 481–488.

Lamb, M. E. Paternal influences on child development: An overview. *In* M. E. Lamb (Ed.), *The role of the father in child development* (Rev. ed.). New York: Wiley, 1981.

Lamb, M. E., and Easterbrooks, M. A. Individual differences in parental sensitivity: Origins, components, and consequences. *In* M. E. Lamb and L. R. Sherrod (Eds.), *Infant social cognition: Empirical and theoretical considerations.* Hillsdale, N.J.: Erlbaum Assoc., 1981.

Lamb, M. E., and Goldberg, W. A. The father-child relatonship: A synthesis of biological, evolutionary and social perspectives. *In* L. W. Hoffman, R. Gandelman, and H. R. Schiffman (Eds.), *Parenting: Its causes and consequences,* Hillsdale, N.J.: Erlbaum Assoc., 1982.

Lamb, M. E., Thompson, R. A., Gardner, W. P., Charnov, E. L., and Estes, D. Security of infantile attachment as assessed in the "strange situation": Its study and biological interpretation. *Behavioral and Brain Sciences*, 1984, *7*, 127–147.

Leventhal, J. M. Risk factors for child abuse: Methodologic standards in case-control studies. *Pediatrics*, 1981, *68*, 684–690.

Lorenzi, M. E., Klerman, L. V., and Jekel, J. F. School-age parents: How permanent a relationship? *Adolescence*, 1977, *12*, 14–22.

McCarthy, J., and Menken, J. Marriage, remarriage, marital disruption and age of first birth. *Family Planning Perspective*, 1979, *11*, 21–30.

Miller, B. C., and Sollie, D. L. Normal stresses during the transition to parenthood. *Family Relations*, 1980, *29*, 459–465.

Moore, K. A., and Hofferth, S. L. *The Consequences of Age at First Childbirth: Family Size*. Washington, D.C.: The Urban Institute, 1978.

Moore, K. A., Waite, L. J., Hofferth, S. L., and Caldwell, S. B. *The consequences of age at first childbirth: Marriage, separation, and divorce*. Washington, D.C.: The Urban Institute, 1978.

Nash, S. C., and Feldman, S. S. Sex role and sex-related attributions: Constancy or change across the family life cycle: In M. E. Lamb and A. L. Brown (Eds.), *Advances in developmental psychology* (Vol. 1). Hillsdale, N.J.: Erlbaum Assoc. 1981.

National Center for Health Statistics. Advance report of final natality statistics, 1979. *Monthly Vital Statistics Report*, 1981, *30*, Suppl. 2.

Offer, D., and Offer, J. B. The offer self-image questionnaire for adolescents. *Archives of General Psychiatry*, 1972, *27*, 529–537.

Owen, M. T., Chase-Lansdale, P. L., and Lamb, M. E. Mothers' and fathers' attitudes, maternal employment, and the security of infant-parent attachment. Unpublished manuscript, 1982.

Parad, H. J., and Caplan, G. A framework for studying families in crises. *In* H. J. Parad (Ed.), *Crises intervention: Selected readings*. New York: Family Service of America, 1965.

Parke, R. D. *Fathers*. Cambridge: Harvard University Press, 1981.

Parke, R. D., Power, T. G., and Gottman, J. Conceptualizing and quantifying influence patterns in the family triad. *In* M. E. Lamb, S. J. Suomi, and G. R. Stephenson (Eds.), *Social interaction analysis: Methodological issues*. Madison: University of Wisconsin Press, 1979.

Pastor, D. L. The quality of mother-infant attachment and its relationship to toddlers' initial sociability with peers. *Developmental Psychology*, 1981, *17*, 326–335.

Radin, N. The role of the father in cognitive, academic, and intellectual development. *In* M. E. Lamb (Ed.), *The role of the father in child development* (Rev. ed.). New York: Wiley, 1981.

Rivara, F. P., Sweeney, P. J., and Henderson, B. F. A study of low socioeconomic status, black teenage fathers and their non-father peers. *Pediatrics*, 1985, *75*, 648–656.

Rutter, M. Why are London children so disturbed? *Proceedings of the Royal Society of Medicine*, 1973, *66*, 1221–1225.

Rutter, M., Cox, A., Tupling, C., Berger, M., and Yule, W. Attainment and adjustment in two geographic areas. I: The prevalence of psychiatric disorder. *British Journal of Psychiatry*, 1975, *126*, 493–509.

Shinn, M. Father absence and children's cognitive development. *Psychological Bulletin*, 1978, *85*, 295–324.

Zelnik, M., and Kantner, J. F. First pregnancies to women aged 15–19: 1976 and 1971. *Family Planning Perspective*, 1978, *10*, 11–20.

10

SOME PSYCHOSOCIAL ASPECTS OF ADOLESCENT SEXUAL AND CONTRACEPTIVE BEHAVIORS IN A CHANGING AMERICAN SOCIETY*

Catherine S. Chilman

INTRODUCTION

Enormous changes in adolescent sexual behaviors and attitudes have occurred between 1965 and 1985. This chapter reviews briefly the nature of these changes together with their probable social and psychological causes. Related topics such as contraception, abortion, and child-bearing are also discussed. In addition, possible future trends in adolescent sexual behaviors are examined. The apparent consequences of these trends are given in another chapter in this volume.

Adolescent sexuality may be defined as including the physical characteristics and capacities of adolescents for specific sex behaviors; psychosocial learning, values, norms, and attitudes toward these behaviors; sex role concepts; and the individual teenager's sense of both gender identity and sex object preference. Thus, adolescent sexuality, like all human sexuality, is affected by the totality of what it means to be a male or a female: by one's past and present experiences and anticipations of the future, the stage of development and life situation, physical and constitutional capacities and characteristics, and the type of society and period of time in which one lives (Chilman, 1980).

Adolescence is defined as that period of life which stretches from the onset of puberty to young adulthood. Puberty refers to the time

*Much of this paper is adapted from other books and articles by the author (Chilman, 1979, 1980, 1983). These publications are mainly based on an analytic summary of social and psychological research concerning adolescent sexuality.

when sexual maturation becomes evident; entrance into young adulthood is less easily defined. For the purposes of this chapter, however, the psychosocial sexual behaviors and attitudes of young people between the ages of 11 or so through ages 19 or 20 will be stressed.

CHANGES IN ATTITUDES TOWARD ADOLESCENT SEXUALITY

ATTITUDE TRENDS

It is no secret that over the past 60 years, most Americans (both adults and adolescents) have become increasingly permissive in attitudes regarding acceptable sexual behavior. Popular acceptance of sex role equality has also grown during this period. The norms favoring sexual freedom and equity between males and females increased notably from the late 1960's through at least the late 1970's, although somewhat more traditional attitudes have seemed to rise in prevalence since 1976.

A more detailed review of attitudes toward adolescent sexuality shows that sharp changes in the United States toward greater sexual liberalism occurred in the early 1900's and were reflected in the more emancipated behaviors of a sizable proportion of middle- and upper-class women in the 1920's. These changes have been documented by the Kinsey research (Kinsey et al., 1948, 1953) and were depicted by numerous novelists and essayists of the period. (For a broader historical perspective on fluctuations in attitudes and behaviors regarding adolescent sexuality over the past 300 years or so, see Chapter 16 by Vinovskis.)

Increasing urbanization and industrialization in the United States, rising employment for women, an increase in women's rights, and greater contact with other cultures (especially in World War I) were partially responsible for these trends. Just as women became more emancipated from earlier puritanical prescriptions, men became more emancipated too, especially in terms of greater freedom to participate in nonmarital relations on a more egalitarian, companionship basis with women in their own reference groups (Reiss, 1960).

It is probable, although formal research is scanty, that further liberalization of attitudes, if not of behaviors, took place between the 1920's and the 1960's, especially as a result of social changes accentuated by World War II. Reiss postulates that, while such changes may have occurred, the 50-year period between 1915 and 1965 mostly represented a time in which cumulative value shifts were being consolidated. By 1965 the United States was changing from an industrial to a postindustrial society and this brought forth a new thrust for extensive social change. The period of the late 1960's included the strong social protest against the Vietnam War and this also involved a push for more sexual freedom and youth autonomy (Reiss, 1976).

Strong double-standard attitudes toward nonmarital sex behavior had been found in various studies from the 1930's through the early 1960's (Terman, 1938; Burgess and Wallin, 1953; Kinsey *et al.*, 1953; Ehrmann, 1959; Reiss, 1967). In general, young women tended to equate sex with love and feel that petting or coitus were unacceptable outside of a love relationship. However, young men were more likely to think that sexual "permissiveness" was acceptable in both love and casual relationships. These attitude differences had declined by the mid-1960's and continued to do so through the 1970's (Packard, 1968; Croake and James, 1973; Sorensen, 1973; Yankelovich, 1974; Hunt, 1974; Reiss, 1976; DeLameter and MacCorquodale, 1979).

In general, attitudes toward nonmarital petting and intercourse became more liberal and egalitarian among high school and college students from the mid-1960's through at least 1979, with the greatest changes occurring for women (Bell and Chaskes, 1970; Robinson *et al.*, 1972; Christensen and Gregg, 1970; Yankelovich, 1974; Glenn and Weaver, 1979; Ferrell *et al.*, 1977; Zelnik and Kantner, 1977).

However, the largest shift toward liberality occurred among high school, compared to college, graduates. Regional differences have been also found, with Southerners being the most conservative and Easterners, as well as Westerners, being the most liberal. Black males were found to be more permissive in their attitudes than any other young group studied in both 1964 and 1973. Moreover, black females were more permissive than white females (Reiss, 1967; Yankelovich, 1974).

PSYCHOSOCIAL FACTORS ASSOCIATED WITH ATTITUDES

As outlined above, attitudes toward sexual behavior tend to vary by time periods, region of the country, educational level, race, age, and sex, although other factors are also important. For instance, Cvetkovich and Grote (1976), among others, found that sexually liberal attitudes are associated with experience in nonmarital intercourse, especially for white girls but somewhat less so far black girls. This is true to a considerable extent for white boys but to a lesser extent for black ones. However, one cannot tell whether these permissive attitudes followed or preceded coital behavior. For instance, many of the white girls said they relented because their boyfriends expected it of them, rather than because they approved of nonmarital coitus for themselves (Cvetkovich and Grote, 1976).

Reiss (1967), Heltsley and Broderick (1969), and Staples (1973) found that conservative sex attitudes were associated with religiosity for whites but not for blacks. The growth of new forms of religion and increased religiosity among a fairly large group of young (and older) people since the late 1960's is probably creating more conservative sexual attitudes among a portion of the population. For instance, such popular movements as the charismatic Christian, Pentecostal, and Evangelical religions are strongly puritinical in character and hold sexual freedoms in deep disfavor. A possible trend toward somewhat more conservative youth attitudes is revealed by a study at a southeastern university. Robinson and Jedlicka (1982) repeated a sex attitude study that had been undertaken some years earlier at this same school. Compared to 1975 data for a group of men and women undergraduates, a higher proportion of men and women in their responses to the 1980 questionnaire said they thought premarital intercourse was immoral, especially with a number of partners (about 40% of the respondents). However, in spite of this change, responses in 1980 showed a far higher proportion of sexually permissive students in that year than in 1965, the first year in which this particular study was carried out.

Additional evidence that sexual permissiveness among youth may be on the decline is furnished by Singh (1980). Analysis by Singh (National Opinion Research Center) for 1972, 1974, 1975, 1977, and 1978, showed that by 1978 a somewhat smaller proportion of men and women between 18 and 25 approved of premarital sexual relations than in 1972 (81.9% in 1978 and 84.3% in 1972). At the same time, data for other age groups, especially for persons between ages 26 and 44, revealed an *increase* in permissiveness, with about 77% of the 26- to 34-year age group and about 60% of these between ages 35 and 44 approving of premarital coitus. Data for aging persons also show an increase in permissiveness, but it is less marked, with about 40% of persons over age 45 expressing approving attitudes in 1978 compared to about one-third in 1972.

SEXUAL BEHAVIORS

TRENDS IN PETTING BEHAVIORS

At least until recently, studies showed that most adolescents, especially young women, move developmentally toward advanced levels of sexual intimacies, such as "heavy petting" and intercourse, through a series of dating and going-steady experiences. A learning period was generally involved during which young people came to know each other better, to develop an affectional relationship, and to respond to each other physically. Kinsey et al. (1953) found that young women seemed to develop their sexual interests through experiencing sexual stimulation in an interpersonal context, whereas young men generally acquired sexual experience earlier, primarily through nocturnal emissions and masturbation. Higher rates of early masturbation among today's females, along with cultural norms of greater sexual permissiveness, and more opportunities for privacy, may predispose contemporary youth to move more quickly into physical intimacies than they did before 1965.

It appears likely that rates of nonmarital petting to orgasm increased somewhat between the early 1920's and the early 1970's, especially for females and younger adolescents (Kinsey *et al.*, 1948, 1953; Ehrman, 1959; Chilman, 1963; Luckey and Nass, 1969; Sorensen, 1973; Robinson *et al.*, 1972; Vener and Stewart, 1974). Until recently, there seems to have been a large numerical gap, especially for females, between those who participated in petting and those who participated in intercourse. For instance, Kinsey *et al.*, (1953) found that about 84% of the females in his study were petting by age 18 but only about 10% were experiencing intercourse. However, Luckey and Nass (1969) found this "erotic gap" to have narrowed by 1968, with almost 70% of the females experiencing petting by age 19 and 43% intercourse.

There has been little research concerning the petting behavior of black adolescents. The little evidence that we have suggests that far fewer have substituted petting for intercourse over the years. Births outside of marriage appear to have been more accepted by blacks than whites, especially in the case of low-income blacks. Thus, petting without subsequent intercourse seems not to have been practised by the majority of black adolescents.

Further evidence along these lines is furnished by Udry (1983) in his recent studies of boys and girls in the 7th, 8th, and 9th grades in selected schools in Raleigh, North Carolina and Tallehassee, Florida. According to the written questionnaire responses of students, the black youngsters report no kissing and petting experiences prior to intercourse. In contrast to findings for the whites, Udry found that the sex behavior differences between the races do not seem to be strongly affected by differences in such intervening variables as reading levels and socioeconomic status of the respondents. Udry writes that, "I suspect the questions I am asking are not the right questions for blacks."

FACTORS ASSOCIATED WITH PETTING EXPERIENCE

Predictably, rates of petting increase with age, largely as a part of normal adolescent development and experience. These changes are reported by Vener and Stewart (1974) and a number of other investigators, including a large Wisconsin study by Delameter and Mac-Corquodale (1979).

Sorenson (1973), like others, found that there was a strong tendency for young people to move into early stages of physical intimacy by age 14 or 15 and progress further by age 16. His findings about the young people with no petting experience (mostly those under age 15 or 16) reveal that most had not yet fully entered the later adolescent stage, with its thrust for independence from parents and for intimate love relationships with peers. However, some of them may have been timid and withdrawn, some may have been late in physical maturation, and a few may have had a homosexual orientation.

In addition, a number of studies show that little or no experience in any stage of petting is often related to "religiosity," which is defined as frequent attendance at religious services (Kinsey et al., 1948, 1953; Reiss, 1967; Robinson et al., 1972; Sorensen, 1973).

Sorensen further found that young people who had engaged in petting but not in intercourse were a midgroup: more conservative in attitude and younger than the "nonvirgins," but less conservative and older than the "beginners." Members of the midgroup were more restless and dissatisfied with their sex lives than either of the other two groups and also reported poorer grades in school. This suggests that many were in a transition stage of middle adolescence and that a number might move toward full intercourse experience in the next few years.

NONMARITAL COITUS

TRENDS

Rates of adolescent nonmarital intercourse appear to have increased even more sharply than those of petting in recent years, with a clear and continuing rise since about 1967. This is particularly true for white females. Data for black females, as well as males, are largely lacking before the 1970's because earlier studies focused on white samples.

By 1973, national studies in varying localities showed that about 35% or more of high school seniors, both male and female, were nonvirgins; by 1979, this figure had risen to 48.5% for females and about 53% for males by age 17 (Zelnik and Kantner, 1980). By contrast, between 1925 and 1965, available research indicated rates of about 10% for white high school senior women and about 25% for white college senior women. Comparable figures for white males were about 25 and 55%. Thus, it appears that between about 1967 and 1974, nonmarital intercourse rates for white females rose by about 300% and for white males about 50%. Somewhat similar trends have been observed in many parts of the world, most notably the industrialized countries and those developing nations in stages of rapid industrialization (George Washington University Medical Center, 1976). We cannot be confident that the rates for non-college youth between the ages of 19 to 21 have risen in similar fashion because adequate data are not available for this group.

Nonmarital intercourse occurred at increasingly younger ages during the 1970's, with about 15% of white females in 1979 having experienced coitus by age 15 and 44% by age 17. Comparable figures for black females were 32 and 73%. By age 19, almost 65% of white females and almost 89% of black females were sexually experienced (Zelnik and Kantner, 1980). Data for both white and black adolescent males are seriously inadequate; this is especially true for black males. A recent study of 533 junior high school students in two southern communities provides provocative information (Udry, 1983). According to questionnaire response, two-thirds of the black males in the 7th grade said they had had intercourse; the proportion rose to 91% by ninth grade. Comparable data for white males are 23% by seventh grade and 51% by the ninth. In general, Udry reports larger proportions of both boys and girls of junior high school age saying they had had coitus than has been found in other studies, including Zelnik and Kantner's nationwide surveys of young women, ages 15–19 (Zelnik and Kantner, 1980). Thus these findings need to be considered with caution, as has been noted by Udry.

After 1965, rates of nonmarital intercourse rose more sharply than those of nonmarital petting, with the probability that, by the early 1970's, heavy petting was far less of a substitute for intercourse than it once was. Inspection of data regarding heavy petting and those for intercourse suggest that, especially for young people over age 18, rates of nonmarital physical intimacy, per se, have not grown as markedly as it would seem, especially for females. It appears as if, compared with the early 1960s, fewer young women limited their sexual experience to heavy petting. Rather, they tended to move on to intercourse. More liberal sex attitudes, plus the greater availability of effective contraceptives and abortion, may account for some of this change. [See Chilman (1979, 1983) for a more comprehensive review of 1920–1979 studies of adolescent coital behaviors.]

AGE, DATING FREQUENCY, AND BEING IN LOVE

A number of studies examine the association between adolescent nonmarital intercourse and other variables. As in the case of petting, the likelihood of nonmarital coitus increases with age. It also is more apt to occur (as one might expect) for those who date frequently, who go steady, or who consider themselves in love (Spanier, 1975; Sorensen, 1973; Reiss, 1976; DeLameter and MacCorquodale, 1979).

SOCIAL REFERENCE GROUPS

Some studies that find a positive correlation between having sexually permissive friends and being sexually active conclude that peers strongly influence sexual behavior (Jackson and Potkay, 1973; Mirande, 1968; Carns, 1971; Spanier, 1975). On the other hand, as in the case of petting, sexually active young people may seek friends who have similar attitudes and behaviors. Clues from a number of studies suggest that males may be more strongly influenced in their sex behavior by their peers than are females (Chilman, 1979; Scales and Beckstein, 1982).

EDUCATION AND ITS EFFECTS

Positive attitudes toward education, higher levels of educational achievement, and clear educational goals appear to make nonmarital intercourse less likely for both white and black females (Gebhard et al., 1956; Udry et al., 1975; Jessor and Jessor, 1975; Zelnik and Kantner, 1980). The association between educational achievement and lower likelihood of nonmarital coitus is doubtlessly tied to interacting socio-economic, social-psychological, and situational variables. For example, the student who does well in school is apt to come from a family background of higher socioeconomic status (SES); to value achievement; to be more controlled, and conforming in orientation; to be more work rather than play oriented; to operate on a higher level of cognitive development; and to be able to foresee and plan for the future (Conger, 1973). These same characteristics may make these youth less likely to engage in nonmarital intercourse during the high school years.

PSYCHOLOGICAL CHARACTERISTICS

Several studies have closely examined psychological characteristics that are significantly associated with nonmarital coitus during the high school years. One investigation found that male and female nonvirgins tended to take a more permissive, risk-taking attitude toward sex relations; fewer of them reported themselves as religious. Sexually active females, furthermore, seemed more likely to espouse a traditional female sex role, saying they participated in intercourse because the male expected it (Cvetkovich and Grote, 1976).

A longitudinal Colorado Study by Jessor and Jessor (1975), showed that nonvirgin adolescents had significantly higher scores for positive evaluation of independence and deviance, permissive attitudes toward sex, parental acceptance of deviance, and acceptance and modeling of deviance by peers. They had lower grade point averages in school, lower acceptance of parental controls, and lower expectations of achievement. Nonvirgin boys, but not girls, had higher measures of self-esteem. On the other hand, nonvirgin girls, but not boys, were more likely to place a high value on affection and to feel they received little parental support. They saw their parents and friends as being in conflict with each other. The nonvirgins girls also were higher in social criticism and alienation and lower in religiosity than virgin girls.

The growth of independence from parents as a significant factor in participating in nonmarital coitus is a major finding in the DeLameter and MacCorquodale study of college students and non-college youth. These investigators stress the importance of moving from dependency on parents, to peer attraction, to involvement with a lover as three basic steps toward nonmarital intercourse (DeLameter and Mac-Corquodale, 1979).

Research by Jessor and Jessor (1975) reports that nonvirgins are more likely than virgins to use drugs and alcohol. Other studies show that promiscuity is associated only with use of hard drugs (Vener and Stewart, 1974; Arafat and Yorburg, 1973). It is probable that there are a number of subgroups within the larger virgin and nonvirgin groups and that differing psychological needs and attitudes characterize these smaller clusters. For example, Sorensen made a useful discrimination between sexual "adventurers" (those with multiple partners) and sexual "monogamists" among his sexually active high school youth. Adventurers (most of them were males) were especially apt to be in poor communication with parents and to have difficulty forming close interpersonal relationships.

FAMILY RELATIONS

A number of studies have found that parent–youth relations make an important difference in adolescent sex behavior. Adolescents are more likely to have nonmarital intercourse if their mothers hold nontraditional attitudes, especially if their mothers fail to combine affection with firm, mild discipline. They are also more likely to have nonmarital intercourse if they perceive themselves to be in poor communication with their parents, to be unhappy at home, and to come from single-parent families (Simon et al., 1972; Jessor and Jessor, 1975; Kantner and Zelnik, 1972; Sorensen, 1973; Reiss, 1967; Bowerman et al., 1966; Ladner, 1971; Fox, 1980; DeLameter and MacCorquodale, 1979; Zelnik et al., 1982; Moore and Burt, 1982).

A number of studies show that at least one-third of the adolescents who are sexually active report anxiety and guilt about their behavior. This is especially true of females (Hunt, 1974; Sorensen, 1973; Bardwick, 1973; Reiss, 1976; Miller, 1974). The degree of guilt is associated, in part, with the attitudes of the peer groups to which the young person belongs (Perlman, 1974). It seems likely that, in a time of change from traditional to nontraditional values, people who engage in the new freedoms would find the transition process disturbing to their belief systems and their sense of self-respect, as well as to their relationships with other significant people in their lives, such as parents. Of course, feelings of guilt and anxiety will vary enormously from person to person depending on her or his early socialization and the attitudes of the person's partner, as well as those of influential close friends. Then too, persons with nonpermissive guilty attitudes are less likely than "sexual liberals" to engage in nonmarital coitus.

There are a number of suggestions in the research that adolescents who participate in sex relations at a very young age (12 or 13) may have special problems. Vener and Stewart (1974) speculate that they have far less internalized guilt about sex relations. Sorensen's group of disturbed youngsters who were promiscuous sex adventurers also tended to have their first coitus at about age 13 (Sorensen, 1973). Stein-hoff (1976) found that young, sexually active adolescent girls were more likely to engage in sex behavior largely to please their boyfriends and did not enjoy it themselves. A later section discusses the impact of a changing society on parental behaviors and the possible effects of these behaviors on adolescent children.

SOCIOECONOMIC STATUS (SES)

It is becoming increasingly clear that low socioeconomic status of parents is strongly associated with early age of nonmarital intercourse for adolescent girls (Zelnik et al., 1982). This is especially true for blacks. For instance, Zelnik and Kantner (1977) found that black females whose fathers were college graduates had nonmarital coitus rates similar to white girls of the same status.

Poverty is also highly associated with single-parent, mother-headed households, and more prevalent among blacks than whites. The relationship of this household composition to child socialization and adolescent behavior patterns is a neglected area of research.

The great majority of urban black adolescents from low-income families eventually become sexually active before marriage (Fursten-berg, 1976; Zelnik and Kantner, 1980; Rainwater, 1970; Staples, 1973; Ladner, 1971). A number of social-psychological factors have been postulated. The adverse life situation, needs for self-expression, the desire to be a "real man or woman," and the self-perceived forces of "fate" have been linked to these behaviors. Economic variables are also significant. Jobs are in short supply and low in both wages and prestige. In 1982, it was estimated that youth unemployment was over 50% in the black urban "ghettos." Schools may be of poor quality, and education often has little demonstrable payoff in terms of future employment.

A recent study of white, blue-collar families shows that many of these families also feel locked into a life of continuing deprivation with little to look forward to in terms of higher education, rewarding jobs, happy marriages, and adequate income. To these families, too, there seems to be little use in deferring gratification and planning for the future. The findings of this study show that nonmarital intercourse during adolescence is prevalent. However, for this white working class group, this is apt to be followed by early marriage, often to legitimate a pregnancy (Rubin, 1976).

BIOLOGICAL FACTORS

Almost none of the social and psychological studies of nonmarital intercourse have considered the age at maturation of the respondents. This issue is discussed in Chapter 7 by Hamburg.

Where data exists, differences in age at maturation seem to have some effect on when individuals become sexually active. For instance, Kinsey et al. (1948) and Chilman (1963) found that early-maturing boys became sexually involved earlier than late-maturing ones. Similar, but less strong, tendencies were found for girls. Presser (1978) found that age at first intercourse appeared to be related to age at puberty for black, but not for white, girls. On the other hand, Udry's (1983) recent study of 533 junior high school students showed that for both sexes and both races, there was a *strong* relationship between age at puberty and age at first intercourse. These contradictory findings indicate that more research is clearly needed.

IMPACT OF SOCIETAL CHANGES

As we have seen, there was a gradual increase in sexually permissive attitudes from 1920 through the mid-1960's, plus a strong upsurge in the incidence of adolescent nonmarital coitus from about 1967 through, at least, 1979. As discussed in the previous section, research shows that a number of individual and familial factors are associated with adolescent coitus. However, studies concerning adolescent sexuality have failed to assess underlying causes associated with behavioral trends for different cohorts of teenagers at different sociohistoric periods of time.

Until recently, the major thrust of contemporary research has also tended to overlook the effects of the larger social, economic, and political environment at different points in time on the attitudes and behaviors of adolescents at various stages of individual development. It is important to add increased awareness of the importance of historical, ecological, and cohort effects to studies of adolescent sexuality. (See also Chapter 15 by Vinovskis.)

As Baltes and others who write of the importance of a multidimensional approach to life span psychology emphasize, adolescence is a particularly vulnerable stage of human development. It is an individual transition period at a time when young people are exploring roles for adulthood. Thus, they are particularly affected by the demographic characteristics of their particular cohort as well as the historical period in which they are living. Furthermore, each adolescent is affected by the particular life events that may occur, such as, a divorce in the family, a physical illness, change in a parent's employment, and the like.

Following the leadership of such researchers as Elder (1975), Baltes et al. (1980), Furstenberg (1976), and others, it is important to investigate the effects of selected social, economic, and political trends during the 1960's and 1970's in order to gain further insight into the impact of society on the revolution in adolescent sexual behaviors of the past 15 years (1967–1982).

The marked increase in permissive adolescent sexual behavior in 1967 and the years following seems to be one aspect of more pervasive, fundamental societal changes during that time. For example, accompanying the upsurge in adolescent coitus (especially among young women), there was a rapidly increasing acceptance of divorce, cohabitation, communes, "open marriages," and the like. Some persons even claimed that families were no longer relevant.

In interpreting the societal change, a number of significant developments of the late 1960's and early 1970's can be identified. There was publication and wide dissemination of *Human Sexual Response* (Masters and Johnson, 1966) with its reports of research showing the essential similarity and equal potential of the male and female sex response. A second Masters and Johnson (1969) publication, *Human Sexual Inadequacy*, reported on effective therapeutic techniques to decrease frigidity in women and premature ejaculation and impotence in men. Through this research the area of sexuality was given further scientific legitimacy and endorsed for public discussion and reassessment.

The United States Department of Health, Education and Welfare adopted a policy in 1966 that made federal funds available to support family planning programs nationwide; this program was extended to adolescents in 1968.

Abortions were declared legal by the Supreme Court in 1973, following the 1967 leadership of Colorado and 15 other states. After this court decision, the Department of Health, Education and Welfare (HEW) made federal funds available for abortion services for low-income women. In 1974, the Attorney General of California issued the opinion that an unmarried teenager under age 18 does not need to obtain her parents' consent for an abortion.

From the mid-1960's, on, advocates of sex education in the public schools became more numerous and committed to their cause. In the early 1970's, a federal ruling forbade schools, on penalty of losing public funds, to exclude pregnant or parenting students from the regular school program.

Public opinion also changed impressively during this period. For instance, although the majority of adults responding to nationwide opinion polls in the mid-1960's had seen unwed motherhood as a serious problem and morally wrong, by the mid-1970's, the majority viewed this condition as a viable style of parenting. Along similar lines in the late 1960's, the majority of parents said they were opposed to cohabitation for their college-age sons and daughters; however, in the 1970's the majority of parents reported this to be acceptable (Yankelovich, 1981).

The feminist movement, building on women's equal rights activities of the past, was reborn in 1967 and continued to gain strength through most of the 1970's. The members of this movement asked for equality between the sexes in many of life's domains, including equally shared parenting and home-making roles; equal rights to sexual fulfillment, both within and outside of marriage; the right to choose parenthood or childlessness; and the right to choose marriage or single status as an acceptable life style for women as well as men. In the late 1950's women who did not marry were usually considered immoral or neurotic. By 1976, however, marriage or non-marriage was generally considered to be a matter of free choice, with either option being acceptable (Veroff et al., 1981).

There were other trends of the late 1960's and 1970's that probably had a strong impact on adolescent sexual behaviors, including: (1) the rising divorce, separation, and remarriage rates, causing more teenagers to live in one-parent or reconstituted stepparent families; (2) continuing inflation and the concurrent entry of more and more mothers into the labor market (three-fourths of the mothers of teenagers); (3) growing "feminization" of poverty, that is, the increasing proportion of female-headed families with mothers obtaining little support from fathers and having limited access to adequate child care resources as well as to steady, well-paid employment (Steiner, 1982); (4) the heightened incidence of youth unemployment, especially for inner-city youth, thereby further reducing both career aspirations and an adequate economic base for marriage.

A consideration of these trends and their probable effects on teenagers is sobering. For example, findings from research show that parental divorce often has severely adverse effects on children, including those who are teenagers (Wallerstein and Kelly, 1980; Hetherington et al., 1979). Divorce is also deeply disturbing to husbands and wives, often distracting them from parenting functions. Adolescents exposed to divorcing or separating parents are apt to become uncomfortably aware of their parents as sexually active persons who often are seeking mates. This can deprive the adolescent of needed stability at a time when hard-to-control sexual needs and interests are increasing.

Then, too, many divorced parents remarry. Adolescents in reconstituted families are apt to be involved in a number of difficult, complex situations with stepparents and stepsiblings (Chilman, 1983).

Zelnik and Kantner (1980) have found that adolescent coitus is most apt to occur during the day in the homes of teenagers while parents are at work. High rates of maternal employment probably mean that a large proportion of teenagers are exposed to the strong temptations of homes where parents are absent for most of the day.

Zelnik and Kantner (1980) also show the greater likelihood of adolescent coitus among teenage girls from one-parent and low-income families. The social, psychological, and economic adversities suffered by women who are single parents are becoming more widely recognized and understood. It seems likely that teenagers in such homes are especially apt to suffer from deprivations that may lead them to seek affection, security, and a sense of significance elsewhere. Thus, these teenagers may turn to escapist sexual intimacies and risk-taking behaviors that include intercourse without contraceptive protection.

The adverse impact of high rates of youth unemployment are related to the above point. When young people perceive that they are unlikely to get a job even if they do manage to graduate from high school, then, quite understandably, their motivation for educational achievement and vocational goal-striving is reduced. A strong argument given to adolescents against early intercourse and contraceptive risk-taking is that such behaviors will bar them from future economic well-being. When there seems to be little hope for this eventual success, arguments against current pleasure-seeking activities lose much of their credibility.

Unmarried parenthood often makes a young woman and her child eligible for Aid for Dependent Children (AFDC) benefits, which can be more adequate than the meager supports that might be available from a young husband who may well be unemployed or working for very low wages. The extent to which welfare availability encourages adolescent childbearing outside of marriage has been widely debated. Research analyses by Ross and Sawhill (1975) and Moore and Caldwell (1977), show that the availability of AFDC seems not to increase adolescent pregnancy but to broaden the options open to a pregnant woman so that she can choose to proceed with her pregnancy or seek an abortion, can keep the baby or place it for adoption, and can marry or not as the opportunity presents itself and as she deems best. More research is needed to provide clearer answers to the important topic of the impact of welfare programs on the behaviors of women and their partners in varying age groups (Moore and Burt, 1982).

Many of the events discussed above occurred against the backdrop of a climate of social unrest that included protests against the war in Vietnam. The period of the late 1960's and early 1970's was characterized by wide spread alienation, social criticism and questioning of traditional social values. However, Yankelovich (1974) writes that liberal political values and individual life style values began to go their separate ways by 1971. The vast majority of college students no longer had a strong identification with the political left but pressed forward for a cultural revolution against the Puritan ethic. By 1973 this drive had also gained many adherents among non-college youth. The largest value shift was in the direction of a desire for more sexual freedom. In 1969, 22% of non-college youth and 43% of college youth asked for this freedom. By 1973, these proportions had changed to 47 and 61%, respectively (Yankelovich, 1974; Chilman, 1983).

As noted earlier, there is some evidence from recent studies that young people, as a group, may have started turning toward somewhat less permissive sexual attitudes in the late 1970's (Robinson and Jedlicka, 1982; Singh, 1980). If this is true, it would be in harmony with the nation's trend toward somewhat more conservative social, political, and economic attitudes (Chilman, 1983).

FERTILITY RATES

Two teenage reproductive rates have increased markedly within recent years: (1) the pregnancy rate (with about one-half of these pregnancies being interrupted through abortion) and (2) the ratio of births outside of marriage: 31% of births to white adolescent mothers and 83% of births to black adolescent mothers in 1979 (Moore and Burt, 1982).

It is interesting to compare the fertility for United States teenagers to those for similar age groups in other countries. According to a recent analysis by Westoff and Calot (1983), the 1979 fertility rates for white American teenagers (221 per 1000 women, ages 14–19, in 1979–1980) were close to the highest rates found for most of the western European nations plus Australia and Canada.

Fertility rates for teenagers in most of the 30 developed nations studied declined between 1971 and 1979, with the rate being least marked in the nations of Eastern Europe (data for Russia were not available). The decline for white American teenagers was somewhat less than the average found for the majority of the 30 developed countries in this study.

A startling finding was obtained by Westoff and Calot: the fertility rates for American black teenagers in both 1971 and 1979 were the highest of all 30 nations surveyed (715 per 1000 women, ages 14–19, in 1971 and 515 per 1000 in 1979–1980). Only the Arab population in Israel approached this rate, with 574 births per 1000 teenagers in 1971 and 376 in 1979. The two groups, however, did show an unusually sharp decline in fertility from 1971 to 1979–1980.

Westoff and Calot (1983) note that the unusually high fertility rates for American black adolescents and Israeli Arabs are not easily understood. The same is true for the finding that the fertility rate for black women in the United States *under* age 18 (237 per 1000 in 1979–1980) is by far the highest of all countries studied. The next highest rate is not that for Israeli Arabs (82 per 1000) but for Hungarian and Roumanian adolescents (103 and 100 per 1000, respectively).

Japan had the lowest teenage fertility with rates of 21 in 1971 and 17 in 1979–1980, as well as only 2 per 1000 women under age 18 in the latter age group. Other nations with markedly low rates included Holland, Switzerland, Sweden, Denmark, and Finland, all with rates of under 100 per 1000 (in the United States the rate was 221 for whites and 515 for blacks, in that year).

Much more information is needed before we can begin to account for the differences in rates in various countries. Contraceptive resources and behaviors among teenagers comprise only part of the picture. An attempt to look at this subject on a world-wide basis is beyond the scope of this chapter.

CONTRACEPTIVE USE

As we have seen, by the late 1970's about one-half or more of young people were engaging in nonmarital intercourse before the age of 18 and this rate probably rose to about 75% or more by age 20 or 21. Only about 45% of sexually active adolescent females studied in 1976 and 1979 said they used any form of contraceptive at their first intercourse. About one-third had never used any form of birth control. Another third said they always used a method of birth control when they had coitus (Zelnik and Kantner, 1980).

TRENDS IN CONTRACEPTIVE USE

Only a few local studies of contraceptive use by males have been made. Cvetkovich and Grote (1976) and Finkel and Finkel (1975) found that 89% of the black and 69% of the white males in their high school study population said they had had unprotected intercourse at least once.

Nationwide surveys by Zelnik and Kantner (1980) revealed that although the proportion of contraceptive users among sexually active 15- to 17-year old girls increased somewhat between 1976 and 1979, the use of effective contraceptives declined. The main method shift was from the "pill" with its superior effectiveness to withdrawal by the male—a far less effective method. This shift in methods plus a rise in the proportion of sexually active young women, resulted in rising rates of adolescent pregnancy between 1971 and 1979, with about 16% of 15- to 19-year-old adolescent women having experienced a pregnancy during that year.

About 40% of sexually active females of both races depended on male methods of contraception in 1979. Because the majority of adolescent males seem to be markedly inconsistent and perhaps unconcerned about contraceptive use, there appears to be a central problem with respect to their attitudes and behaviors and the reliance of so many adolescent girls on the contraceptive vigilance of boys (Sorensen, 1973; Finkel and Finkel, 1975; Kantner and Zelnik, 1973; Zelnik and Kantner, 1980; Brown et al., 1975). If the few available studies are correct in their findings and can be generalized, a particular problem seems to reside with the contraceptive behavior of black males (Cvetkovich and Grote, 1976; Finkel and Finkel, 1975).

Variables associated with the failure of adolescents to use contraceptives at all or to use effective contraceptives consistently are revealed in a number of studies made during the 1970's and early 1980's (Goldsmith et al., 1972; Zelnik and Kantner, 1977, 1980; Shah et al., 1975, 1980; Cvetkovich and Grote, 1975; Finkel and Finkel, 1975; Furstenberg, 1976, 1980; Ladner, 1971; Miller, 1976; Luker, 1975; Lindemann, 1974; Rosen et al., 1976; Hornick et al., 1979; Jorgenson et al., 1980; Presser, 1977; DeLameter and McCorquodale, 1979; Fox and Inazu, 1980; Zelnik et al., 1982; Mindick and Oskamp, 1982; Rogel et al., 1980; Flaherty et al., 1982). (For a detailed review of these studies, see Chilman, 1983.)

A number of factors are associated with failure to use effective contraceptives:

1. *Demographic variables*—age lower than 18; single status; lower socioeconomic status; minority group membership; nonattendance at college; fundamentalist Protestant affiliation.

2. *Situational variables*—not being in a steady, committed relationship; not having experienced a pregnancy; having intercourse sporadically and without prior planning; contraceptives not available at the moment of need; being in a high-stress situation; not having ready access to a free, confidential family planning service that does not require parental consent; lack of communication with parents regarding contraceptives.

3. *Psychological variables*—desiring a pregnancy–high fertility values; ignorance of pregnancy risks and of family planning services; attitudes of fatalism, powerlessness, alienation, incompetence, trusting to luck; low educational achievement and goals; passive, dependent, traditional female role attitudes; high levels of anxiety—low ego

strength, low self-esteem; lack of acceptance of the reality of one's own sex behavior—thinking coitus will not occur; poor parent–youth and couple communication skills about sex and contraceptives; low levels of communication with parents and poor parent–youth relationships; disturbed family situation; risk-taking, pleasure-oriented attitudes; fear of contraceptive side effects and possible infertility; lack of knowledge of parents' experience with contraceptives; adverse physical side effects experienced but often strongly associated with negative, fatalistic attitudes; incorrect assumptions about the "safe time" of the menstrual cycle; immature level of cognitive development; lack of planful attitudes and poor problem-solving skills; attitudes and experiences of peer groups, including presence of friends and siblings who have become adolescent mothers.

Space limitations prevent a more detailed discussion of the meaning and impact of these factors. However, it can be seen that contraceptive behavior, like coital behavior, is affected by many social and psychological variables that go far beyond such "common-sense" considerations as the ready availability of contraceptive services (important as that may be) and education about sexuality, reproduction, and contraception. In respect to the latter, there is only limited research support for the effectiveness of sex education in preventing adolescent pregnancy and promoting contraceptive use (Chilman, 1983; Zelnik and Kim 1982).

Although much emphasis has been placed by human service professionals (among others) on the importance of teaching teenagers the techniques of "rational decision-making and contraceptive problem-solving skills" (Libby and Carlson, 1973; Gilchrist and Schinke, 1983) available research evidence, plus numerous theoretical concepts of the dynamics of human behavior, argue against such an essentially mechanistic, intellectualized approach as the solution to problems of adolescent sexual behavior. Such a rational, skill-oriented concept may well be effective in working with some teenagers, especially those who are in favorable familial, school, and community situations and who, thereby, are strongly motivated toward behavior that will, supposedly, help them reach such generally desirable long-range goals as advanced education, vocational success, economic security, marital and parental satisfactions, and the like.

However, as shown by the above research summaries, many teenagers engage in early nonmarital coitus and fail to use adequate contraceptives consistently partly because their total life situation and developmental experiences provide little support for their opportunity to achieve "successful" adulthood. For these types of adolescents, more comprehensive service programs, together with more basic social system changes seem indicated—a topic that far exceeds the present discussion.

ABORTION BEHAVIORS

There was a rapid increase in the rate of adolescent abortions during the 1970's. For example, between 1972 and 1975 the abortion rate among teenagers rose by more than three-fifths and this rate nearly doubled for girls under age 15 (Baldwin, 1976). For this age group, there were more abortions than live births from 1974 to 1976. Although in previous years abortion seemed to be more aceptable to white than to black women, national data for 1973–1977 showed that the abortion rates for blacks had increased markedly (Forrest et al., 1979). The high incidence of abortion among adolescents during the 1970's largely accounts for the decline in the birth rate for teenagers, despite the increased incidence of pregnancy for this age group.

According to the few studies that were available, abortion was more often chosen by young women whose parents were of higher socio-economic status, who did well in school, who were employed, and who were in a long-term, positive dating relationship with the putative father. Abortion tends not to be chosen by pregnant adolescents who desire a child, who have role models of adolescent parenthood among friends and relatives, nor is it chosen by those who hold anti-abortion attitudes (Olson, 1980; Klerman et al., 1982; Fischman, 1977; Rosen, 1980). Additional characteristics of adolescents who choose to carry their pregnancies to term are provided in a report of the National Center for Population Research (1983). According to a number of recent studies, more adolescents who delivered, rather than choosing to terminate their pregnancies "were below grade level in school, had poor or failing grades, had no plans for post-high school training or education, had fewer parental expectations for post-high school training or education, and did not think a baby interfered with their educational plans. Girls who delivered were less likely to have ever had a paid job, less likely to identify any future job, and more likely to receive welfare. More adolescents who delivered perceived their mothers and fathers as clearly supportive of the pregnancy. They also had more support from their boyfriends and had more girlfriends who had babies. These delivery and abortion groups were matched on many characteristics and did not differ in measures of "self-esteem, sex-role attitudes or nine emotional factors including depression, anxiety and hostility" (Center for Population Research, pp. 31–32).

Although there is little, if any, research evidence that shows negative social and psychological effects of abortion on adolescents (especially when the alternatives to an early, unplanned pregnancy are considered) (Klerman et al., 1983), it surely seems preferable to further develop programs and policies that help to prevent such pregnancies in the first place.

However, it is important that high-quality, confidential abortion services remain available to young people who experience an unwanted pregnancy. In this connection, more research is clearly needed concerning the longitudinal effects of abortion and its alternatives on the lives of teenagers, their parents, and any children that the young people may have.

SUMMARY AND CONCLUSIONS

American attitudes toward human sexuality, in general, became increasingly permissive in the years between 1920 and 1980. This trend affected adolescents as well as adults. Equality between the sexes in all aspects of life, including those of sexual behavior, was a central theme. The double-standard of sex morality is fading gradually, its decline hastened by the sweeping social and psychological upheavals of the 1960's and 1970's, but aspects of this standard linger on into the 1980's.

Remaining a "technical virgin" was an important value for young women before the mid-1960's. Of course, this value had its pragmatic aspects in that the newer "intercourse-independent" contraceptives were not developed until that time. However, more fundamental factors probably account for the normative turn around years of 1967 and 1968—years in which a number of behaviors that had previously been considered deviant moved into the realm of social acceptability. These behaviors included a sharp increase in nonmarital coitus for adolescents. According to a number of small studies of white populations, rates of intercourse by age 17 jumped from about 10% for young women and 30% for young men in 1965 to about 35% for young women and 40% for young men in 1967 (Chilman, 1979). Large national studies carried out by Kantner and Zelnik (1972) showed that rates of coitus continued to climb, though less rapidly, during the 1970's and involved progressively younger age groups. By 1979, about 65% of young white women and 88% of young black women reported they had experienced coitus by age 19 (Zelnik and Kantner, 1980).

Through various federal governmental actions, free or low-cost contraceptive services became available to adolescents in most localities by the early 1970's. Although a number of high-quality family planning programs were developed for teenagers (among others), at least 50% of adolescent women failed to use effective contraceptives at first coitus and many continued their risk-taking behavior over a period of months or years. By 1979, many sexually active adolescent women had changed from the oral contraceptives to less effective male methods, including withdrawal.

The result of increased rates of adolescent intercourse among adolescents during the 1970's and non-use or poor use of contraceptives was a rise in the proportion of sexually active teenagers who became pregnant: over 16% in 1979. The rising rates of early unplanned pregnancies were accompanied by growing numbers of abortions obtained by this age group. In fact, for younger pregnant teenagers (under age 16) the abortion rate exceeded the birth rate (Baldwin, 1976).

Although the birth rate to teenagers declined during the 1960's and 1970's from the "boom years" of 1948–1958, the rate of births to unmarried adolescents increased. In 1979, this rate was 31% of all babies born to white mothers and 83% of all babies born to black mothers. A recent paper by Westoff and Calot (1983) analyzes adolescent fertility rates for 30 developed countries. It reveals that the fertility rate for black teenagers in the United States is by far the highest of all nations studied. However, this rate has shown a particularly sharp decline between 1971 and 1979.

A number of studies indicate that clusters of demographic, situational, social, psychological, and economic variables are associated with adolescent coital and contraceptive behaviors. Although the ready availability of free or low-cost confidential family planning services is important in promoting "responsible sexuality," many other variables need to be taken into account in understanding the family planning (or nonplanning) behaviors of different kinds of adolescents. These variables are far more complex and extensive for many teenagers than such relatively simplistic (and frequently endorsed) ones as the presence or lack of sex education and "decision-making skills."

As shown above, the 1960's and 1970's were a period of profound societal changes which included a revolt against many traditional, generally conservative, attitudes toward sexuality in its many aspects. Shifts toward more permissive adolescent sexual attitudes and behaviors were one aspect of these overall societal upheavals. These upheavals exacted their costs as well as their benefits in expanded individual freedoms and greater equality between the sexes. The costs include rising divorce rates, the "feminization of poverty" through the increase in female-headed households, a rise in adolescent pregnancies and nonmarital births, and increased use of abortion.

By the early 1980's many sectors of the populace were expressing growing concern about adolescent sexuality and pregnancy. These concerns have taken several forms. On the one hand, there has been a demand by some groups for more readily available, confidential contraceptive and abortion services for adolescents. On the other hand, moral conservatives and administrators of the Reagan presidency have called for such measures as a ban on abortions, restriction of contraceptives for teenagers, prevention of sex education in the schools, and cuts in the Aid to Families of Dependent Children programs.

Young people entering adolescence in the early 1980's face a quite different world than was the case for the cohorts of the immediately preceding decades. Partly in response to a changed society, these young people may well form different sexual attitudes and engage in different sexual behaviors than was true for their older siblings. For instance, it is possible that many of them will become more conservative in their behavior and more or less return to earlier norms. On the other hand, if they follow the pattern set by Scandinavian youth, rates of nonmarital coitus and nonmarital childbearing will continue to rise.

Present knowledge about adolescent sexuality is limited by various problems in past investigation of this topic, although there has been a marked improvement in pertinent research methodologies in recent years. However, even if past research had been well nigh perfect, we would still need new studies to provide information about the present and future lives of today's adolescents, including the sexual aspects of their lives.

We also need a renewed commitment to humane values and creative explorations for more effective ways of reducing the numerous societal problems that so deeply affect the lives of all people, including the sexual lives of today's—and tomorrow's—adolescents.

REFERENCES

Arafat, I., and Yorburg, B. Drug use and the sexual behavior of college women. *Journal of Sex Research*, 1973, 9, 21–29.

Baldwin, W. Adolescent pregnancy and childbearing-growing concerns for Americans. (Population Reference Bureau), Vol. 31, 1976. Washington, D.C., 1976.

Baltes, P., Reese, H., and Lipsitt, R. Life span developmental psychology. *Annual Review of Psychology*, 1980, pp. 65–110.

Bardwick, J. Psychological factors in the acceptance and use of oral contraceptives. *In Psychological aspects of population*. James Fawcett (Ed.), New York: Basic Books, 1973.

Bell, R., and Chaskes, J. Premarital sexual experience among coeds, 1958 and 1968. *Journal of Marriage and the Family*, 1970, 32, 81–84.

Bowerman, C., Irish, D., and Pope, H. *Unwed motherhood: Personal and social consequences*. Institute for Research in Social Sciences, University of North Carolina, Chapel Hill, NC, 1966.

Brown, S., Lieberman, J., and Miller, W. *Young adults as partners and planners: A preliminary report on the antecedents of responsible family formation."* Paper presented at 103rd Annual meeting of the American Public Health Association, Chicago, IL, 1975.

Burgess, E., and Wallin, P. *Engagement and marriage*. New York: Lippincott, 1953.

Cannon, K., and Long, R. Premarital sex behavior in the '60's. *Journal of Marriage and the Family*, 1971, *33*, 37–49.

Carns, D. Talking about sex: Notes on first coitus and the double standard. *Journal of Marriage and the Family*, 1971, 33, 37–49.

Center for Population Research, National Institute of Health and Human Development. Progress Report, January. Bethesda, MD, 1983, 31–32.

Chilman, C. The educational-vocational aspirations and behaviors of un-married and married undergraduates at Syracuse University. Unpublished study, 1963.

Chilman, C. Some psychosocial aspects of female sexuality. The Family Co-ordinator, 1974, 23, 123–131.

Chilman, C. Adolescent sexuality in a changing American society: social and psychological perspectives. Washington, D.C.: U.S. Government Printing Office, 1979.

Chilman, C. Adolescent pregnancy and childbearing: Findings from research. U.S. Dept. of Health, and Human Services, NIH Publication No. 81-2077, Washington, D.C.: U.S. Government Printing office, 1980.

Chilman, C. Adolescent sexuality in a changing society (2nd ed). New York: Wiley, 1983.

Christensen, H., and Gregg, C. Changing sex norms in America and Scan-danavia. Journal of Marriage and the Family, 1970, 32, 616–627.

Clayton, R., and Bokemaier, J. Premarital sex in the seventies. Journal of Mar-riage and the Family, 1980, 42, 750–775.

Conger, J. Adolescence and youth. New York: Harper and Row, 1973.

Croake, J., and James, B. A four year comparison of premarital sexual attitudes. Journal of Sex Research, 1973, 9, 91–96.

Cvetkovich, G. and Grote, B. Psychological factors associated with adolescent premarital coitus. Paper presented at the National Institute of Child Health and Human Development, Bethesda, MD, May, 1976.

DeLameter, J., and MacCorquodale, M. Premarital sexuality: Attitudes, rela-tionships, behaviors. Madison, WI: University of Wisconsin Press, 1979.

Ehrmann, W. Premarital dating behavior. New York: Holt, Rinehart & Winston, 1959.

Elder, G. Adolescence in the life cycle: An introduction. In J. Adelson (Ed.), Handbook of Adolescent Psychology. New York: Wiley, 1975, pp. 1–22.

Ferrell, M., Tolone, W., and Walsh, R. Maturational and societal changes in the sexual double standard. Journal of Marriage and the Family, 1977, 39, 225–271.

Finkel, M., and Finkel, D. Sexual and contraceptive knowledge, attitudes and behaviors of male adolescents. Family Planning Perspectives, 1975, 7, 256–260.

Fischman, S. Delivery or abortion in inner-city adolescents. American Journal of Orthopsychiatry, 1977, 47, 127–133.

Flaherty, E., Maracek, J., Olsen, K., and Wilcove, G. Psychological factors associated with fertility regulation among adolescents. Final Report. Contract # NO1-HD-82883-NICHD, Bethesda MD, 1982.

Forrest, J., Sullivan, E., and Tietze, C. Abortion in the United States. Family Planning Perspectives, 1979, 11, 329–341.

Fox, G. The mother-adolescent daughter relationship as a sexual socialization structure: A research review. Family Relations, 1980, 29, 21–28.

Fox, G., and Inazu, J. Patterns and outcomes of mother-daughter communi-cation about sexuality. Journal of Social Issues, 1980, 36, 7–29.

Furstenberg, F. Jr. Unplanned parenthood: The social consequences of teenage childbearing. New York: Free Press, 1976.

Furstenberg, F. Jr. The impact of early childbearing on the family. Journal of Social Issues, 1980, 36, 64–87.

Gebhard, P., Pomeroy, W., Martin, C., and Christensen, C. Pregnancy, birth, and abortion. New York: Harper and Bros., 1956.

George Washington University Medical Center. Adolescent Fertility Risks and Consequences. *Population Reports*, Series J (July), J-157-175, 1976.

Gilchrist, L. and Schinke, S. Sexuality counseling with adolescents and their parents. *In* C. Chilman (Ed.), *Adolescent sexuality in a changing society (2nd ed.)*. New York: Wiley, 1983.

Glenn, N., and Weaver, C. Attitudes toward premarital, extramarital and homosexual relations in the U.S. in the 1970's. *Journal of Sex Research*, 1979, *15*, 108–118.

Goldsmith, S., Gabrielson, M., and Gabrielson, I. Teenagers, sex and contraception. *Family Planning Perspectives*, 1972, *4*. pp. 32–38.

Heltsey, M., and Broderick, C. Religiosity and premarital sexual permissiveness: Reexamination of Reiss's traditionalism proposition. *Journal of Marriage and the Family*, 1969, *31*, 441–443.

Hetherington, M., Cox, M., and Cox, R. The aftermath of divorce. *In* J. Stevens and M. Matthews (Eds.), *Mother-child, father-child relations*. Washington, D.C.: National Association for Education of Young Children, 1979.

Hornick, J., Doran, L., and Crawford, S. Premarital contraceptive behaviors among young male and female adolescents. *Family Coordinator*, 1979, *28*, 181–190.

Hunt, M. *Sexual behavior in the 1970's*. Chicago: Playboy Press, 1974.

Jackson, E., and Potkay, C. Pre-college influences on sexual experiences of coeds. *Journal of Sex Research*, 1973, *9*, 143–149.

Jessor, S., and Jessor R. Transition from virginity to nonvirginity among youth: A social-psychological study over time. *Developmental Psychology*, 1975, *11*, 473–484.

Jorgenson, S., King, S., and Torrey, B. Dyadic and social network influencing an adolescent exposure to pregnancy risk. *Journal of Marriage and the Family*, 1980, *42*, 141–155.

Kantner, J., and Zelnik, M. Sexual experiences of young unmarried women in the U.S. *Family Planning Perspectives*, 1972, *4*, 9–17.

Kinsey, A., Pomeroy, W., and Martin, C. *Sexual behavior in the human male*. Philadelphia, PA: Saunders, 1948.

Kinsey, A., Pomeroy, W., Martin, C., and Gebhard, P. *Sexual behavior in the human female*. Philadelphia, PA: Saunders, 1953.

Klerman, L., Bracken, M., Jekel, J., and Bracken, M. The delivery abortion decision among adolescents. *In* I. Stuart and C. Wells (Eds.), *Pregnancy in Adolescence*. New York: van Nostrand Reinhold, 1982, pp. 219–235.

Komarovsky, M. *Dilemmas of masculinity: A study of college youth*. New York: W. W. Norton, 1976.

Ladner, J. *Tomorrow's tomorrow: The black women*. Garden City, N.J.: Doubleday, 1971.

Lewis, R., and Burr, W. Premarital coitus and commitment among college students. *Archives of Sexual Behavior*, 1975, *4*, 73–79.

Libby, R., and Carlson, J. A theoretical framework for premarital sexual decisions in the use of contraceptives. *Archives of Sexual Behavior*, 1973, *2*, 365–378.

Lindemann, C. *Birth control and unmarried young women*. New York: Springer, 1974.

Luckey, E., and Nass, G. A comparison of sexual attitudes and behavior of an international sample. *Journal of Marriage and the Family*, 1969, *31*, 346–379.

Luker, K. *Taking chances: Abortion and the decision not to contracept*. Berkeley, CA: University of California Press, 1975.

Masters, W., and Johnson, V. *Human sexual response*. Boston, MA: Little, Brown, 1966.

Masters, W., and Johnson, V. *Human sexual inadequacy*. Boston, MA: Little, Brown, 1969.

Miller, W. Relationships between the intendedness of contraception and wantedness of pregnancy. *Journal of Nervous and Mental Diseases*, 1974, *59*, 396–406.

Miller, W. *Some psychological factors predictive of undergraduate sexual and contraceptive behavior*. Paper presented at the 84th Annual Convention of American Psychological Association, Washington, D.C., Sept., 1976.

Mindick, B. and Oskamp, S. Individual differences among adolescent contraceptors: Some implications for intervention. *In* I. Stuart and C. Wells (Eds.), *Pregnancy in adolescence*. New York: Van Nostrand Reinhold, 1982, 140–176.

Mirande, A. Reference group theory and adolescent sexual behavior. *Journal of Marriage and the Family*, 1968, *30*, 572–577.

Moore, K., and Caldwell, S. Out of wedlock childbearing. Washington, D.C.: The Urban Institute, 1977.

Olson, L. Social and psychological correlates of promancy resolution among young adolescent women: A review. *American Journal of Orthopsychiatry*, 1980, *50*, 432–445.

Packard, V. *The sexual wilderness*. New York: David McKay, 1968.

Perlman, D. Self-esteem and sexual permissiveness. *Journal of Marriage and the Family*, 1974, *36*, 470–474.

Playboy. What's really happening on campus. *Playboy*, 1976, *23*, 128–169.

Presser H. Guessing and misinformation about pregnancy risks among urban mothers. *Family Planning Perspectives*, 1977, *9*, 234–236.

Presser, H. Age at menarche, socio-sexual behavior and fertility. *Social Biology* 1978, *2*, 94–101.

Rainwater, L. *Behind ghetto walls: Black families in a federal slum*. Chicago: Aldine, 1970.

Reiss, I. *Premarital sex standards in America*. Glencoe, Illinois: Free Press, 1960.

Reiss, I. *The social context of sexual permissiveness*. New York: Holt, Rhinehart & Winston, 1967.

Reiss, I. *Family systems in America* (2nd ed.) Hinsdale, IL: Dryden Press, 1976.

Reiss, I., and Miller, B. Heterosexual permissiveness: A theoretical analysis. *In* W. Burr, R. Hill, I. Nye, and I. Reiss (Eds.). *Contemporary Theories about Family* (Vol. I). New York: The Free Press, 1979, pp. 57–100.

Robinson, I., King, K., and Balswick, J. The premarital sexual revolution among college females. *Family Coordinator*, 1972, *21*, 189–194.

Robinson, I., and Jedlicka, D. Change in sexual attitudes and behavior of college students from 1965–1980: A research note. *Journal of Marriage and the Family*, 1982, *44*, 237–240.

Rogel, M., Zuehlke, M., Petersen, A., Tobin-Richards, M., and Shelton, M. Contraceptive behavior in adolescence: A decision-making perspective. *Journal of Youth and Adolescence*, 1980, *9*, 491–506.

Rosen, R., Martindale, L., and Grisdela, M. *Pregnancy study report*. Wayne State University, Detroit, MI, March, 1976.

Rosen, R. Adolescent pregnancy decision-making: Are parents important? *Adolescence*, 1980, *15*, 43–54.

Ross, H., and Sawhill, I. *Time of transition: The growth of families headed by women*. Washington, D.C.: The Urban Institute, 1975.

Rubin, L. *Worlds of pain.* New York: Basic Books, 1976.

Scales, P., and Beckstein, D. From macho to mutuality: Helping young men make effective decisions about sex, contraception, and pregnancy. *In* I. Stuart and C. Wells (Eds.), *Pregnancy in adolescence.* New York: Van Nostrand Reinhold, Van Nostrand Reinhold, 1982, pp. 264–289.

Shah, F., Zelnik, M., and Kantner, J., Unprotected intercourse among unwed teenager. *Family Planning Perspectives,* 1975, 7, 39.

Simon, W., Berger, A., and Gagnon, J. Beyond anxiety and fantasy: The coital experience of college youths. *Journal of Youth and Adolescence,* 1972, *1* (3), 203–222.

Singh. B. Trends in attitudes toward premarital sexual relationships. *Journal of Marriage and the Family,* 1980, *42,* 387–394.

Sorensen, R. *Adolescent sexuality in contemporary America.* New York: World Publishing, 1973.

Spanier, G. Sexualization and premarital sexual behavior. *Family Coordinator,* 1975, *24,* 33–41.

Staples, R. *The black woman in America: Sex, marriage and the family.* Chicago: Nelson-Hall Co., 1973.

Steiner, G. *The futility of family policy.* Washington, D.C.: The Brookings Institution, 1982.

Steinhoff, P. *Premarital pregnancy and first birth.* Paper presented at the Conference on the Birth of the First Child and Family Formation, Pacific Grove, Calif, March, 1976. Report of larger study, *Hawaii Pregnancy, Birth Control, and Abortion Study,* University of Hawaii.

Terman, L. *Psychological factors in marital happiness.* New York: McGraw-Hill, 1938.

Udry, J. Bauman, K., and Morris, N. Changes in premarital coital experience of recent decades of birth cohorts of urban America. *Journal of Marriage and the Family,* 1975, *37,* 783–787.

Udry, J. Socialization of adolescent sexual behavior. Carolina Population Center, University of North Carolina, Chapel Hill, N.C., 1983.

Vener, A., and Stewart, C. Adolescent sexual behavior in middle America revisited: 1970–1973. *Journal of Marriage and the Family,* 1974, *36,* 728–735.

Veroff, J., Douvan, E., and Kulka, R. *The inner American.* New York, Basic Books, 1981.

Wallerstein, J., and Kelly, J. *Surviving the break-up: How children and parents cope with divorce.* New York, Basic Books, 1980.

Westoff, C. and Calot, G. Teenage fertility in the developed nations in the 1970's (draft). Princeton University, Princeton, N.J., February, 1983.

Yankelovich, D. A world turned upside down. *Psychology Today,* 1981, pp. 35–91.

Yankelovich, D. *The new morality: A profile of American youth in the 1970's.* New York: McGraw-Hill, 1974.

Zelnik, M., and Kantner, J. Sexual and contraceptive experience of young married women in the United States, 1966–1971. *Family Planning Perspectives,* 1977, *9,* 55–73.

Zelnik, M., and Kantner, J. Sexuality, contraception and pregnancy among young unwed females in the United States. *Research Reports Vol. I.* Commission on Population Growth and the American Future. Washington, D.C.: U.S. Government Printing Office, 1980.

Zelnik, M., Kantner, J., and Ford, K. *Adolescent pathways to pregnancy.* Beverly Hills, CA: Sage Public., 1982.

Zelnik, M., and Kim, Y. Sex education and its association with teenage sexual activity, pregnancy and contraceptive use. *Family Planning Perspectives,* 1982, *14,* 117–125.

11

FAMILY COMMUNICATION AND CONTRACEPTIVE USE AMONG SEXUALLY ACTIVE ADOLESCENTS

Frank F. Furstenberg, Jr.
Roberta Herceg-Baron
Judy Shea
David Webb

INTRODUCTION

Over the past decade the proportion of sexually active adolescents has increased dramatically, creating a climate of concern in American society (Zelnik and Kantner, 1980). The gap between the onset of intercourse and the timing of marriage has widened considerably because young women (and probably young men as well) are initiating sexual relations much earlier than they ever had in the past and are marrying, on the average, a good deal later than has been the custom in recent generations. Accordingly, the risk of premarital pregnancy has risen sharply, resulting in some increase in abortion and elevated rates of out-of-wedlock childbearing among the teenage population (Furstenberg et al., 1981; Zelnik et al., 1981).

In the 1950's early marriage, adoption, and illegal abortion masked the number of premarital pregnancies among adolescents. Today, young women who become pregnant before marriage are not as likely to resort to any of these "solutions." Consequently, teenage sexual activity and pregnancy are far more visible than they were a generation ago, and are made even more so by the availability of national health statistics and social surveys. What was once discretely concealed is now openly revealed.

The heightened visibility of teenage sexuality, pregnancy, and childbearing generated much interest in preventive policies and services in the 1970s. After a brief but spirited debate, federal funding was provided to make family planning services available to sexually active adolescents. This effort seems to have had some qualified success in limiting the increase of pregnancies in the teenage population. A substantial number of adolescents—one and a half million in 1979—obtain birth control from federally funded programs that have prevented an estimated 367 thousand unplanned pregnancies (Torres et al., 1981). Unfortunately, research also reveals that adolescents experience a great deal of difficulty in using the birth control methods they obtain (Ager, et al., 1982; Mendick and Oskamp, 1982). This had led to a consideration of measures that might enhance contraceptive use.

One significant barrier to getting teenagers to use contraception effectively arises from their fear of being detected by their family. Most girls believe, probably with good reason, that their parents would strongly disapprove if they discovered that they were sexually active. Several studies have reported that teenagers use birth control less often and less effectively when their parents did not know that they are having sexual relations and that parents would have disapproved if this information had been disclosed (Furstenberg, 1971; Fox and Inazu, 1980a). Consequently, some experts have suggested that one value to increasing contraceptive practice was to break down the wall of silence between adolescents and their parents (Ooms, 1981). If parents were better informed, they might accept, albeit reluctantly, the need for contraceptive services and might therefore more openly endorse their use. In turn, teenagers could feel free to practice contraception without the fear of being discovered.

In the past several years, a number of proposals have been advocated for promoting greater communication between adolescents and their parents. These have ranged from voluntary programs of public education and family counseling to the recent proposal of HHS to mandate parental notification. The controversy over the latter policy, the so-called "squeal rule," exposed a number of practical problems to involving parents as a matter of routine. Beyond the programmatic considerations of implementing a notification procedure, the debate over the "squeal rule" revealed that our empirical research on the relationship between family communication and contraceptive practice is extremely sparse. There is generally a paucity of information on the process of sexual socialization within the family, and very little of the data collected speaks directly to the issues of how teenage sexual practices are affected by their parents' attitudes and actions.

The idea of involving parents more directly in service programs in an effort to build support for contraceptive practice has aroused considerable controversy. Even most proponents are aware of the practical problems of involving parents as a matter of routine. It is well documented that the patient confidentiality currently offered by family planning clinics is highly valued by adolescents (Coughlin and Perales, 1978; Herold and Goodwin, 1979). Mandatory measures of achieving parental involvement, such as notification, might deter a significant proportion of adolescent clients from seeking services (Torres et al., 1980).

This chapter briefly reviews some of the relevant research on the topic of family communication about sex and birth control and reports findings from a recent study examining the impact of family communication on contraceptive use among a sample of adolescents who sought services from family planning clinics in the Philadelphia and surrounding county areas of southeastern Pennsylvania. We shall try to draw some lessons from our study for the current policy debate over how to involve parents in family planning services by providing data on how adolescents and parents communicate about sex and birth control and the consequence of such communication on birth control practice.

RESEARCH ON FAMILY COMMUNICATION AND CONTRACEPTION USE

Existing studies of sexual socialization in the family do not provide a clear or consistent picture of how adolescent sexual practices are shaped by parental attitudes and sanctions (Shea, 1983). Many previous studies on this topic are plagued by methodological difficulties. First, there is a reckless tendency to generalize from research on special samples. Findings from college samples cannot be extended to more youthful populations or to teens in different social strata. Second, researchers often infer parental influence from poorly measured or poorly conceived indicators. Data collected only from adolescents, who are asked to supply information on their parents' views, cannot be used as a proxie for the actual views of parents as previous research has difinitively demonstrated that teenagers are frequently mistaken about their parents' views (and vice versa). A final fault in most of the current studies is that cross-sectionally designed studies do not examine the issue of causality and leave open the question of how associations are to be explained when they occur. For example, if parental communication is positively related to adolescent contraceptive use, it is not at all clear that teenagers use contraception at the urging of their parents or are merely more willing to communicate with their parents because they are already committed to using contraception.

Two excellent reviews have sifted through the available evidence in an effort to derive lessons from the data that are relevant for public policy. They also point to several important areas for future research. Fox (1981) carefully weighed findings from previous investigations of the family's role in shaping adolescent sexual behavior and reached the following conclusions: (1) There is very little direct communication from parents to children; (2) what little there is generally occurs between mothers and daughters; (3) findings from a variety of studies seem to suggest that the impact of communication may have a marked effect on behavior, forestalling the transition to nonvirginity and promoting more effective contraceptive practices. The latter conclusion, however, is only tentatively drawn by Fox, who observes, in the absence of longitudinal studies, that researchers have not yet demonstrated a causal connection between parental communication and adolescent sexual behavior.

In another review of fertility-related socialization, Philliber (1980), relating her own research to that of others, discovered that communication about sex and birth control, even between mothers and daughters, is often accompanied by strain and uncertainty. Although parents and children both report conversations about contraceptive use, the conversations are generally oblique; sometimes mother–daughter pairs do not even agree on the occurrence of discussions. These results agree with the findings of an earlier study by Furstenberg (1971), who discovered that a high proportion of adolescents and their mothers did not agree when asked whether birth control had been discussed. Philliber's findings also reinforce the results of a more recent study by Fox and Inazu (1980b) showing that when conversations occur between mothers and daughters about contraception, they are much more frequently perceived as uncomfortable by daughters than by mothers. Fox and Inazu did find, nonetheless, that frequent conversation was related to the daughter's receptivity to birth control. Philliber concurs with Fox that more research is needed on the way that both direct and indirect sexual communication in the family influences adolescent behavior.

The present study grew out of an interest in exploring whether and how family communication is related to adolescent contraceptive use. It also resulted from an experiment attempted by several federally funded family planning agencies affiliated with the Family Planning Council of Southeastern Pennsylvania. The service program was designed to facilitate more open communication between teenage clients and family members about the fact that they were sexually active and seeking contraceptive services from the clinics. The larger research project tested the hypothesis that through a planned intervention it would be possible to increase the level of communication between the sexually active adolescent and her family and that by producing a more open climate of communication, adolescents would receive and perceive more support for contraceptive practice. This project came to be known as the "Kinship Study."

DATA AND METHODS

THE SAMPLE

The Kinship Study was funded in 1979 by a grant from the Office of Family Planning, Bureau of Community Health Services. Adolescent participants in the project were drawn from six federally funded family planning agencies operating nine separate clinic sites. The participating agencies included those that had a large proportion of teenage clients and expressed a willingness to cooperate in the research by expanding their programs for parental involvement. The agencies represented a mix of settings, including three Planned Parenthood affiliates, two hospital programs, and one neighborhood health center. They served adolescents from urban, suburban, and semi-rural areas, who were racially diverse and came from families distributed across economic strata. Table 11.1 presents a portrait of the characteristics of the sample.

The sample is evenly divided between whites and non-whites. Almost all of the participants in the study were currently enrolled in school when they entered the study. Approximately one-third was 17, one-third was 16, and one-third was 15 years or younger. For nearly all of the respondents, it was their first visit to a family planning clinic. However, 85% had been sexually active before they came for services, and more than one-third had initiated intercourse at least a year before the clinic visit. About one-fifth had been pregnant previously and 10% were already teenaged mothers at the beginning of the study. All but four of the young women were single.

About one-half of the participants were living with two parents at the time of the initial clinic visit, and most of the others were living with a single biological parent. All but 9% were residing with their biological mothers. The educational level of the parents was widely distributed. Taking the education level of the parent who was best educated, one-sixth had not graduated from high school, one-half had completed high school but had gone no further, and the remaining third had received some college or postsecondary technical training.

In examining the results of this study, it is important to bear in mind that the sample is confined to adolescents who have sought services from a federally funded family planning clinic. As noted earlier, only a minority of all sexually active adolescents obtain birth control from family planning clinics (Torres et al., 1981). Our study does not reflect the experiences of adolescents who obtain contraception from private

TABLE 11.1. Selected Characteristics of the Adolescent
Sample at Time of the Initial Interview[a]

Characteristic	N	%
Race		
White	142	49.5
Black	145	50.5
	287	100
Age		
15 and under	88	30.4
16	90	31.1
17	111	38.4
	289	100
Marital status		
Never married	285	98.6
Divorced/separated	0	0
Married	4	1.4
	289	100
Pregnancies		
Never pregnant	229	79.5
One or more pregnancies, now mother	30	10.4
One or more pregnancies, no children	29	10.1
	288	100
Time of first intercourse		
Never had intercourse	40	14.2
First intercourse within one year before clinic visit	136	48.2
First intercourse one year or more before clinic visit	106	37.6
	272	100
Guardians		
Biological mother and father	176	60.9
Biological mother and stepfather	31	10.7
Biological mother only	55	19.0
Other	27	9.3
	289	100
Parents' education[b]		
Less than high school	43	15.9
High school	141	52.0
Some college or technical school	87	32.1
	271	100

[a] Totals reflect the number of respondents who completed all three interviews (289) less the number for which information was missing or invalid.

[b] Based on parent with highest education.

physicians (probably a small figure for women under the age of 18), who rely on nonprescriptive methods which can be obtained at a pharmacy, or who do not use contraception at all. Moreover, ours was not a representative sample, even from the geographical area from which it is drawn. In comparison to the larger population of 13,000 teenaged clients served by family planning agencies in the Southeast Pennsylvania Council, whites were slightly overrepresented in the study, although the age distributions, pregnancy, and parenting experiences of the sample closely resembled those of all adolescent clients.

THE DESIGN OF THE STUDY

During a period of 20 months from January 1980 to September 1981, we invited new adolescent family planning clients who visited the nine clinics to participate in the study programs. Of those approached, nearly 90% agreed to participate in the study, resulting in a sample of 417 participants. Adolescents were assigned on a random basis to one of two experimental groups or to serve as a control in the study. Approximately 24% of the sample were invited to receive a family-oriented counseling service provided by family planning counselors specially trained by an experienced family therapist. The family counseling program has been described in some detail elsewhere (Furstenberg et al., 1981). Another 18% received periodic support for contraceptive use from one of the members of the research team. This intervention was designed to occur at about the same time that family counseling took place in order to compare effects. The periodic support was conducted by telephone while the family counseling was delivered at the clinic. The remainder of teens (58%) received routine clinic services and participated in the study as controls. By design, some of these adolescents were initially interviewed then and reinterviewed 6 months later by telephone, as were the participants who received family or periodic support. Other members of the control group were contacted only at 15 months, when we made our final assessment of all participants to determine the effects of the special programs. The results of this aspect of the program are presently being analyzed and will be reported in a subsequent paper.

We had a high degree of success in retaining adolescents in the study. Among those who agreed to participate and who completed an initial interview, 88% were reinterviewed at 6 months and 85% completed the second follow up, an average of 15 months after the initial visit. Only 7% refused to participate in the final interview, while 8% could not be located by the end of the project. There was some selectivity to the attrition. Dropouts were more likely to be younger teens and black. Furthermore, we suspect that those who dropped out were less likely to be continuous contraceptive users and probably also somewhat less likely to have extensive communication with their families. Consequently, our findings may slightly inflate the proportion of continuous birth control users and overstate the amount of communication in the family. Even so, because the loss to follow up was so small, the distortion in our results cannot be very substantial.

The purpose of the interviews was to evaluate the effects of the special program, so that we have fairly extensive information on the scope of family communication about sex and birth control at the three points of data collection. Adolescents were asked how much they discussed sexual matters in their family, to whom they spoke, how comfortable they felt, and what was disclosed or discovered about their use of clinic services. As the study proceeded, we realized we needed more qualitative information about the content of discussions, and in the final interview, we attempted to capture greater details of the context in which disclosure about the clinic visit took place.

Since the interviews were, by necessity, intended to be brief (20–30 minutes each), the information in our study does not overcome the limitations of collecting information on such an intimate area through survey research. However, it does supply more information than any previous longitudinal study on changing patterns of sex-related communication among adolescents and their parents. Moreover, the usefulness of the data is improved by supplementary interviews with 95 mothers of the adolescents. A subsample of adolescents gave us permission to invite their mothers to participate in an interview which contained a parallel set of questions designed to measure mothers' perceptions of family sexual communication. At certain points in this analysis, we shall introduce data from this small corroborative survey of 95 mothers and some of the qualitative case study data which was collected in the course of preparing the mother interview schedule. The supplementary data help to overcome the bias inherent in relying only on the reports of the adolescent participants.

The analysis which follows builds upon and expands a preliminary report of the study which described the changing patterns of family communication over the period from the initial interview to the 6-month follow up (Herceg-Baron and Furstenberg, 1982). Several important findings emerged from that prior investigation of the data. First, most adolescents stated that there was at least one member of their family with whom they could discuss sex and birth control. The adolescent's confidante was usually her mother, a sister, or occasionally both; only rarely were sexual matters discussed with a male in the family. Significantly, communication with female siblings rose between the two interviews, but reliance on the mother for information or support remained constant. While they were not more likely to become sexual confidantes, more mothers did learn of the clinic visit by the second interview. Left unexplored in the initial phase of the study was how the mothers found out about the clinic visit and how they responded to the disclosure.

The most striking result of the preliminary analysis was that neither communication about sex and birth control nor knowledge of the clinic visit was strongly related to adolescent use of contraception. Adolescents were somewhat more likely to use contraception continually when they reported that they could communicate with their mothers at the 6-month follow up, but the direction of the causal link is unclear, especially since communication at the initial interview was unrelated to subsequent birth control practice. The more plausible interpretation appeared to be that adolescents who used contraception regularly were somewhat more willing to speak openly with their mothers about sex and birth control.

As mentioned earlier the data from the second follow up, conducted about 15 months after the initial visit, gathered additional information about the amount and type of communication, repeating items from the previous interviews as well as including some new questions which delved into the content of conversations about the clinic visit. In the following section we review some of the results on the patterns of communication over the duration of the study, beginning with comparable information drawn from the initial and two follow-up interviews. We will make some effort to chart the evolving course of communication and identify some of the major demographic and social characteristics of families with high and low communication. In this analysis, we confine our attention to communication with the mother (or female guardian), reserving for a later paper a discussion of patterns of communication with siblings. There are too few fathers who discussed sex and birth control to include them in the analysis. After we have introduced the data on patterns of mother–daughter communication, we shall then turn to the question of whether and how communication is linked to contraceptive use.

PATTERNS OF MOTHER–DAUGHTER COMMUNICATION ABOUT SEX AND BIRTH CONTROL

There is a high degree of congruence between our findings and the research results referred to earlier showing that, when they communicate at all, many sexually active teenagers experience discomfort or delays in sharing information about sex and birth control with their mothers. Table 11.2 displays the various items from each of the three interviews which tap the extent of mother–daughter communication as reported by the adolescent.

It seems that the majority of teenagers at the first visit generally have

TABLE 11.2. Measures of Family Communication[a]

Numbered item[b]		At initial interview	At 6-month follow up	At 15-month follow up
1. Mom knows of clinic visit (N = 279)	Yes	41	58	72
	No	60	42	28
2. Usually discuss sex and birth control with mom (N = 282)	Yes	39	37	38
	No	62	63	62
3. Never discuss sex and birth control with mom (N = 282)	True	15	17	16
	Not true	85	83	84
4. Told mom about sex (N = 282)	Yes	18		
	No	82		
5. Mom is someone R does not want to know about clinic (N = 282)	True	22		
	Not true	78		
6. Learned of clinic from mom (N = 282)	Yes	10		
	No	90		
7. Discussed sex and birth control with mom in last 4 weeks (N = 274)	Yes			25
	No			76

228

8. R's use of birth control

Mom doesn't know 31
Mom knows, R feels uncomfortable 39
Mom knows, R feels comfortable 30
  (N = 278)

9. Mom and R talk about birth control

Less often 37
About the same 27
More often than others 37
  (N = 271)

---

[a] Data in percentages.

[b] Variables were constructed from the adolescents' responses to the following set of interview questions:

(1) Who, if anyone from your family, knows that you have come here to (this clinic)?

(2) Who, if anyone in your family, do you usually talk with about sex and birth control?

(3) Who, if anyone in your family, do you never talk to about sex and birth control?

(4) Who, in your family, have you told that you are having or planning to have sexual intercourse?

(5) Who, if anyone in your family, do you *not* want to know about (visit to this clinic)?

(6) How did you learn or hear about this clinic?

(7) Who in your family have you talked to in the last 4 weeks about sex and birth control?

(8) Does your (female guardian) know you are currently using birth control or have used it before? And, at the time when you first talked about it with her, how did you feel?

(9) When it comes to talking about using birth control, would you say you and your (female guardian) have talked more often, about the same, or less often than most of your girlfriends and their mothers have talked?

rather limited communication with their mothers about their transition to sexuality and decision to visit a family planning agency for contraception even though most teenagers in our study reported having fairly good overall relations with their mothers. More than two-fifths say that they would be most likely to discuss a personal problem with their mothers (not shown), but when it comes to sexual topics, they are clearly more reticent. At the time of the initial interview, less than one-fifth had told their mothers that they were sexually active, although close to another one-third conjectured that their mother might know anyhow (not shown). This seems likely since two-fifths reported that their mother was aware of their visit to the family planning clinic. In addition, slightly more than one-third indicated that they had been able to discuss sex and birth control with their mothers. Although the majority expect that their mothers would approve of their decision to visit the clinic, close to one-quarter expressed the belief that their mother would not approve (not shown) and about the same proportion indicated that they did not want their mothers to learn of their clinic visit. Only a small minority (10%) had been informed about and directed to the clinic by their mothers.

The impression we get from the initial interview is that at the time of their first clinic visit many teenagers are reluctant to confide in their mothers. They prefer not to talk directly to their mothers about being sexually active although some are willing to have their mothers find out indirectly. A sizable minority took considerable pains not to have their mothers know. These data are consistent with anecdotal information we collected in the course of the field work. Some teenagers, who had not informed their parents of their clinic visits were still willing to have us contact them at home for the interviews even though we alerted them to the possibility that their parents might learn of their contact with the clinic. Others denied us permission to call them at home and worked out other arrangements for completing the interviews.

We asked fewer communication questions at the 6-month follow up. Nonetheless, it is clear that substantive communication with mothers did not greatly change after the initial clinic visit. Roughly the same proportion as in the first interview replied that their mother was someone that they were able to talk to about sexual matters and birth control. A similar proportion replied at the second interview that they would never discuss these subjects with their mother. On the other hand, there was a distinct rise in the proportion of teenagers who said that their mothers knew about the clinic visit by the second interview. Apparently, this fact comes to light even though the mother–daughter communication relationship is unchanged.

As Table 11.2 reveals, the proportion of teenagers who said that their mothers knew about the clinic visit continued to rise, and by the 15-month follow up a substantial majority of the mothers had learned that their daughters received birth control services. Nevertheless, this information does not signify enhanced communication between the teenagers and their mothers. Just about the same proportion as in earlier interviews had discussed sex and birth control with their mothers and roughly the same percentage stated that they would never share these topics with their mother. The preponderance of respondents at both the initial and concluding interviews revealed that they are more likely to talk to a friend or someone outside their family than a parent or sibling abou sex and birth control, and the proportion of those who would confide in a family member remained stable over the course of the study (not shown in Table 11.2).

Most informative of all were the responses to a question in the 15-month interview which asked adolescents whose mothers knew they were using contraception, how comfortable they felt about having shared that information. Among the adolescents who replied that their mothers were aware that they were using birth control, just over one-half (56%) said that they felt somewhat or very uncomfortable talking to their mothers about their contraceptive use. Only 16% reported that they felt completely comfortable in their communications with their mothers.

In the 15-month follow up, adolescents were also asked an open-ended question concerning how their mothers learned they were using contraception. Two-fifths of the teens reporting that their mothers knew they had received contraceptive services indicated that they had volunteered the information. For example, one respondent replied:

> I told her about the clinic visit a couple of weeks before. I just felt she should know. She approved. She thought I should go to the clinic.

Of the respondents one-quarter indicated that their mothers encouraged them to obtain birth control and about one-tenth were accompanied to the clinic by their mothers.

> She took me up there. . . . She thought it was a good idea for me to go because the boy I was going with—he got one girl pregnant.

In another one-fourth of the cases, the mothers found out indirectly when they discovered contraception around the house, were told by someone else, or learned through some other means. Many adolescents reported that this discovery led to a direct inquiry by their mothers, who sometimes expressed anger or sometimes relief at making the discovery. It was not unusual for the teenagers to report that their mothers expressed a mixture of emotions.

I write poetry and I had a notebook sitting on the porch. It was my diary and she read it. She was mad that I don't confront her with it but she was happy I was getting protection.

Not counting the 78 adolescents who reported at the final interview that their mothers still did not know of their clinic visit, the majority of teenagers (56%) indicated that their mothers found out before or at about the time of the initial clinic visit. Still, as we learned earlier, a substantial number of mothers only became informed after the 6-month interview. Although we cannot say for certain, it does not appear from the open-ended comments that girls whose revelations occurred earlier had more extensive discussions with their mothers. Judging from the replies, most adolescents who disclosed the information, whether willingly or unwillingly, earlier or later, received relatively little feedback from their mothers. Few teenagers reported that they had lengthy conversations or received much reenforcement from their mothers, although about four out of five who indicated their mothers' responses to the news perceived that their mothers ultimately approved of the clinic visit.

The accounts from the small number of mothers from whom we had corroborative information seem to bear out the teenager's perceptions about their mothers' support for contraception. The mothers generally supported birth control use if their daughters were sexually active. Still, there is little evidence of open and direct communication in the family, even though the subsample of mothers is biased in the direction of including more mothers who openly communicate with their daughters. Most mothers believe teenagers should learn about sex and birth control in the home. However, one-third of the mothers did not know that their teenagers were sexually active and less than one-third had actually discussed their teenager's sexual activity with them. Similarly, while two-thirds of the mothers knew that one of their teenagers had used a family planning clinic, only one-half of these knew because of direct communication; the remainder inferred that they used contraception from the teenager's behaviors and general conversations. Consistent with reports from teens, mothers generally learn of the clinic visit from their daughters, usually after the fact, although one-third had accompanied their daughters to the clinic on at least one occasion.

When we examined the mother–daughter pair of reports on sex-related communication, we discovered only a modest level of correspondence in the accounts of the two. Mothers apparently believe that they are more communicative and comfortable about discussing sex and birth control than their daughters perceive. Considering that the mothers in the study were only interviewed if their daughters consented to their being contacted, the level of consensus was surprisingly low and the extent of communication, far from ample.

What conditions within the family are associated with high or low levels of communication? In order to answer this question, we took the items listed in Table 11.2 and constructed three indexes of communication, pooling the various measures available from daughters at each interview point. The internal reliability measures of the indexes were quite acceptable (alphas ranged from .64 to .70) and there was a strong association among the three indexes, suggesting that teenagers who reported high or low communication tended to be consistent in their accounts over time.

None of a number of demographic factors was strongly related to the extent of communication in the family. In the initial interview, blacks were more likely to report higher levels of communication, in large part because their mothers more often knew of the clinic visit (59 compared to 21% for whites). This difference in overall levels of communication diminishes over time, as white mothers learn of the news, although even by the final interview, substantial differences persisted between the proportions of black and white teenagers reporting their mothers knew of the clinic visit (86 and 56%, respectively). The socioeconomic status of the parents seems to have little effect on the amount of communication at any time during the study. Finally, we discern little differences in the patterns of communication among older and younger adolescents. Moreover, adolescents who had a prior history of pregnancy or who initiated sex earlier were also not any more likely to report higher levels of communication with their mothers.

Our inability to identify determinants of communication within the family parallels a finding reported by Fox (1981), who also was frustrated in a search for sources of communication within the family. In our study, part of the problem may stem from the fact that we are studying a population of family planning clinic users. Generally, we might expect that girls who seek services probably have better communication about sex and birth control than sexually active teenagers who do not visit clinics. On the other hand, some research suggests that extensive family communication may lead to delay of sexual activity among college-aged women (Lewis, 1973; Spanier, 1977), although this fact remains poorly documented in an adolescent population. If this were true, however, it might limit the variability of communication in our sample of sexually active teenagers in just the opposite direction but with the same effect of hampering our ability to identify the influences of communication. Nevertheless, there is a fairly wide range in the measures of communication, and it is surprising not to be able to account for the patterns of communication.

COMMUNICATION AND CONTRACEPTIVE USE

In a previous paper describing the impact of communication among both mothers and siblings on contraceptive practice at the 6-month follow up, we found little support from our data for our expectation that adolescents who were less secretive about their sexual activity and use of birth control would practice contraception more effectively (Herceg-Baron and Furstenberg, 1982). This finding came as both a surprise and a disappointment.

In view of the fact that our study was still underway at the time we took this initial reading, we advised caution in drawing any firm conclusion from those results. We pointed out that the findings might look different when we examined a longer time interval for a larger sample. Although we had found that communication at the initial interview was not related to birth control practice at 6 months, there was a modest relationship between communication with mothers reported at 6 months and the adolescents' contraceptive use during that interval. While this link probably indicated that communication was a consequence rather than a cause of effective contraceptive practice, we pointed out that the second follow up would provide a better test of our hypothesis that communication in the family promotes and reinforces contraceptive practice. We speculated that the effect of family communication may become more salient over time, when the immediate impact of clinic services begins to fade. At the time, we surmised that as initial motivation wanes, family communication, most particularly the reinforcement provided by the mothers, may become a more critical ingredient for helping the teenager to maintain her commitment to use contraception.

To test the communication hypothesis with our greatly expanded data base, we drew upon the variety of items measuring the extent and type of communication between the mother and daughter presented in Table 11.2. In the analysis which follows, we examined each item separately and pooled sets of items into three indexes of mother–daughter communication about sex and birth control at each of the three interview points. Thus, we could examine the influence of communication both at the initial and 6-month follow up on subsequent contraceptive patterns as well as the current association between communication and birth control practice at the final interview.

Since birth control practice can be tapped in a variety of ways, a good deal of effort was invested in designing the most sensitive and refined measure of contraceptive continuation. Elsewhere we have described the effort to construct a measure which takes into account the problems of reliably capturing the adolescent's behavior (Furstenberg et al., 1983). When data from the 6- and 15-month follow up were contrasted, we discovered that adolescents frequently failed to recall periods of non-use or provide inconsistent accounts of their contraceptive practice. The same question asked at different points in time produced variant responses and different questions posed at the same time also yielded a certain amount of inconsistency.

Our resulting measure of birth control use is a stringent one, for to be counted as a continuous user, an adolescent had to always report use of an effective method during the times she was sexually active, and we removed from the continuous category adolescents who reported imperfect use on *any* of the birth control items included in the two follow ups. Thus, we did not give the respondents the benefit of doubt if they gave us reason to suspect their responses. Once these discrepencies were resolved, we divided the user population into three subgroups: "continuous users" were those who report that they have used effective birth control methods continuously at both follow ups, "intermittent users" were those who report regular but imperfect use, and "ineffective users" were those who reported using birth control irregularly or not at all.* Of the 289 adolescents for whom we had complete histories throughout the study, we discovered that 3% had never initiated sexual activity. Of those who had, 43% had used birth control continuously with no lapses, 23% used birth control most of the time, and the remaining 34% were ineffective users.

Table 11.3 shows the trichotomy of contraceptive use by the array of communication measures at each interview point. While a few of the findings reveal slight differences in the predicted direction showing enhanced contraceptive use among adolescents who report greater communication with their mothers and some differences tend in the opposite direction, none is significant. The overall pattern does not indicate the existence of a link between communication and contraceptive use. Since the individual measures are highly intercorrelated, we examined the association between the three indexes of communication, representing the sum of items at each interview, and contraceptive continuation. Again, evidence in the support of the hypothesis is lacking. None of the indexes of communication was significantly related to contraceptive use.

Reasoning that communication did not necessarily produce the same impact on all adolescents, we introduced some of the demographic variables in order to see if the effect of communication was greater for certain subgroups of the population. Among our data there is some indication that communication may have a greater effect for white ad-

---

*An adolescent was classified as a "continuous user" if she indicated that she began using a reliable method (pill, IUD, diaphragm, or condom) within 1 month of the clinic visit, and continued to use a reliable method all of the time she was sexually active for the duration of the study. An adolescent was classified as an "intermittent user" if she used a reliable method most of the time for the length of the study; that is, if she indicated that she was protected for 80% of the months and 80% of the time during those months that she was sexually active. If an adolescent did not meet these criteria, she was classified as an "ineffective user." Most of those in this group, in fact, used birth control only occasionally or not at all. Those girls who said that they were not sexually active during the study period were excluded from the analysis.

TABLE 11.3. Measures of Family Communication and Birth Control Use[a]

	(1)[a] Mom knows of clinic visit		(2) Usually discussed sex and birth control with mom		(3) Never discussed sex and birth control with mom		(4) Has told mom about sex		(5) R does not want mom to know	
	Yes	No	Yes	No	True	Not true	Yes	No	True	Not true
Initial interview										
Continuous users	38	46	45	41	43	43	47	42	39	44
Intermittent users	26	22	23	24	33	22	22	24	24	23
Ineffective users	36	32	32	35	25	36	31	35	37	33
(N)	(110)	(164)	(105)	(169)	(40)	(234)	(49)	(225)	(59)	(215)
6-month follow up										
Continuous users	44	41	47	41	45	42				
Intermittent users	23	24	22	24	28	23				
Ineffective users	34	35	31	35	28	35				
(N)	(158)	(116)	(99)	(175)	(47)	(227)				
15-month follow up										
Continuous users	44	39	46	40	41	43				
Intermittent users	23	23	21	24	28	22				
Ineffective users	34	39	33	36	30	35				
(N)	(194)	(78)	(106)	(172)	(46)	(232)				

	(6) R Learned of Clinic from mom		(7) R recently discussed sex or birth control with mom		(8) Mom's knowledge of R's birth control use			(9) Mom and R talk about birth control		
	Yes	No	Yes	No	Does not know	Knows/ R feels uncomfortable	Knows/ R feels comfortable	Less often	About the same	More often
Initial interview										
Continuous users	44	43								
Intermittent users	22	24								
Ineffective users	33	34								
(N)	(27)	(247)								
6-month follow up										
Continuous users			44	40						
Intermittent users			23	24						
Ineffective users			33	36						
(N)			(67)	(207)						
15-month follow up										
Continuous users					40	45	42	44	47	37
Moderate users					22	23	24	20	26	23
Ineffective users					38	32	34	35	27	39
(N)					(86)	(109)	(83)	(99)	(73)	(99)

[a] Data in percentages.
[b] Refer to Table 11.2 for list of source questions.

olescents than for blacks. Among whites, the proportion of teenagers using contraception continuously is higher for those who report that they can talk to their mothers about birth control and that their mothers knew of their decision to attend the clinic. Among blacks, we could not even find a trace of evidence that communication was linked to contraceptive use. We caution against relying too much on these racial differences, however, since they are not large enough to result in a statistically significant finding. Without additional evidence, we cannot dismiss the possibility that the small differences we observed are due to random variation.

One additional test was made of the effect of communication on contraceptive use to determine if adolescents might have been given greater support and encouragement to use contraception, directly or indirectly, when their mothers knew about their clinic visit and had spoken to them about contraception. For the two items that were repeated in each of the three interviews, we examined the contraceptive patterns for girls who had continuously high or low patterns of communication compared to those who increased their communication with mothers during the course of the study (no adolescents reported *decreased* communications). While the differences are not large, teenagers who increased their communication had higher levels of continuous use than those who did not (49 vs. 40%, respectively). Interestingly, however, girls who were low at both points in time were not significantly less likely to use birth control effectively than those who were consistently high. Again the findings do not indicate that communication counts for very much. Furthermore, it seems more plausible that communication follows rather than precedes contraceptive use (cf. Fox and Inazu, 1980a). This interpretation is supported by the fact that teenagers were just as likely to use contraception effectively if they improved their communication between the first and second follow up as between the initial interview and first follow up. This finding suggests that girls who were using contraception regularly eventually divulged the secret, but they are just as likely to do it later than sooner; whether they do it later or sooner does not seem to affect their use of contraception.

Thus far we have relied exclusively on the reports of the adolescents to gauge the level of family communication. As mentioned earlier, data were also collected from 95 mothers who constituted a subsample which is distinctly biased in the direction of including mothers who have higher levels of communication with their teenagers. Nevertheless, as we discussed earlier, many of these mothers had limited communication with their adolescent children. Therefore, it is possible to examine the relationship between the mothers' reports about communication and the daughter's use of contraception. If communication matters, we might expect to find that mothers who feel freer to talk to their teenagers and who report knowledge of their visit to the clinic would encourage more effective contraceptive practice.

We examined a series of questions from the mothers' interview measuring the extent of communication with their children about sex and birth control. None of the items was significantly related to the daughter's birth control performance. Once again, we are led to the conclusion that communication between mothers and daughters does not significantly alter an adolescent's ability to practice contraception effectively.

Before rejecting our hypothesis, we must consider one additional contingency to which we alluded earlier. The level of communication would be less influential than the emotional tone of the conversations or the specific message conveyed by the mother. As we observed in the preceding section, not all mothers who communicate with their adolescents do so in a style which supports or reinforces use of birth control. The initial interview and first follow up did not contain sufficient information to measure the content of communication other than an item asking adolescents who had confided in their parents whether or not they approved of their use of birth control and their decision to attend the clinic. Both of these item were unrelated to subsequent patterns of contraceptive use.

In the final interview, we probed more deeply about the nature of communication, asking a retrospective question about how the mother learned of the clinic visit. This open-ended question was coded to tap the degree to which the mother actively initiated the conversation and whether she was perceived by the adolescent to support her visit to the clinic. Neither of these dimensions of communication related to contraceptive continuation.

If contraceptive use by the adolescent does not seem to be affected by the amount and type of communication, it is still possible that the mother's influence is visible in other ways. Given the difficulties many teenagers have in using contraception and the possible concerns that parents might express about the health and safety of birth control methods, perhaps we ought to look elsewhere to detect the guidance of the parent. If parental input matters, then we might expect to discover that adolescents who had more open and active communication with their mothers would be more likely to return to family planning visits for a check up within the recommended time.

Data on clinic return visits, extracted from the records maintained by the clinics, were added to the data file, enabling us to examine the relationship between family communication and clinic continuation. We ran the analysis in a variety of ways, considering both the number of return visits and the timing of such visits. No significant association appeared between the mother–daughter communication or the mother's knowledge of the clinic visit at either the initial interview or 6-month follow up and the pattern of clinic use. There was a slight relationship between timeliness of return visits and the mother's knowledge of clinic use at the 15-month follow up. However, the evidence again points to the interpretation that communication is a consequence rather than a cause of clinic attendance. Adolescents who return on time are often more likely to share the information with their parents, but adolescents who share the information before or soon after visiting the clinic for the first time are not significantly more likely to return for a check up.

DISCUSSION AND CONCLUSIONS

A popular but untested belief among both policy makers and some practitioners is that adolescents will be more likely to use birth control effectively if their parents, especially their mothers, have knowledge of their need for services and support their decision to visit a family planning clinic. We specifically tested and found no support for the assumption that a mother's knowledge of the clinic visit enhances a teenager's ability to use contraception effectively, although in our study the information about the clinic visit was volunteered by the adolescent. It seems unlikely that a policy of notifying her parents about adolescent clinic visits will produce any more positive results.

We also discovered that knowledge of the clinic visit, although associated with greater communication in the family, frequently occurred in the face of little or no discussion between mother and daughter. The proportion of adolescents who said that their mothers knew that they had received contraceptive services, rose from 41 to 72 during the course of the study but the number of teenagers who reported that they could talk to their mothers about sex and birth control did not change at all. Clearly, in most families, the information that the adolescent is using birth control does not stimulate greater involvement with the mother.

Even when discussions do occur, they seem to contribute very little if at all to the adolescent's ability to practice contraception effectively. Using a variety of measures, we looked for evidence that communication with mothers influenced the patterns of birth control use or return to the family planning clinic. We were repeatedly led to the conclusion that communication with parents is not very significant in promoting contraception compliance among sexually active teenagers.

Why this is so remains an intriguing question. Based on discussions we have had with parents of adolescents, we suspect that there are several different reasons the influence of parents is so slight. First, it appears as though most parents do not want to get directly involved and, certainly, most teenagers are reluctant to encourage involvement.

Most parents would prefer that their teenagers defer sexual activity, but seem resigned to the fact that their views are not likely to be the single determining factor. Recognizing that sexual activity is likely to take place, parents want to be sure that their daughters avoid pregnancy. Consequently, many are relieved to discover that their teenagers are obtaining contraception. Beyond that, it seems that most are either willing or prefer to respect the adolescent's privacy. In any event, few feel equipped to become directly involved in monitoring the adolescent's sexual behavior.

Parents acknowledge either directly or implicitly that their teenagers are more likely to consult with peers or other adults for advice about sexual relationships. Many more of the teens in our study shared information with their sisters than with their parents, and even more consulted with their girlfriends. Whether one believes this pattern is appropriate or undesirable, the parents we talked with were generally realistic about how much influence they can exert (Herceg-Baron and Shea, 1982). As Fox (1981) has so perceptively observed, most parents shift from acting as protector to serving as guides when their children enter adolescence. They attempt to forestall the sexual transition, but when it occurs, are forced to adopt a different strategy. At best, they can provide resources in the form of information and advice to their children, but they are probably incapable of regulating their behavior. Our results seem to support Fox's description of the changing role of parents when their children pass from virginity to non-virginity.

Does this mean that family planning agencies ought not to attempt to involve parents in their service programs? We continue to support the burgeoning efforts of many programs to reach out to parents, particularly parents of their adolescent clients. Our discussions with parents reveal that many want and need information which may equip them to act more authoratively in providing sexual guidance to their children. Some parents want to communicate more comfortably with their teenagers, others want to marshall as much information as they can to try to dissuade their adolescents from engaging in sexual activity, and others only want to know enough to direct their teenagers to outside agencies for services. Clearly, one preventive program approach with a single message will not satisfy the diverse needs of parents.

We believe that parents have a desire to be better informed about adolescent sexuality and communication techniques and that public and private health care and social service agencies should assume a more active role in educating and working with parents—family planning services are no exception. They have a special obligation to assist parents, in general, and parents of adolescent clients, in particular, who want to expand their educational and supportive role. Family planning agencies are designing and offering programs to direct more attention to parents and community education, but these efforts can only be part of a comprehensive strategy. One promising approach which has hardly been developed is wider use of mass media, especially radio, television, and home video cassettes. We anticipate tremendous change in the receptivity of the mass media to sex educational programs directed at parents and teenagers.

In the meantime, we hold out little hope for the effectiveness of efforts to mandate parental involvement. The data from our study, which is admittedly not the final word, provides compelling evidence that compulsory notification of parents whose adolescents enroll in family planning services is not likely to be beneficial to teenagers, at least in regard to their improved use of contraception. There is nothing in our analysis that warrants changing the conclusion we reached from our earlier analysis of the data. We said then and we reiterate now that it appears far wiser to adopt a flexible approach to involving parents in family planning agencies by experimentation and evaluation of a variety of family-oriented programs than to mandate rigid and bureaucratic solutions that are untested and probably unworkable.

REFERENCES

Ager, J. W., Shea, F. P., and Agronow, S. J. Method discontinuance in teenage women: Implications for teen contraceptive programs. In I. R. Stuart and C. F. Wells (Eds.), Pregnancy in adolescence: Needs, problems, and management. New York: Van Nostrand Reinhold Company, 1982.

Coughlin, D., and Perales C. Family planning and the teenager: A service delivery assessment. Report to the Secretary of Health, Education, and Welfare, New York, November, 1978.

Fox, G. L., and Inazu, J. K. Patterns and outcomes of mother-daughter communication about sexuality. Journal of Social Issues, 1980, 36, 7–29. (a)

Fox, G. L., and Inazu, J. K. Mother-daughter communication about sex. Family Relations, 1980, 29, 347–352. (b)

Fox, G. L. The family's role in adolescent sexual behavior. In T. Ooms (Ed.), Teenage pregnancy in a family context. Philadelphia: Temple University Press, 1981.

Furstenberg, F. F., Jr. Birth control experience among pregnant adolescents: The process of unplanned parenthood. Social Problems, 1971, 19, 192–203.

Furstenberg, F. F., Jr., Herceg-Baron, R., Jemail, J. Bringing in the family: Kinship support and adolescent contraceptive behavior. In T. Ooms (Ed.), Adolescent pregnancy in a family context. Philadelphia: Temple University Press, 1981.

Furstenberg, F. F., Jr., Lincoln, R., and Menken, J. Teenage sexuality, pregnancy, and childbearing. Philadelphia: University of Pennsylvania Press, 1981.

Furstenberg, F. F., Jr., Shea, J., Allison, P., Herceg-Baron, R., and Webb, D. Patterns of contraceptive use among adolescent clients in family planning clinics: A longitudinal study. Paper presented at the annual meeting of the Population Association of America, Pittsburgh, April, 1983.

Herceg-Baron, R., and Furstenberg, F. F., Jr. Adolescent contraceptive use: The impact of family support systems. *In* G. L. Fox (Ed.), *The childbearing decision: Fertility attitudes and behavior.* Beverly Hills: Sage Publications, 1982.

Herceg-Baron, R., and Shea, J. *Mother-daughter sex-related communications: Implications for family planning providers.* Report submitted to Bureau of Community Health Services, Office of Adolescent Pregnancy Prevention, December, 1982.

Herold, E., and Goodwin, M. Why adolescents go to birth control clinics rather than to family physicians. *Canadian Journal of Public Health*, 1979, *70*, 317–319.

Jessor, S. L., and Jessor, R. Transitions from virginity to nonvirginity among youth: A social psychological study over time. *Developmental Psychology*, 1975, *11*, 473–484.

Lewis, R. A. Parents and peers: Socialization agents in the coital? Behavior of young adults. *Journal of Sex Research*, 1973, *9*, 157–170.

Mendick, B., and Oskamp, S. Individual differences among adolescent contraceptors: Some implications for intervention. *In* I. R. Stuart and C. F. Wells (Eds.), *Pregnancy in adolescence: needs, problems, and management.* New York: Van Nostrand Reinhold Company, 1982.

Ooms, T. (Ed.). *Adolescent pregnancy in a family context.* Philadelphia: Temple University Press, 1981.

Philliber, S. Socialization for childbearing. *Journal of Social Issues*, 1980, *36*, 30–44.

Shea, J. *An annotated bibliography of family involvement.* Prepared for the Office of Adolescent Family Life Program, Washington, D.C., 1983.

Shea, J., Herceg-Baron, R., and Furstenberg, F. F., Jr. *Clinic and contraceptive use of adolescent clients.* Paper presented at the annual meeting of the National Family Planning and Reproductive Health Association, Washington, D.C., March, 1983.

Spanier, G. B. Sources of sex information and premarital sexual behavior. *Journal of Sex Research*, 1977, *13*, 73–88.

Torres, A., Forrest, J. D., and Eisman, S. Telling parents: Clinic policies and adolescents' use of family planning and abortion services. *Family Planning Perspectives*, 1980, *12*, 284–292.

Torres, A., Forrest, J. D., and Eisman, S. Family planning services in the United States, 1978–1979. *Family Planning Perspectives*, 1981, *13*, 132–141.

Zelnik, M., and Kantner, J. F. Sexual activity, contraceptive use and pregnancy among metropolitan-area teenagers: 1971–1979. *Family Planning Perspectives*, 1980, *12*, 230–237.

Zelnik, M., Kantner, J. F., and Ford, K. *Sex and pregnancy in adolescence.* Beverly Hills: Sage Publications, 1981.

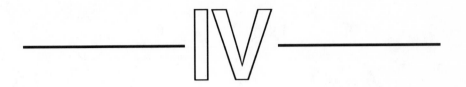

COMPARATIVE DIMENSIONS: SPECIES, HISTORY, AND CULTURE

12

ADOLESCENT PREGNANCIES IN NON-HUMAN PRIMATES: AN ECOLOGICAL AND DEVELOPMENTAL PERSPECTIVE

Jeanne Altmann

INTRODUCTION

From the standpoint of natural selection, reduction in age of first reproduction potentially will have major advantages, both by increasing the number of offspring and by reducing generation time. All other things being equal, we would expect any heritable trait that reduced age of first reproduction to spread in a population over successive generations. What, we might then ask, limits the reduction of reproductive onset in primates, human and non-human, and why might "all other things" not be equal? Anthropoid primates, monkeys and apes, have an unusually long prereproductive period for mammals of their size and there is higher mortality risk for first offspring than for ones born later. These facts suggest that primates may be pushing the limits of the cost/benefit balance of accelerating reproductive onset. Our recognition among humans of a category of pregnancies that we refer to as "adolescent pregnancies" suggests that there are some special characteristics of pregnancies that occur to unusually young females. I shall focus, below, on the thesis that adequate adult functioning, including successful reproduction, depends on maturation of a number of different somatic and behavioral systems and that these various systems differ in the conditions and degree to which they are subject to acceleration. Whether reproductive acceleration is advantageous or disadvantageous will depend on the extent to which other critical developmental processes are also accelerated under those conditions that accelerate attainment of reproductive maturity.

247

What do we mean by adolescent pregnancies? Do they exist in non-human primates? Most people agree on what pregnancies fall within the category of adolescent pregnancies—at least while we restrict our discussion to humans, to our own culture, and to recent times. As soon as we expand our perspective, however, we suddenly realize that our intuitive idea rests on a number of implicit assumptions about the time course of normal development and the potential consequences of deviation. We find that these assumptions may be difficult to explicate and that they may be more culturally, historically, and species bound than we thought (see Chapter 2 by Lancaster, Chapter 3 by Eveleth, Chapter 6 by Worthman, Chapter 14 by Whiting *et al.*, and Chapter 15 by Vinovskis). By expanding our time frame and the populations that we examine, we are forced to consider what the basic issues are that lead us to single out, and be concerned about, adolescent pregnancy.

Researchers have always categorized as an adult any monkey female who has given birth to an infant. In fact, the presence of a pregnancy that has been carried to term is taken as prima facie evidence that the female is no longer just an adolescent who is experiencing menstrual cycles, but rather that she is an adult. We might note that the other monkeys seem to make the same distinction as the human observers do. That is, there seems to be an implicit assumption that reproductive maturity is appropriately coupled with other aspects of physical maturity and with psychological and social maturity as well, and that a monkey has completed the essential aspects of her "school of life" as well as having achieved internal maturation by the time she gives birth to her first infant.

It is the assumption of this synchrony of development that seems to be at the core of any consideration of adolescent pregnancy. Adolescent pregnancies are those that occur as a result of some degree of developmental dyssynchrony, those pregnancies that occur before other aspects of development are as complete as usual, or as is considered to be desirable for both the parent and the infant. What, then, do we know of normal developmental synchrony in non-human primates; what are the conditions under which reproduction is accelerated; and what are the consequences of this acceleration and of any developmental dyssynchrony or new synchronies that result? These are the questions explored in the several sections below, starting first with a brief overview of patterns of maturation and reproduction in anthropoid primates.

REPRODUCTION AND PREADOLESCENT MATURATION

Relative to other mammals of comparable size, anthropoid primates might be considered as poor reproducers: in ecological jargon they are characterized as K-selected (Mc Naughton and Wolf, 1973). That is, monkeys and apes have relatively long gestations and long infant and juvenile stages, small litter size (usually only one), and a long interval between successive births (Sacher and Staffeldt, 1974; Western, 1979; Eisenberg, 1981). Although these reproductive deficits, both later onset of reproduction and lower rate of reproduction, may be partially compensated for by a somewhat longer adult span (Sacher, 1978), the primary compensation probably must occur through mortality reduction at earlier life stages. Infancy is the period of highest mortality in non-human primates as it is in humans and most other mammals (Caughley, 1966). Features of a parent's physical, psychological, and social condition may be particularly important to offspring survival in primates.

We shall take as our baseline, or norm, the patterns of reproduction and development that are found in wild, unprovisioned animals that are living with a sufficiently normal complement of predators or other natural hazards that the population is approximately stable in age-sex distribution and stationary in total size. We shall then explore conditions that diverge from this and consider the developmental consequences of the divergence. The available data for these explorations are predominantly from the larger, primarily ground-dwelling monkeys, the macaques of Asia, and the baboons of Africa, and, to a lesser extent from chimpanzees. Because the author's work is on savannah baboons, *Papio cynocephalus*, and because some of the most extensive available developmental data are for this species, these animals will be used for illustration.

Baboons and macaques, like most anthropoids other than the small, monogamous monkeys who provide extensive paternal care, give birth to a single offspring (Schultz, 1948; Leutenegger, 1979). In Amboseli National Park where we have conducted a longitudinal study of baboons since 1971, over one-hundred pregnancies have resulted in only one instance of live-born twins and one other of stillborn twins. The single primate young has a tenacious grip (Hines, 1942) that enables it to ride close against its mother's ventrum. There, a baboon infant obtains warmth, access to the nipple, and transportation as its mother spends three-quarters of the daytime walking and feeding to obtain nutrition for them both (Altmann, 1980). Among savannah baboon species, an adult male, usually the one within the multi-male social group who is likely to be the infant's father, will probably provide some active as well as passive care for the infant (see e.g., Altmann, 1978; Packer, 1979; Stein, 1984). However, the burden of most care falls to the mother in this as well as other nonmonogamous species.

Possible maternal weight loss during the months of infant care (e.g., Whichelow, 1976, for humans and a review for several mammalian species in Widdowson, 1976) and effects of nursing on prolactin levels

(Konner and Worthman, 1980, for humans), results in a prolonged postpartum amenorrhea, which lasts anywhere from 6 to 18 months in Amboseli baboons. Thereafter, the infant or young juvenile still depends on individuals and on the group as a whole for occasional care, warmth at night, learning opportunities, and predator warning and defense. By 1–1½ years of age a youngster can obtain its own nutrition (S. Altmann, unpublished data) and has a fairly good chance of survival without maternal care (J. Altmann, 1980). A long juvenile period follows—a fascinating developmental stage for which there has been a paucity of research (but for illuminating exceptions see Lancaster, 1971 for vervet monkeys; Owens 1975a,b and Pereira 1984 for baboons). Although mortality remains high for young juvenile baboons, the later juvenile years, from about age 3–5 for females and 5½ or 6 for males is one of low mortality, relative independence, much play, and changing dominance relationships accompanied by relatively frequent aggressive interactions (Altmann, 1980; Pereira, 1984; Altmann et al., unpublished data).

ADOLESCENCE

The transition from the juvenile period to that of adolescence is delineated in many species by the presence of externally visible indicators of reproductive maturation. For females this usually means presence of sex skin swellings or particular other skin swellings or coloration, externally visible menstruation, or onset of estrous behavior. For males, descent or enlargement of testes or changes in skin coloration are diagnostic features of adolescence or "subadulthood."

In seasonally breeding macaques, the females usually first become pregnant in the breeding season the year after the one in which they first exhibit estrous behavior, coloration, and swelling (see review in Lancaster, Chapter 2, this volume). In savannah baboons, in which breeding is not restricted to a single season, first pregnancy occurs 6–15 months after the first menstrual cycle (Altmann et al., 1977, 1981; Scott, 1984). This is approximately four cycles after the components of the female's menstrual cycle (Altmann et al., unpublished data), and other characteristics of the cycle (Scott, 1984) are the same as those for fully adult females. In the great apes, too, there is a period of adolescent subfertility; 2–3 years elapse between onset of cycles and first pregnancy in wild chimpanzees (Tutin and McGinnis, 1981) and gorillas (Harcourt et al., 1980; Fossey, 1982). The duration of adolescent subfertility among baboon and macaque females is at least partially physiological. In addition, there may also be a social component because fully adult males do not form consorts with these adolescents until their cycles are indistinguishable, by our external daily observations (Altmann *et al.*, unpublished data), from those of adults (see also similar results in Scott, 1984).

For adolescent males, social factors appear to be even more important in preventing reproduction. Macaques and baboons, like most primates, are sexually dimorphic and to some extent polygynous. Males are in competition with each other for access to fertile females. Adolescent males are appreciably smaller than adult males, have not yet fully developed secondary sexual characteristics, and are subordinate to the adult males in the dominance hierarchy. Although juvenile males occasionally mate briefly with fertile adult females without much reaction from adult males, for the most part adolescent males are actively prevented from mating. In Amboseli, it is not until the end of adolescence, when the male is within the size range of fully adult males, has fully developed canines, and achieves a rapid rise in dominance, that he can successfully compete with adult males for reproductive access to fertile adult females (Altmann *et al.*, in press). Before that time, his matings are almost exclusively with females who are also adolescents (see also Rostal and Eaton, 1983, for captive macaques and Scott, 1984, for another population of baboons) or with adult females at times that they are not likely to conceive.

Adolescence, then, encompasses an extended period that spans the transition from partial to complete reproductive competence. In addition, it is also a period during which other aspects of maturation proceed. For both males and females it is a period of continued growth (Watts and Gaven, 1982). It is during adolescence that most of the sexual dimorphism in weight develops. Apparently this is partially due to steeper weight velocity curves in males, but is also as a result of weight gain that continues until age 8–10 among baboon males, for example, and only until about age 6 or 7 for baboon females.

Adolescence, like the late juvenile period, is one of high survivorship. Adolescent males and females probably continue to acquire knowledge and skills during this period, the benefits of which may not be seen until several years later when females must simultaneously care for themselves and a neonate and when young males of most species leave their natal group to survive alone, if sometimes only briefly, and to make their way into a new group where they will live and reproduce as an adult.

Social maturation also proceeds during adolescence. Some data are available regarding attainment of dominance relationships in wild baboons. For baboon males, adolescence may be a period of temporary stability in dominance relationships. Baboon males are dominant to most or all adult females by the onset of adolescence, and they do not challenge adult males until the end of the period (Hausfater *et al.*, unpublished data). Among females, during adulthood, dominance relationships change only rarely and, during maturation, daughters achieve dominance over members of families to whom their mothers were dominant (Hausfater *et al.*, 1982). Most of this transition occurs before the onset of menstrual cycles (Walters, 1980; Scott, 1984), but some relationships remain unstable until the end of adolescence.

In a number of species, it has been reported that older juvenile and adolescent females play and fight less than do their male peers and interact with infants more than do the males (e.g., Lancaster, 1971; Pereira and Altmann, 1985, and references therein). However, major questions about adolescent behavior remain unanswered. For no wild primates do we have measures of the magnitude, sources, or consequences of the variability in performance of these behaviors, either among individuals, between sexes, or among populations or species; the data for provisioned and captive animals also remain limited (see review in Caine, 1985).

In summary, the period of adolescence in anthropoid primates is one of growth and maturation, physical and behavioral. Although the very limited available behavioral data pertain to social interactions, there is every reason to believe that individual skill attainment and other aspects of behavioral development are as important a feature of this period as those more obvious characteristics that have been reported.

REPRODUCTIVE ACCELERATION

It has recently become well-documented, particularly for savannah baboons and for Japanese macaques, that captivity, or even artificial food provisioning in the wild, results in greater weight gains throughout maturation, in lower age of onset of adolescence, and in earlier age of first reproduction (Altmann *et al.*, 1977, 1981; Coe *et al.*, 1979; Mori, 1979; Harcourt *et al.*, 1980; Sugiyama and Ohsawa, 1982; Nicolson, 1982). In addition, interbirth intervals (essentially the duration of infancy) are shorter, and average annual survivorship for both infants and adults is increased. For baboons, a schematic diagram of these dramatic differences appears in Fig. 12.1.

The main comparative studies of Japanese macaques are a result of different amounts of food provisioning, or absence of provisioning, in otherwise either wild or at least free-ranging animals (e.g., Mori, 1979; Sugiyama and Ohsawa, 1982). These authors have usually studied the effects of different feeding regimes on the same groups of animals. Additional data are available from captive animals. The data for baboons result from comparisons of wild savannah baboons with those in captivity (e.g., Snow, 1967; Altmann *et al.*, 1977, 1981; Nicolson, 1982; Coehlo, 1985). Limited data are also becoming available for ba-

BABOONS

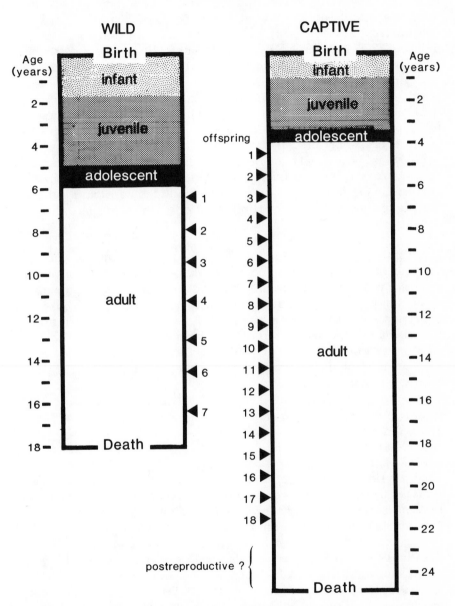

FIGURE 12.1. Schematic diagram of differences in reproductive patterns between wild and captive baboons.

boons under conditions of varying food availability, natural or human-produced, in the wild (Strum and Western, 1982; Altmann *et al.*, unpublished data). The data for chimpanzees come from wild animals with limited and varying amount of food provisioning and from captive animals (Coe *et al.*, 1979; Tutin and McGinnis, 1981, Pusey, 1983). It is often the case that data pertaining to a particular issue or to changes in a certain variable are not available for each species. Where comparable data are available for several species, they are in at least qualitative agreement, with the exception that Chism *et al.* (1984) found no difference in reproductive parameters between captive and wild patas monkeys, *Erythrocebus patas*.

Below, is constructed a tentative scenario for the effects of food provisioning or a high nutritional plane on the time course of development. This has been done by pooling and piecing together data for these various species and conditions and by making extrapolations and predictions from the limited data base.

1. *From birth, weight gain is greater in food-supplemented conditions than otherwise and the difference in weight between the two conditions increases with age.* This has been a consistent finding, for several taxa, of the many studies that have been previously cited. Anatomical and physiological constraints on prenatal development and parturition probably limit the possible variability in birth weight itself (see Schultz, 1969, and Napier and Napier, 1970, for anatomical constraints, and Riopelle and Hale 1975 for reduction in gestation length when full-term weight is reached earlier).

2. *Weight is more accelerated than skeletal growth and skeletal growth more than tooth eruption* (Mori, 1979; Altmann *et al.*, 1981; Sigg *et al.*, 1982).

3. *Menarche occurs earlier in food-enriched situations, perhaps as a result of greater weight or of body fat accumulation but age, or some other physical variable that is less food-sensitive than weight, is also a factor in determining age of menarche, resulting in attainment of reproductive functioning at a lower weight in low-nutrition than in high-nutrition animals.* Among primates, the importance of minimal weight or fat accumulation has been best studied for humans (e.g., Frisch and Revelle, 1969, and sequelae; see also discussion in Lancaster, this volume, Chapter 2). The non-human evidence comes primarily from the studies of Mori (1979) and of Sugiyama and Ohsawa (1982) on Japanese macaques. Mori discusses the fact that older low-weight females for whom menarche has been delayed do reach menarche after a few years delay, despite low weight.

4. *Age of first conception is also accelerated in food-enriched situations (references as previously noted). However, this seems to be pri-*

*marily a result of earlier attainment of menarche, that is, the length
of adolescent subfertility is less reduced than is the age of menarche.*
The data are primarily the same as those for menarche but the period
of subfertility is not itself usually reported. It appears that the duration
of subfertility is at least partially a function of the time needed for full
hormonal developmental and coordination which is not food-limited
in the ecological sense (e.g., McNaughton and Wolf, 1973). See, for
example, Reiter, Chapter 4 this volume, for a review of the human
data.

5. *If the food enrichment is through provision of a concentrated
source, social differences favoring early and more successful reproduction in high-ranking animals are exaggerated relative to their occurrence in unprovisioned, lower-nutrition conditions.* The evidence
for this is primarily from the work on Japanese macaques cited above.
An important point for future research is the need to distinguish the
effects of food enrichment at the group level and the extent to which
food enrichment is equally available to all members of the group. This
distinction is important whether the enrichment is human-produced or
otherwise. Some natural foods may be readily monopolizable, such as
fruiting trees; others such as grass corms are not (e.g., Wrangham,
1980). Likewise, although human-produced food enrichment usually
results in concentrated resources to which high-ranking animals have
greater access, this need not necessarily be the case. One would expect
these two types of changes in overall food abundance to have different
effects on social-class differences in reproduction.

6. *Food provisioning or other human-enrichment situations tend to
produce higher survival rates as well as high reproductive rates, population growth, a larger proportion of immature animals in the population, at least in the short run, and larger kin groups and maturing
age cohorts* (e.g., Altmann and Altmann, 1979; Southwick et al., 1980;
Berman, 1980). These social factors may interact with the direct nutritional effects, perhaps magnifying them through social facilitation (e.g.,
Vandenbergh and Drickamer, 1974; Vandenbergh, 1977; models in Silk
and Boyd, 1983). However, at high animal densities the social effects
may produce reproductive delay or other suppression, particularly for
low-dominance status animals (e.g., Dunbar and Dunbar, 1977; Dunbar, 1984; see also review of reproductive facilitation and suppression
in McClintock, 1981).

7. *Infant survivorship may not be as great for first-born infants in
high-nutrition situations as would be predicted based on the improved
survival for later-born offspring* (see review in Lancaster, this volume,
Chapter 2). The data are, as yet, quite inadequate on this point but it
may be that there is higher risk from inadequate skeletal development
and from the greater social pressures that occur particularly for low-

ranking females in the high-density, often captive, situations in which high nutrition studies have been conducted.

As tentative or speculative as some of the preceding conclusions are, most arise fairly directly from existing data, albeit limited in some cases. In the next section, however, it will be necessary to move further from existing data as we consider potential consequences of differential changes in developmental rates.

DEVELOPMENTAL DYSSYNCHRONY AND ADOLESCENT PREGNANCIES

If all aspects of physical, psychological, and social development occurred apace, population biologists, cross-cultural anthropologists, and students of historical change would still surely find the acceleration of interest, but the question of adolescent pregnancies would not arise. It is the situation of differential effects on aspects of development, in particular the situation in which first pregnancies occur at an earlier stage relative to other aspects of development, that leads us to consider some mothers as still being adolescents and to speculate on the possible detrimental consequences for them and for their offspring.

With respect to dyssynchrony of physical development, the data suggest that under conditions of food enrichment a monkey female will give birth to her first infant not only at a younger age but at a smaller skeletal size and less complete dental development than she would otherwise. Consequently, although a higher nutritional plane could result in less competition between a mother and her fetus or offspring for nutrients, and probably does for older mothers, adolescent mothers and their offspring may be in greater competition over nutrients, particularly those nutrients, such as calcium, that are in high demand for skeletal growth. Thus, food enrichment probably results in better nutrition and better health for both high parity mothers and their infants but it may put adolescent primiparous females at higher risk. One would expect this relationship to be some U-shaped function of nutrition rather than a linear one.

Laboratory data suggest that first-born infants have a lower birth weight than infants born later (e.g., Broadhurst and Jinks, 1965; see also Lancaster, Chapter 2, this volume). Although this may put the infants at greater risk as in humans (Van Valen and Mellin, 1967; also see Garn, this volume), low birth weight may also have the positive effect of facilitating parturition in a mother whose skeletal development is less complete. If one were able to increase infant birth weight it might be at the cost of greater problems at parturition, at least in many of the monkeys which, like humans, have potential problems of infant "fit" during birth, and in contrast to the great apes that do not (Schultz, 1969). These birth and infant survival problems would be greatest for those monkeys, such as squirrel monkeys, that naturally have the greatest birth-proportion problems. Moreover, anthropoid species seem to vary in the stage of growth at which they reach menarche and at which they first reproduce (Rowell, 1977; Watts, 1985). Cross-species predictions and comparative studies should be highly informative for understanding the range of physical developmental synchrony and its consequences.

As little as is known about dyssynchrony in physical development, it is still greater than the information available on factors that accelerate behavioral development, both individual and social, and the potential dyssynchronies that might arise when reproductive maturation is accelerated. One obvious concern is whether the time needed for learning about foods and the home range, and the time necessary for development of foraging skills, and social skills used in grooming, aggression, mating, and care of infants can be reduced, and whether it is reduced under conditions that accelerate reproductive maturation. It is quite possible that learning can be, and is, appropriately accelerated because abundant food supply reduces the time spent foraging and frees more time for leisure activities (Altmann, 1980; Lee, 1984; Brennan *et al.*, 1984; Altmann *et al.*, unpublished data), but this has not been studied.

Another potentially important kind of dyssynchrony arises when we consider the attainment of adult dominance rank. As discussed above, for example, Amboseli baboons have attained their usually permanent dominance rank by the time they conceive their first infant. If reproductive maturation is accelerated, is attainment of dominance rank comparably accelerated? If not, does this result in detrimental levels of stress and disruption for the female and her infant if these rank-change interactions occur after reproduction begins? It is unknown.

Two factors appear to be potentially important in determining whether a consequential dyssynchrony results from reproductive acceleration. The first is related to the reduction in time needed to obtain and process food that usually occurs in high-nutrition situations. If this time is used to increase the rate and time spent in social and other behavioral activities whose development would otherwise be relatively retarded, and if an increased density of these activities within a shorter period and at an earlier age can result in the same level of maturation, then dyssynchrony may not occur; otherwise it probably will. Second, there is probably a range of synchrony, not just a particular set amount, that is within the animals' range of response without any detriment to functioning. The amount of reproductive acceleration or variability that normally occurs as a result of temporal and spatial variability in food available to different groups or populations or to successive age cohorts may well be within the animals' range of response; that due to major upheavals or change such as coming in contact with human-provided food sources may not be. An understanding of both of these factors would contribute considerably to a basic understanding of developmental plasticity as well as to the specific questions of interest here.

CONCLUSION

An exploration of issues involved in adolescent pregnancies in nonhuman primates raises many questions about the meshing of developmental events. These have not been the subject of investigation in primate studies, neither for normal development nor with respect to situations that change the developmental time course. This is an example of a situation in which study of an important human problem leads us to interesting basic questions about non-humans. However, the benefit is potentially in the other direction as well. The very fact that this sometimes culture-bound and emotional topic contains elements that are of general developmental importance across species, suggests that non-human primates might also provide useful animal models for the study of adolescent pregnancies, with contributions both from comparative studies of well-chosen contrasting primate species and from in-depth investigations of developmental variability within a single species or even population.

Finally, we should bear in mind that we have considered only one situation in which *relative* acceleration of reproduction can occur, albeit probably the one most common in human and non-human primates. Reproductive maturation will also occur early in the life cycle relative to other aspects of maturation if there is delay of other aspects of physical, or, more likely behavioral maturation, for example, by increasing demands for skills that a functioning adult needs in a complex society. The dyssynchronies that result are likely to have some, but not all, features in common with those that have already commanded our attention.

ACKNOWLEDGMENTS

Many of the ideas for this manuscript were developed as a direct result of the SSRC Conference on Adolescent Pregnancies. I am grateful to the conference organizers and to the other participants. My research in Kenya is conducted under the sponsorship of the Institute of Primate Research, National Museums of Kenya. Thanks are due to the Institute and the other individuals and agencies in Kenya who facilitate our work there. The Amboseli Baboon Research Project has benefited from the financial support of the Harry Frank Guggenheim Foundation, the Spencer Committee of the University of Chicago, the National Institutes of Health, and the National Science Foundation. Assistance with literature sources and with manuscript preparation were provided by Victoria Drake and Carolyn Johnson. Jane Lancaster made helpful comments on an earlier draft.

REFERENCES

Altmann, J. Infant independence in yellow baboons. In G. Burghardt and M. Bekoff (Eds.), The development of behavior. New York: Garland STPM Press, 1978, pp. 253–277.

Altmann, J. Baboon mothers and infants. Cambridge, Mass.: Harvard University Press, 1980.

Altmann, J., Altmann, S.A., Hausfater, G., and McCuskey, S. Life history of yellow baboons: physical development, reproductive parameters, and infant mortality. Primates, 1977, 18, 315–330.

Altmann, J., Altmann, S.A., and Hausfater, G. Physical maturation and age estimates of yellow baboons, Papio cynocephalus. American Journal of Primatology, 1981, 1, 389–399.

Altmann, J., Altmann, S.A., and Hausfater, G. Determinants of reproductive success in savannah baboons (Papio cynocephalus). In T. Clutton-Brock (Ed.), Reproductive success. Chicago: University of Chicago Press, 1985, in press.

Altmann, S.A., and Altmann, J. Demographic constraints on behavior and social organization. In I.S. Bernstein and E.O. Smith (Eds.), Primate ecology and human origins. New York: Garland STPM Press, 1979, pp. 47–63.

Berman, C.M. Mother-infant relationships among free-ranging rhesus monkeys on Cayo Santiago: a comparison with captive pairs. Animal Behaviour, 1980, 28, 860–873.

Brennan, J., Else, J., Altmann, J., and Lee, P. Ecology and behaviour of vervet monkeys in a tourist lodge habitat. International Journal of Primatology, 1984, 5, 324 (Abstr.).

Broadhurst, P.L., and Jinks, J.L. Parity as a determinant of birth weight in the rhesus monkey. Folia Primatologica, 1965, 3, 201–210.

Caine, N.G. Behavior during puberty and adolescence. In J. Erwin and G. Mitchell (Eds.), Comparative primate biology, Vol. IIa: Behavior and ecology, New York: A.R. Liss, 1985.

Caughley, G. Mortality patterns in animals. Ecology, 1966, 47, 906–918.

Chism, J., Rowell, T., and Olson, D. Life history patterns of female patas monkeys. In M. Small (Ed.), Female primates: Studies by women primatologists. New York: A.R. Liss, 1984, pp. 175–190.

Coe, C.L., Connolly, A.C., Kraemer, H.C., and Levine, S. Reproductive development and behavior of captive female chimpanzees. Primates, 1979, 20, 571–582.

Coelho, A.M., Jr. Baboon dimorphism: growth in weight, length and adiposity from birth to 8 years of age. In E.S. Watts (Ed.), Nonhuman primate models for growth and development. New York: A.R. Liss, 1985, pp. 125–159.

Dunbar, R.I.M. Reproductive decisions: An economic analysis of gelada baboon social strategies. Princeton, N.J.: Princeton University Press, 1984.

Dunbar, R.I.M., and Dunbar, P. Dominance and reproductive success among female gelada baboons. Nature (London), 1977, 266, 351–352.

Eisenberg, J.F. *The mammalian radiations.* Chicago, IL.: University of Chicago Press, 1981.

Fossey, D. Reproduction among free-living mountain gorillas. *American Journal of Primatology Suppl.,* 1982, *1,* 97–104.

Frisch, R., and Revelle, R. Variation in body weights and the age of the adolescent growth spurt among Latin American and Asian populations, in relation to caloric supplies. *Human Biology,* 1969, *41,* 185–212.

Harcourt, A.H., Fossey, D., Stewart, K.J., and Watts, D.P. Reproduction in wild gorillas and some comparisons with chimpanzees. *Journal of Reproduction and Fertility Suppl.,* 1980, *28,* 59–70.

Hausfater, G., Altmann, J., and Altmann, S.A. Long-term consistency of dominance relations among female baboons *(Papio cynocephalus). Science,* 1982, *217,* 752–755.

Hines, Marion. The development and regression of reflexes, postures, and progression in the young macaque. *Contributions to Embryology,* 1942, *196,* 155–209 + 4 plates.

Konner, M., and Worthman, C. Nursing frequency, gonadal function, and birth spacing among !Kung hunter-gatherers. *Science,* 1980, *207,* 788–791.

Lancaster, J.B. Play-mothering: the relations between juvenile females and young infants among free-ranging vervet monkeys *(Cercopithecus aethiops). Folia Primatologica,* 1971, *15,* 161–182.

Lee, P.C. Ecological constraints on the social development of vervet monkeys. *Behaviour,* 1984, *91,* 245–262.

Leutenegger, W. Evolution of litter size in primates. *American Naturalist,* 1979, *114,* 525–531.

McClintock, M. Social control of the ovarian cycle and the function of estrous synchrony. *American Zoologist,* 1981, *21,* 243–256.

McNaughton, S.J., and Wolf, L.L. *General ecology.* New York: Holt Rinehart & Winston, 1973.

Mori, A. Analysis of population changes by measurement of body weight in the Koshima Troop of Japanese monkeys. *Primates,* 1979, *20,* 371–397.

Napier, J.R., and Napier, P.H. (Eds.), *Old World monkeys. Evolution, systematics and behavior.* New York: Academic Press, 1970.

Nicolson, N. *Weaning and the development of independence in olive baboons.* Ph.D. Thesis. Cambridge, Mass.: Harvard University, 1982.

Owens, N.W. A comparison of aggressive play and aggression in free-living baboons, *Papio anubis. Animal Behaviour,* 1975, *23,* 757–765. (a)

Owens, N.W. Social play behavior in free living baboons, *Papio anubis. Animal Behaviour,* 1975, *23,* 387–408. (b)

Packer, C. Male dominance and reproductive activity in *Papio anubis. Animal Behaviour,* 1979, *27,* 37–46.

Pereira, M.E. *Age changes and sex differences in the social behavior of juvenile yellow baboons (Papio cynocephalus).* Ph.D. Thesis. Chicago: The University of Chicago, 1984.

Pereira, M.E., and Altmann, J. Development of social behavior in free-living nonhuman primates. In E.S. Watts (Ed.), *Nonhuman Primate models for growth and development.* New York: A.R. Liss, 1985, pp. 217–309.

Pusey, A.E. Mother-offspring relationships in chimpanzees after weaning. *Animal Behaviour,* 1983, *31,* 363–377.

Riopelle, A.J., and Hale, P.A. Nutritional and environmental factors affecting gestation length in rhesus monkeys. *American Journal of Clinical Nutrition,* 1975, *28,* 1170–1176.

Rostal, D.C., and Eaton, G.G. Puberty in male Japanese macaques *Macaca fuscata*). *American Journal of Primatology*, 1983, *4*, 135–141.

Rowell, T.E. Variation in age at puberty in monkeys. *Folia Primatologica*, 1977, *27*, 284–296.

Sacher, G.A. Evolution of longevity and survival characteristics in mammals. *In* E.L. Schneider (Ed.), *The genetics of aging*. New York: Plenum, 1978.

Sacher, G.A., and Staffeldt, E.F. Relation of gestation time to brain weight for placental mammals: implications for the theory of vertebrate growth. *American Naturalist*, 1974, *108*, 593–615.

Schultz, A.H. The number of young at birth and the number of nipples in primates. *American Journal of Physical Anthropology*, 1948, 6 [N.S.], 1–23.

Schultz, A.H. *The life of primates*. New York: Universe Books (London: Weindenfeld & Nicolson Natural History), 1969.

Scott, L.M. Reproductive behavior of adolescent female baboons *(Papio anubis)* in Kenya. *In* M. Small (Ed.), *Female primates: Studies by women primatologists*. New York: A.R. Liss, 1984, pp. 77–100.

Sigg, H., Stolba, A., Abegglen, J.-J., and Dasser, V. Life history of hamadryas baboons: Physical development, infant mortality, reproductive parameters and family relationships. *Primates*, 1982, *23*, 473–487.

Silk, J., and Boyd, R. Cooperation, competition, and mate choice in matrilineal macaque groups. *In* S.K. Wasser (Ed.), *Female vertebrates*. New York: Academic Press, 1983, pp. 316–349.

Snow, C.C. *The physical growth and development of the open-land baboon, Papio doguera*. Ph.D. Thesis, University of Arizona, 1967.

Southwick, C.H., Richie, T., Taylor, H., Teas, H.J., and M.F. Siddiqi, N.F. Rhesus monkey populations in India and Nepal: patterns of growth, decline, and natural regulation. *In* M.N. Cohen, R.S. Malpass, and H.G. Klein (Eds.), *Biosocial mechanisms of population regulation*. New Haven: Yale Univ. Press, 1980, pp. 151–170.

Stein, D.M. Ontogeny of infant-adult male relationships during the first year of life for yellow baboons *(Papio cynocephalus)*. *In* D.M. Taub (Ed.), *Primate paternalism*. New York: Van Nostrand Reinhold, 1984, pp. 213–243.

Strum, S.C., and Western, J. Variations in fecundity with age and environment in olive baboons *(Papio anubis)*. *American Journal of Primatology*, 1982, *3*, 61–76.

Sugiyama, Y., and Ohsawa, H. Population dynamics of Japanese monkeys with special reference to the effect of artificial feeding. *Folia Primatologica*, 1982, *39*, 238–263.

Tutin, C.E.G. and McGinnis, P.R. Chimpanzee reproduction in the wild. *Reproductive biology of the great apes*. New York: Academic Press, 1981, pp. 239–264.

Van Valen, L., and Mellin, G.W. Selection in natural populations. 7. New York babies (Fetal Life Study). *Annals Human Genetics London*, 1967, *31*, 109–127.

Vandenbergh, J.G. Social influences on reproduction in rhesus monkeys. *In* M.R.N. Prasad and T.C. Arand Kumar (Eds.), *Use of nonhuman primates in biomedical research*. New Delhi: Indian National Science Academy, 1977, pp. 174–182.

Vandenbergh, J.G., and Drickamer, L.C. Reproductive coordination among free-ranging rhesus monkeys. *Physiology and Behavior*, 1974, *13*, 1–4.

Walters, J. Interventions and the development of dominance relationships in female baboons. *Folia Primatologica*, 1980, *34*, 61–89.

Watts, E.S. Adolescent growth and development of monkeys, apes and humans. *In* E.S. Watts (Ed.), *Nonhuman primates models for growth and development.* New York: A.R. Liss, 1985, pp. 41–65.

Watts, E.S., and Gavan, J.A. Post-natal growth of nonhuman primates: the problem of the adolescent spurt. *Human Biology,* 1982, *54,* 53–70.

Western, D. Size, life history and ecology in mammals. *African Journal of Ecology,* 1979, *20,* 185–204.

Whichelow, M.J. Success and failure of breast-feeding in relation to energy intake. *Proceedings of the Nutrition Society,* 1976, *35,* 62A.

Widdowson, E.M. Changes in the body and its organs during lactation: nutritional implications. *Breast-feeding and the mother.* Ciba Found. Symp. 45 (NS). Amsterdam: Elsevier, 1976, pp. 103–118.

Wrangham, R.W. An ecological model of female-bonded primate groups. *Behaviour,* 1980, *75,* 262–300.

13

School-Age Parenthood in Different Ethnic Groups and Family Constellations: Effects on Infant Development

Tiffany Field
Susan Widmayer
Sherilyn Stoller
Mercedes de Cubas

School-age parenthood is considered a high-risk factor for the development of the teenager's offspring as well as for her own socioeconomic condition. The effects of teenager parenthood may vary, however, as a function of cultural variation in child-rearing attitudes, variable family support systems, and whether or not the teenage mother is the primary caregiver of the child. The importance of these variables has recently been highlighted by a series of cross-cultural studies in which infant development was notably different across different cultures possibly because patterns of relating to the infant vary across cultural groups (Field et al., 1981). It is conceivable that some infants reared by school-age mothers in some ethnic groups and family constellations may be at lesser risk for developmental delays.

EVIDENCE FOR SCHOOL-AGE PARENTHOOD AS A RISK FACTOR

Most of the research on the effects of school-age parenthood has compared infants and children who were born to teenage mothers versus adult mothers of the same ethnic group and socioeconomic status. This literature generally suggests a number of developmental problems for the offspring of school-age mothers and some undesirable socioeconomic consequences for the mothers themselves (c.f. the volume edited by Scott et al., 1980). Infants of teenage versus adult mothers are noted to receive less verbal stimulation (Field, 1979; Osofsky and Osofsky, 1970) and to experience developmental delays (Broman, 1979; Field et al., 1980). Some of these delays have been attributed to school-age mothers having relatively limited knowledge and unrealistic expectations regarding developmental milestones, as well as punitive child-rearing attitudes (Delissovoy, 1973; Field et al., 1980). As pre-schoolers, a number of children parented by teenagers perform less competently (Furstenberg, 1976), and as school-age children they are frequently unable to maintain grade-appropriate reading levels (Oppel and Royston, 1971). Data from larger-scale studies in New York City (Dryfoos and Belmont, 1979) and Great Britain (Record et al., 1969) suggest that, holding socioeconomic status constant, maternal youth is a significant contributor to deflated childhood IQ scores. In most of these studies the lesser education of the teenage mother, her less viable so-cioeconomic status, and her negative attitudes toward child rearing have been implicated as correlates of her child's unfavorable developmental outcome. These reports coupled with those showing lower levels of education and greater dependence on public assistance among school-age mothers (Furstenberg, 1976) have highlighted school-age parenthood as a risk factor in the development of young children.

Other variables which were not investigated in these teenage-adult parenthood studies but might differentially affect outcomes are cultural variation in child-rearing attitudes, the family support available to the teenage mother, and whether or not she is the primary caregiver.

VARIATION IN ETHNIC GROUPS

The studies on teenage parenthood often feature samples of Hispanic and black teenage mothers, probably because the incidence of teenage parenthood is higher among these cultures (Scott, 1981). However, until recently cross-cultural comparisons were not made (Lester et al., 1982). In this study by Lester and his colleagues the outcome for neonates born to Puerto Rican teenage mothers was superior to that of infants born to mainland teenage mothers (principally black mothers) of equivalent socioeconomic status. One of the interpretations offered for this difference was that the Puerto Rican mothers were more often married and thus possibly received more support or experienced less stressful pregnancies. Differences in the infants' development might be expected to persist beyond the neonatal period not only because of the different support systems of those cultures but also because of their different attitudes toward child rearing.

Child-rearing attitudes and practices are notably different between Hispanic and black mothers and between different Hispanic mothers such as Puerto Ricans and Cubans (Field and Widmayer, 1981). We have conducted research that focused on the two cultures of primary interest, the blacks and Cubans. A number of differences have been noted between the adult mothers of these cultures (Field and Widmayer, 1981). For example, Cuban mothers generally indulge their infants as well as talk to them almost excessively. In contrast, black mothers frequently expressed concerns about not spoiling their infants by giving them too much attention. Black mothers with such concerns talked very little to their infants. In a study by Field and Widmayer (1981) the face-to-face interactions of Cuban mothers and their infants were more effective than those of black mother–infant dyads, in part because the Cuban mothers and infants were more attentive and responsive to each other and engaged in more verbal interaction. Thus, different child-rearing attitudes appeared to contribute to different interactions which, in turn, might be expected to contribute to differential development of their infants (Field et al., 1982).

VARIATIONS IN FAMILY CONSTELLATIONS

The question of the optimal family constellation for child rearing has rarely been investigated, despite the recent increase in single parenting. Within the last generation, the proportion of children raised in single-parent families has doubled (Bronfenbrenner, 1975). The incidence of single parenting (currently at 18%), may be inflated among teenage mothers: approximately 27% in a sample of black, hispanic, and caucasian teenage mothers (Cannon-Bonventre and Kahn, 1979). This may not be surprising inasmuch as the current welfare system is frequently experienced by the teenage mother as favoring the single-parenting family situation by advancing public assistance payments to her for the support of her child. Although it is unreasonable to assume that single-parenting must have "harmful" consequences for young children, studies on father absence suggest that the children reared by single parents are at some disadvantage. Most of the single-parenting studies (because single parents are often mothers) have focused on the effects of father absence. Physically, the greater consequences of father absence are reported for the child under three than for older children (Burton, 1962). While single-parent families headed by the mother often have fewer economic resources than two-parent families, father absence has been noted to have an effect on child development that goes beyond that which is attributable to socioeconomic factors alone (Deutsch and Brown, 1964).

Although a two-parent family may, in general, be at lower risk for parenting and child development problems, it is not clear that two-parent families are at lesser risk than one-parent families when the parents are teenagers. While the average annual income of teenage nuclear families is reportedly twice that of the single teenager mother (Cannon-Bonventre and Kahn, 1979), it is not clear whether the fathers of the two-parent families surveyed were also teenagers or adults. Some have expressed concern that if the teenage mother marries a teenager, the undesirable socioeconomic consequences may then exist for both the teenage mother and father, since the teenage father assumes the additional burden of supporting a wife and family without himself having completed high school or had adequate training to find employment. Nonetheless, the presence of a father may facilitate the teenage mother's role by providing her social support, and the child's development may be enhanced by those forms of playful stimulation frequently attributed to fathers (Clarke-Stewart, 1978; Kotelchuk, 1976; Pederson et al., 1979).

Despite these considerations, most teenage mothers in our sample and in those of other teenage parenthood studies (Badger, 1979; Hardy et al., 1980) have remained in their extended families. Assessing the effects of the extended family network on a child's development is particularly complex in the case of the teenage parent who often lives under the same roof with an average of nine others under age 20 and three others over age 20 (Field et al., 1980). One positive feature of extended families is the presence of older siblings (in this case, the infants of aunts and uncles) who provide companionship and role models (Dunn and Kendrick 1979; Lamb, 1978; Sutton-Smith and Rosenberg, 1970). Another is the presence of grandparents. Anecdotal reports on grandparents who are prominent in the lives of teenage parents and their children vary; some suggest that grandparents may compensate for the sometimes inadequate parenting by the teenage mother (Field et al., 1980), and others claim that the grandparents, particularly the grandmother, compete with the teenage mothers for the child-rearing control of her children (Badger, 1979; Levenson et al., 1978). The extended family may have negative effects on a child's development by sheer family size alone. This concept is most clearly stated in the controversial confluence model of Zajonc and Markus (1975) supported by data from Dunn and Wooding (1979) whereby each additional child in the family is viewed as "diluting" the intellectual environment of the home to a degree depending on the spacing between siblings. In summary, then, the literature on optimal family constellations is equivocal at best.

THE SCHOOL-AGE MOTHER VERSUS OTHER PRIMARY CAREGIVERS

The relative effects of being reared by a school-age mother versus being cared for by someone else (usually the grandmother, another relative, or a childcare center) are unknown. Very little is known, for example, about the comparative benefits of grandmothers versus school-age mothers serving as primary caregivers. It is often assumed that the grandmother would be the superior caregiver by virtue of her greater experience. However, a comparison of the interactions of school-age mothers and grandmothers playing with the same infants yielded very few differences, and those few favored the school-age mothers (Field, 1982). Teenage mothers engaged in more teaching behavior and ignored their infants less frequently than the grandmothers (Field, 1983).

There is also very little literature on the effects of day-care as the primary caregiving arrangement. Those studies generally show very minimal differences between children who remained at home with their mothers during the early years versus those who attended day-care (c.f. Hoffman, 1979 for a review of those studies).

Thus the development of infants reared by school-age mothers may vary in different ethnic groups, different family constellations, and depending on whether the mother or someone else is the primary caregiver. In the next section we will discuss some findings from a study in which we explored the differences in infants who were reared by Cuban and American black school-age mothers, some of whom were single, married, or lived with their extended family and some of whom were the primary care givers.

DIFFERENCES IN INFANTS REARED IN DIFFERENT ETHNIC GROUPS AND FAMILY CONSTELLATIONS

Differences in the development of infants reared in different ethnic groups and family constellations were studied in a sample of Cuban and black school-age mothers in Miami. Although our sample appeared to be representative of the school-age parent population in Miami, it might not be as representative of school-age parents in other areas of the country. The sample was comprised of 164 lower-income school-age mothers and their infants. The mothers averaged 16 years of age and completed 10 years of schooling. Of this sample, 112 were black and 52 were Cuban. The family constellations of these women varied, with 111 living in extended families (the teenage mother's family), 30 in nuclear families (the teenage mother and her husband/boyfriend), and 23 in single-parent families.

The mothers were interviewed using a series of questionnaires on her current support system, her child-rearing attitudes and practices, and her own as well as her child's temperament. The infants' cognitive and motor development was assessed using the Bayley Scales of Infant Development (Bayley, 1969). Observations were also made of the child's home environment (Caldwell et al., 1966), family interaction, and mother—infant play interaction patterns.

This cross-cultural comparison between Cuban and black teenage mother–infant dyads yielded data that are consistent with those reported for adult mothers and infants of the same cultures (Field and Widmayer, 1981). The data on child-rearing attitudes, home observations, and the mother–infant play interactions suggest that the Cuban teenage mothers, like their adult counterparts, are more indulgent and provide more social stimulation for their infants. Black teenage mothers behave in a more restrictive/punitive and less stimulating way which is consistent with their fears of "spoiling the child" and their expectations for earlier autonomy of their offspring. Thus, the behaviors of these mothers appear to reflect the child-rearing attitudes and expectations held by their cultures, highlighting the importance of considering cultural differences in teenage parenting.

While the socioeconomic status of these two groups was roughly equivalent, the Cuban mothers experienced greater social support. This may have contributed to their being more involved socially with their infants. Their infants were also more sociable during interactions which is not surprising since mothers who show more affective and talkative behavior generally have infants who are more sociable and talkative (Field, 1982). The Cuban infants were more fussy possibly because of being overstimulated by their mothers. This may also explain the absence of cultural differences in infant development and language production we noted at 2 years of age. One might expect infants who have received more social stimulation to perform better on developmental assessments and to show more highly developed language production. The Cuban teen-age mothers, like Cuban mothers of preterm infants reported in other studies (DiVitto and Goldberg, 1979; Field, 1979), however, may have been overstimulating their infants, thus attenuating the expected acceleration in their infants' development. Overstimulation by the Cuban teenage mothers may affect infant development in ways that are similar to the effects of low levels of stimulation, as were noted in the results with black teenage mothers. An alternative possibility is that the differential stimulation provided by mothers may have "sleeper"effects and, as in a transactional model, those effects may emerge only later in childhood (Field and Dempsey, 1982; Sameroff and Chandler, 1975; Siegel, 1982; Sigman and Parmelee, 1979).

The comparisons of teenage mother–infant dyads living in single-parent, nuclear, and extended families generally favored the nuclear family constellation. Consistent with other reports (Cannon-Bonventre and Kahn, 1979), the teenage nuclear families of this sample had a higher socioeconomic status (SES) than the single parents or extended families, at least at the time of this study. Nonetheless, even after controlling for SES differences, the nuclear family mothers and infants fared better socially. Perhaps, as for the Cuban mothers, the nuclear family mothers who felt they had a stronger social support network were able to be more interactive with their infants, having more emotional energy to do so. In turn, their infants were more interactive. In addition, the nuclear family mothers felt they had more control over their lives. This may have contributed to greater confidence in their own parenting skills. Single parents reported the least amount of social support and had the most unreasonable developmental expectations for their infants. On some level they may have wished for faster development of their infants so they might serve as social companions or, at the very least, achieve early autonomy so the mother would have the freedom to pursue socially supportive relationships.

Surprisingly, few differences were noted for primary versus secondary caregivers or their infants. Those that did emerge related to the mother's child-rearing attitudes and practices. The primary caregiver mothers' views of child rearing were less positive than the views of mothers who left care-giving responsibilities to someone else. The primary caregivers also considered their infants' temperaments as being more difficult, their homes were less organized, and were more restrictive and punitive. Generally, this might describe any mother who remains at home all day assuming the primary responsibility for the care of her child without much relief time for herself. However, several authors have suggested that the school-age mother may have even less tolerance for care-giving activities because of her own youth, egocentrism, and dependency needs, and may be more readily frustrated and resort to punitive child-rearing practices (Delissovoy, 1973; Field et al., 1980).

Overall downward trends were observed in developmental assessment and language production scores of the infants during their second year of life. These were noted in each of the ethnic, family constellation, and type of care-giving groups, suggesting that school-age parenthood in each of these contexts may have negative consequences for infant development. These trends are consistent with those noted in other school-age mother samples (Broman, 1979; Field et al., 1980) except when intervention is provided and may relate to a decrease in stimulation provided by the mothers during play interactions with the infants during their second year of life.

In summary, the effects of being reared by a Cuban mother living in a nuclear family and being a secondary care giver appeared to be positive when considering mothers' social support systems and child-rearing attitudes and the mother–infant dyads' play interaction behaviors. However, the downward trend in mothers' stimulation and infants' development and language production scores over the second year of life for the sample at large suggests that teenage parenting may have negative consequences irrespective of context variables like child-rearing culture and family constellation. Nonetheless, the emergence of strong effects for these context variables on mothers' attitudes and mother–child play highlights the importance of further investigation of these school-age parenthood context variables.

ACKNOWLEDGMENTS

We would like to thank all the mothers and infants who participated in this study. This research was funded by the National Foundation/March of Dimes and the Administration of Children, Youth and Families, and by an NIMH Research Scientist Development Award to T. Field.

REFERENCES

Badger, E. Effects of parent education on teenage mothers and their offspring. In K. Scott, T. Field, and E. Robertson (Eds.), Teenage parents and their offspring. New York: Grune & Stratton, 1979.

Bayley, N. Manual for the Bayley scales of infant development. New York: Psychological Corp., 1969.

Broman, S. Seven year outcome of 4,000 children born to teenagers in the U.S. In K., Scott, T. Field, and E. Robertson (Eds.), Teenage parents and their offspring. New York: Grune & Stratton, 1979.

Bronfenbrenner, U. The challenge of social change to public policy and development research. Paper presented at the biennial meeting of the Society for Research in Child Development, Denver, April, 1975.

Burton, R.V. Cross-sex identity in Barbados. Developmental Psychology, 1962, 6, 365–374.

Caldwell, B.M., Heider, J., and Kaplan, B. The inventory of home stimulation. Paper presented at the meeting of the American Psychological Association, New York, September 1966.

Cannon-Bonventre, K., and Kahn, J. R. The ecology of help-seeking behavior among adolescent parents. Executive summary of final report prepared for the Department of Health, Education and Welfare, Administration for Children, Youth and Families, Jan. 1979.

Clarke-Stewart, K. Alison. And daddy makes three: The father's impact on mother and child. Child Development, 1978, 49, 466–478.

Delissovoy, V. Child care by adolescent parents. Children Today, 1973, 2, 22–25.

Deutsch, M., and Brown, B. Social influences in negro-white intelligence differences. Journal of Social Issues, 1964, 20: 24–35.

Divitto, B., and Goldberg, S. The effects of newborn medical status on early parent-infant interactions. In T. Field et al. (Eds.), Infants born at risk. New York: Spectrum, 1979.

Dryfoos, J., and Belmont, L. Longterm development of children born to New York City teenagers. In K. Scott, T. Field, and E. Robertson (Eds.), Teenage parents and their offspring. New York: Grune & Stratton, 1979.

Dunn, J., and Kendrick, C. Interaction between young siblings in the context of family relationships. In M. Lewis, and L. Rosenblum (Eds.), The child and its family. New York: Plenum Press, 1979.

Dunn, J., and Wooding, C. Play in the home and its implications for learning. *In* B. Tizard, and D. Harvey (Eds.), *The biology of play*. London: Heineman Medical Books, 1977.

Field, T. Interaction patterns of preterm and term infants. *In* T. Field, A. Sostek, S. Goldberg, and H. Shuman (Eds.), *Infants born at risk*. NY: Spectrum, 1979.

Field, T. Interactions of high-risk infants: Quantitative and qualitative differences. *In* D. Sawin *et al.* (Eds.), *Current perspectives on psychosocial risks during pregnancy and early infancy*. New York: Bruner/Mazel, 1980. (a)

Field, T. Interactions of preterm and term infants with their lower and middle class teenage and adult mothers. *In* T. Field, S. Goldberg, D. Stern, and A. Sostek (Eds.), *High-risk infants and children: Adult and peer interactions*. New York: Academic Press, 1980. (b)

Field, T. Affective displays of high-risk infants during early interactions. *In* T. Field, and A. Fogel (Eds.), *Emotion and interactions*. Hillsdale, NJ: Erlbaum Assoc., 1982.

Field, T. Social interactions between high-risk infants and their mothers, fathers and grandmothers. *In* B. B. Lahey and A. Kazdin (Eds.), *Advances in clinical child psychology*. New York: Plenum, 1983.

Field, T., Demsey, J. and Shuman, H. H. Five-year follow-up of preterm respiratory distress syndrome and postterm postmaturity syndrome infants. *In* T. Field and A. Sostek (Eds.), *Infants born at risk: Physiological and perceptual development*. New York: Grune & Stratton, 1982.

Field, T., and Widmayer, S. Mother-infant interaction among SES Black, Cuban, Puerto Rican and South American immigrants. *In* T. Field, P. Sostek, P. Vietze, and A. H. Liederman (Eds.), *Culture and early interaction*. Hillsdale, New Jersey: Erlbaum Assoc., 1981.

Field, T., Widmayer, S., Stringer, S., and Ignatoff, E. Teenage, lower-class, black mothers and their preterm infants: An intervention and developmental follow-up. *Child Development*, 1980, *51*, 426–436.

Field, T., Sostek, P., Vietze, P., and Liederman, A. H. (Eds.). *Culture and early interaction*. Hillsdale, New Jersey: Erlbaum Assoc., 1981.

Field, T., Widmayer, S., Greenberg, R., and Stoller, S. Effects of parent training on teenage mothers and their infants. *Pediatrics*, 1982, *69*, 703–707.

Furstenberg, F. F. The social consequences of teenage pregnancy. *Family Perceptives*, 1976, *8*, 148–164.

Hardy, J., King, T.M., Shipp, D.A., and Welcher, D. W. A comprehensive approach to adolescent pregnancy. *In* K. Scott, T. Field, and E. Robertson (Eds.), *Teenage parents and their offspring*. New York: Grune & Stratton, 1980.

Hoffman, L. W. Maternal employment: 1979. *American Psychologist*, 1979, *34*, 859–865.

Kotelchuck, M. The infant's relationship to the father: Experimental evidence. *In* M. E. Lamb (Ed.), *The role of the father in child development*. New York: Wiley, 1976.

Lamb, M. Interactions between eighteen-month-olds and their preschool aged siblings. *Child Development*, 1978, *49*, 51–59.

Lester, B. M., Coll, C.T.E., and Sepkoski, C. A cross cultural study of teenage pregnancy and neonatal behavior. *In* T. Field, and A. Sostek (Eds.), *Infants born at risk: Perceptual and physiological processes*. New York: Grune & Stratton, 1982.

Levenson, P., Atkinson, B., Hale, J., and Hollier, M. Adolescent parent education. A maturational model. *Child Psychiatry and Human Development*, 1978, *9*, 104–118.

Oppel, W., and Royston, A. B. Teenage births: Some social, psychological and physical sequelae. *American Journal of Public Health*, 1971, *61*, 751–756.

Osofsky, H., and Osofsky, J. Adolescents as mother: Results of a program for low-income pregnant teenagers with some emphasis upon infants' development. *American Journal of Orthopsychiatry*, 1970, *40*, 825–834.

Pederson, F., Yarrow, L., Anderson, B., and Cain, R., Jr. Conceptualization of the father influences in the infancy period. *In* M. Lewis and L. Rosenblum (Eds.), *The child and its family* (Vol. 2). New York: Plenum, 1979.

Record, R. G., McKeown, T., and Edwards, I. G. The relation of measured intelligence to birth order and maternal age. *Annals of Human Genetics*, 1969, *33*, 61–69.

Sameroff, A. J., and Chandler, M. J. Reproductive risk and the continuum of caretaking casualty. *In* F. D. Horowitz, M. Hetherington, S. Scarr-Salapatek, and G. Siegel, (Eds.), *Review of child development research* (Vol. 4). Chicago, IL: Univ. of Chicago Press, 1975.

Scott, K.G. Epidemiologic aspects of teenage pregnancy. *In* K. G. Scott, T. Field, and E. Robertson (Eds.), *Teenage parents and their offspring*. New York: Grune & Stratton, 1981.

Scott, K., Field, T., and Robertson, E. (Eds.). *Teenage parents and their offspring*. New York: Grune & Stratton, 1980.

Siegel, L. A five-year developmental follow-up of high-risk infants. *In* T. Field, and A. Sostek (Eds.), *Infants born at risk: Physiological and perceptual processes*. New York: Grune & Stratton, 1982.

Sigman, M., and Parmelee, A. M. Longitudinal evaluation of the preterm infant. *In* T. Field, A. Sostek, S. Goldberg, and H. H. Shuman (Eds.), *Infants born at risk*. New York: Spectrum, 1979.

Sutton-Smith, B., and Rosenberg, B. G. *The sibling*. New York: Holt, Rinehart & Winston, 1970.

Zajonc, R. B., and Markus, G. B. Birth order and intellectual development. *Psychological Review*, 1975, *82*, 74–83.

14

THE DURATION OF MAIDENHOOD ACROSS CULTURES*

John W. M. Whiting
Victoria K. Burbank
Mitchell S. Ratner

INTRODUCTION

Every society has cultural rules and customary strategies whose intent is to ensure reproductive continuity from generation to generation. Viable methods of infant care, child rearing, and mate selection during adolescence are necessary for such continuity. We have chosen to investigate the strategies adopted by various cultures to ensure that a young woman is married at the right time to the right husband. We assume that a limited set of strategies have been devised over the course of social evolution and that their choice is predictable.

Since menarche marks the onset of female fecundity and a wedding legitimates motherhood, the interval between these two events, which we have called MAIDENHOOD, will be the focus of this chapter. In the United States, where the median age of menarche is 12.8 years and the median age of marriage is 20.6 years, maidenhood lasts for almost 8 years. In contrast, for most preindustrial societies the period is less than 3 years and in some in which girls marry at or before they first menstruate there is no period of maidenhood at all.

In order to investigate the various strategies regarding maidenhood that have been used over the course of human social evolution two samples will be discussed. The first, shown in Table 14.1, is a set of modern national cultures for which survey data on the age of menarche

---

*Revision of a paper presented at a conference sponsored by the Social Science Research Council on School-Age Pregnancies and Parenthood, Elkridge, Maryland, May 23–26, 1982.

273

TABLE 14.1. Duration of Maidenhood and Ages at Menarche and Marriage

Country	Duration of maidenhood	Mean age of menarche	Mean age of marriage
Japan	11.8	12.9	24.7
Switzerland	10.7	13.1	23.8
Sweden	10.1	13.1	23.2
Hong Kong (Chinese)	9.5	12.8	22.3
Netherlands	9.8	13.4	23.2
England and Wales	9.8	13.0	21.8
Finland	9.6	13.2	22.8
France	9.3	13.2	22.5
Belgium	9.2	13.1	22.3
Norway	9.0	13.2	22.2
Denmark	9.0	13.2	22.2
New Zealand	8.7	13.0	21.7
Australia	8.5	13.2	21.7
Canada	8.6	13.1	21.7
Israel	8.2	13.2	21.4
Hungary	7.6	13.4	20.7
Singapore	7.8	12.7	20.5
United States	7.8	12.8	20.6
Czechoslovakia	6.9	14.2	21.1
Malaysian Chinese	6.4	14.2	20.6
Iraq	6.1	14.0	20.1
Turkey	6.0	13.2	19.2
Iran	5.8	13.3	19.1
Tunis	5.2	14.0	19.2
Pakistan	3.8	13.9	17.7
Bangladesh (Hindu)	2.7	15.9	18.6
India	2.4	14.4	16.8
Bangladesh (Muslim)	1.8	15.6	17.4

(Eveleth and Tanner, 1976) and on the age of marriage (Dixon, 1971) were available for the same time period—1960–1975. The median duration of maidenhood is taken as the difference between these two values.

The second sample, shown in Table 14.2, is a subset of the "standard cross-cultural sample" (Murdock and White, 1969). It is largely preindustrial and is based on ethnographic community studies. Each of the communities in this sample are part of a distinct culture and for the most part speak a language of a distinct family. For those societies that were socially stratified, customs relating to the middle class or commoners rather than nobles or slaves were taken as a basis of judgment. In societies undergoing rapid modernization, the earliest reliable reports describing the culture were chosen.

The cases in Table 14.2 are arranged by maidenhood strategies, e.g., the duration of maidenhood and the rules governing premarital sex. Each strategy is identified by the name of a society that exemplifies it. These type cases were chosen on the basis of the adequacy of the available ethnographic description of maidenhood.

Since most of the cases in this preindustrial sample are preliterate and lack a calendar, chronological age could rarely be used to estimate the duration of maidenhood. People in these societies do, however, recognize critical maturational stages. In many societies menarche is celebrated by a public festival which marks status change and is often accompanied by a change of costume or hairstyle. In societies that do not celebrate menarche the appearance of secondary sex characteristics is often noted and used as a marker for change of status. In fact, many preindustrial peoples use an approximation of the Tanner scale for measuring the development of secondary sex characteristics (see Buckler, 1979) to judge the transition from girl- to womanhood. Communities included in the Standard Sample for which neither chronological nor adequate maturational data were obtainable were omitted from our analysis.

In order to understand maidenhood strategies the probability of pregnancy occurring during the period must be determined. This depends not only on the duration of maidenhood but on two other factors (1) postmenarcheal subfecundity and (2) the rules governing premarital sex. If females are married at or before menarche in a given culture, the probability of premarital pregnancy is minimal even when sexual intercourse is permitted or encouraged. Furthermore, even when marriage occurs several years after menarche, the probability of premarital pregnancy is low due to postmenarcheal subfecundity.

For the most part, the research on postmenarcheal subfecundity in humans has been carried out with samples drawn from modern societies in which maidenhood is prolonged and premarital chastity is expected (see Ashley Montague, 1979). Estimates from these studies may not be appropriate for our preindustrial sample. The Maasai of Kenya, a case in our sample with a very brief maidenhood, provide a more appropriate estimate. Girls in this society are initiated during the year they first menstruate, and as initiation is customarily the first step in the Maasai wedding ceremony, most women move into their husband's hut soon after. It can be assumed that the median interval between menarche and the beginning of marital intercourse is approximately 1 year. Lewellyn-Davies (unpublished field notes, 1972) obtained data on both the date of initiation and the date of the first child on a sample of 67 Maasai women. Since the Maasai do not practice contraception and place a high value on large families, it is possible to estimate from these data the average interval between menarche and first pregnancy. The results are presented below in Table 14.3.

The fact that only 77% of the sample had borne a child after 10 years

Table 14.2. Ethnographic Sample by Type of Maidenhood Strategy

Maidenhood strategy[a]	Society name	Ethno. present	Standard sample no.	Ethnographic atlas region
Very long— restricted	Irish	1932	051	Circum-Mediterranean
	Russians	1955	054	Circum-Mediterranean
	Romanians	1980	000	Circum-Mediterranean
	Japanese	1936	117	East Eurasia
Long— restricted	Mbundu	1980	005	Africa
	Kikuyu	1900	011	Africa
Medium— encouraged	Azande	1905	028	Africa
	Gond	1938	060	East Eurasia
	Toda	1900	061	East Eurasia
	Lolo	1910	067	East Eurasia
	Andamanese	1860	079	East Eurasia
	Trobrianders	1914	098	Insular Pacific
	Marquesans	1800	105	Insular Pacific
	Samoans	1829	106	Insular Pacific
	Marshallese	1900	108	Insular Pacific
	Ifugao	1910	112	Insular Pacific
	Yukaghir	1850	120	East-Eurasia
	Comanche	1870	147	North America
	Carib	1932	164	South America
	Tupinamba	1550	177	South America
Short— restricted	Alorese	1938	089	Insular Pacific
	Kapauku	1955	094	Insular Pacific
	Kwoma	1937	095	Insular Pacific
	Papago	1910	151	North America
Short— permitted	Mbuti	1980	013	Africa
	Tallensi	1934	023	Africa
	Lesu	1930	097	Insular Pacific
	Kaska	1900	129	North America
	Siriono	1942	173	South America
	Timbira	1915	176	South America
Absent— permitted	!Kung San	1970	002	Africa
	Maasai	1970	034	Africa
	Aranda	1896	091	Insular Pacific
	Gilyak	1890	119	East Eurasia
	Cooper Eskimo	1915	124	North America
	Paiute	1870	137	North America
	Gros Ventre	1880	140	North America
	Havasupai	1918	150	North America
	Yanomamo	1965	163	South America
	Jivaro	1920	169	South America
	Techuelche	1870	185	South America

continued

Table 14.2. *Continued*

Maidenhood strategy[a]	Society name	Ethno. present	Standard sample no.	Ethnographic atlas region
Absent—	Wolof	1950	021	Circum-Mediterranean
prohibited	Hausa	1900	026	Circum-Mediterranean
	Amhara	1953	037	Circum-Mediterranean
	Egyptians	1950	043	Circum-Mediterranean
	Turks	1950	047	Circum-Mediterranean
	Gheg	1910	048	Circum-Mediterranean
	Kurd	1951	057	Circum-Mediterranean
	Micmac	1650	126	North America
	Cuna	1940	158	South America

[a]Definition of maidenhood strategies. The code for duration of maidenhood is as follows: Very long–more than 5 years; long–about 4 years; medium–about 3 years; short–about 2 years; very short–less than 1 year; absent–at or before menarche.

The code for premarital sex roles is as follows: prohibited, premarital sex taboo, virginity highly valued; restricted, premarital sex approved only with contraception; permitted, premarital sex allowed but not encouraged; encouraged, premarital sex positively valued.

of marriage indicates a relatively low level of fertility for the adult population. This is probably due to a high incidence of venereal disease. For this reason the values in the table are probably somewhat too low.

The theoretical maximum probability of premarital pregnancy can be estimated for societies with various durations of maidenhood by using the above figures and adjusting for the low fertility of the Maasai.

TABLE 14.3. Cumulative Percentages of
Maasai Women Whose
First Pregnancy Was
During the Indicated
Interval After Menarche[a]

Years between menarche and first pregnancy	Cumulative percentages
0–1	6
0–2	30
0–3	48
0–4	53
0–5	62
0–10	77

[a]The data on postmenarcheal subfecundity reported by Reiter (Chapter 4) in this volume is strikingly similar to the results reported in this table.

The probability should approximate zero in societies with no maidenhood no matter whether premarital sex is permitted or not. If premarital sex is freely permitted, the probability of pregnancy should be about 30% in societies with the maidenhood lasting from 1 to 2 years, somewhat less than 50% in societies with a maidenhood of 2 to 3 years, and about 60% when maidenhood lasts from 3 to 4 years.

Whereas many societies depend entirely on subfecundity to govern premarital pregnancy, others do so by imposing restrictive rules governing premarital sex. These rules vary widely in the societies of the ethnographic sample. In some, sex is strictly taboo and it is believed that the hymen should be intact at marriage; often a bloody sheet must be publicly displayed after the wedding night by the bride's relatives to prove this. Others are more concerned with premarital pregnancy than an intact hymen and permit or sometimes even encourage sexual intimacy if proper contraceptive measures are used. Still other societies ignore the sexual behavior of adolescents if it is done with proper decorum or permit sex under certain circumstances and forbid it in others. Finally, a substantial set of societies actively encourage premarital sex believing that it is a necessary part of premarital courtship.

The judgments of the duration of maidenhood and the rules governing premarital sexual behavior were combined to define a number of maidenhood strategies and classify the cases in the ethnographic sample. The grouping of the ethnographic sample by maidenhood strategy and the criteria of inclusion are both presented in Table 14.2.

CASE ILLUSTRATIONS

To provide a more concrete understanding of the different strategies listed in Table 14.2, one or more exemplars of each type is described below. (As an aid to cross reference, the standard sample identification number follows the name and date of each exemplar.)

VERY LONG—RESTRICTED STRATEGY

For this category maidenhood extends for 5 years or more; restrictive rules govern premarital sex. This strategy of prolonged maidenhood beyond the period of postmenarcheal subfecundity is, as can be seen from Table 14.2, characteristic of modern European and far Eastern societies. Only four examples were included in the ethnographic sample—the Irish of County Clare with an estimated maidenhood of 14 years, the Russian village of Viratiano with a maidenhood of 5 years duration, Suye Mura, a Japanese community with a 7-year maidenhood, and Baisoara, a Romanian village with 7 years of maidenhood. All these societies ideally believe in premarital chastity but they do not

go so far as to have tests of virginity and, if proper contraceptive measures are used, premarital sex is sometimes condoned.

Since one of the authors has recently made a study of adolescent
life in a Romanian village (Ratner, unpublished fieldnotes) it will be
used as an example of this type.

Romania (000). Baisoara is a Romanian village with a population
of 1200, located in the foothills of the inner Carpathians of western Romania. Traditionally, the village economy was based on agriculture
and animal husbandry, supplemented with income derived from forest
work, carting, and seasonal labor. In 1965, however, an iron mining
complex opened nearby and for the first time it became possible for
many to obtain the benefits of industrial employment without migrating
from the village. By the late 1970's Baisoara had become, by Romanian
standards, a fairly prosperous peasant-worker village. The great majority of the households had at least one member working at the mining
complex or with some other form of permanent wage employment.

Among the adolescent girls studied in 1981, the mean age of menarche was 14 years, 3 months. In past generations, first menstruation
was the primary and necessary criteria for becoming a FATA MARE (big
girl). As a FATA MARE the young girl could fully participate in the village's
Sunday afternoon dance, could openly court, and theoretically was
eligible for marriage. More recently, however, menstruation, per se,
has become less important as institutional criteria have increased their
role. For example, various social activities, such as participation in
coed school dances, are keyed to school grade, rather than maturational age. In addition, regardless of maturational age, most parents
discourage a girl's interest in boys and courting until after her schooling
is completed. At the earliest this occurs at 16 years of age, after the
compulsory 10th grade. For many, however, it does not occur until the
completion of high school at 18 or 19 years of age.

In spite of parental opposition, many of the young girls develop an
active interest in boys and courting well before they are considered to
be eligible for marriage. Many of the 8th and 9th graders, 14 and 15
years of age, have already developed a special relationship to a particular, usually older, boy.

As the girls enter their late teens, a certain amount of sexual activity
is expected. For example, when a boy accompanies a girl home from
the Sunday dance, there will often be some necking at the gate of the
girls home, or in some other secluded spot. However, the limits of social
permissiveness do not extend to intercourse. Village norms clearly state
that a young girl should be a virgin when she marries. The generally
accepted village perspective is that there are two types of girls, "hon-
orable girls" who retain their virginity and "whores" who do not. For
the most part, the social pressure is effective: young girls greatly fear

the social disapproval that would accompany discovery of the act and pregnancy.

However, for various reasons the social pressure is not always effective. In Baisoara and in other nearby villages there are young girls who, for more or less good reason, have reputations for having been sexually free with a number of young men. Often, it is with these girls that young men will have their first sexual experience, although they would never consider them as marriage prospects.

Not encompassed in the the popular dichotomy of "good girl" and "whore" are some of the older adolescent girls who discretely carry on sexual relations with young men they intend to marry. Not infrequently, because of the lack of effective birth control measures, the outcome of these affairs is a pregnant bride.

Aside from marriages more or less necessitated by an unwanted pregnancy, villagers recognize two basic ways of arranging a marriage. "Marriages of interest" are arranged by parents to maintain or boost the families' social status or material base. (Traditionally and currently, it is generally a son and his wife who are an elder couples' old age security.) "Love marriages" are arranged by the young people themselves and are based on mutual attraction. The 20th century trend has been away from "marriages of interest," especially of the more blatant type in which the bride hardly knows the groom and has little to say in the matter. Nonetheless, there is still often in the background a controlling parent who is steering the young person away from certain partners and toward others.

In recent years, the median and most common age of marriage has been 22 years, although some girls have married as early as 16 or 17. Available evidence suggests that although the reasons for delaying marriage have changed over the last 60 years, from land to school pressure, the median age of marriage has changed little.

LONG—RESTRICTED STRATEGY

A maidenhood of 4 to 5 years is characteristic of this strategy. Premarital sex without penetration is encouraged. These societies employ a strategy for coping with maidenhood that is widespread among Bantu-speaking peoples of East and South Africa. Premarital sex is actively encouraged as long as penetration is avoided. Girls and boys are expected to sleep together, frequently changing partners, for several years.

Kikuyu of Kenya (1900, 1980) (011). Ngeca, a Kikuyu village 20 miles north of Nairobi, was one of the panel communities of the Child Development Research Unit of the University of Nairobi from 1968 to 1975, and was intensively studied by John and Beatrice Whiting, John Herzog,

Thomas Landauer, Herbert Liederman, and others. Carol Worthman continued the research from 1979 to 1980, focusing on adolescents.

Before the advent of the British at the turn of the century, the Kikuyu were a maize-farming group with patrilocal residence and descent, polygyny, and a highly developed age grade system into which both boys and girls were initiated at puberty. Initiation consisted of elaborate rites involving a genital operation for each sex. It was believed that in order to become a woman, a girl must have the tip of her "male" clitoris removed and the boy, to become a man, must have his "female" prepuce excised. The purpose of Kikuyu clitoridectomy has little in common with the practice of infibulation customary in some of the societies in the Sudan whose purpose was to ensure virginity.

Kikuyu girls were carefully observed by their mothers as soon as their breasts began to form, so that they could be initiated just before they first menstruated. Shortly after initiation one authority (Lambert, 1956) states that a girl must have full sexual intercourse in order to ritually remove the effects of the operation. This should take place before first menstruation so there is minimal chance of pregnancy. This is not mentioned by Kenyatta (1939) or Leakey (1977), who state that a girl should have an intact hymen at the time of marriage.

Soon after the initiation was completed, girls were carefully instructed by members of the next older age set on how to sleep with a man without getting pregnant, a practice called NGWEKO, which Kenyatta translates as "platonic love and fondling." She was told to always keep her pubic apron in place and shown how to intertwine her legs with those of her lover so that sex without penetration might be enjoyed. Young men were given similar instructions. In order to advertise her sexual attractiveness and get a high bride price, she was expected to entertain the young men from neighboring villages who came to visit her older brothers by spending the night with one of them in one of the boy's houses. Kenyatta (1979, pp. 151–152) describes the procedure.

> Girls may visit the "thingira" (boy's house) at any time, day or night. After eating, while engaged in conversation with the boys, one of the boys turns the talk to the subject of "ngweko". If there are more boys than girls, the girls are asked to select whom they want to have as their companion. The selection is done in the most liberal way. . . . It is not necessary for the girls to select their own intimate friends, as this would be considered selfish and unsociable. Of course, this does not mean that the girls do not sometimes have "NGWEKO" with those whom they are especially fond of, but generally they follow the rules of exchanging partners.

In 1968 Ngeca girls were being initiated between the ages of 13 and 14 and married between 19 and 20 (Whiting, Whiting, and Herzog, n.d.). Since menarche usually occurs about a year after initiation, the duration of maidenhood is about 6 years during which time a young Ngeca woman can select a compatible mate. Worthman (1982) reports that by 1980–1981 modernization had greatly changed their strategy for maidenhood. Christian missionaries have convinced the people of Ngeca that the elaborate initiation rites are pagan and godless, and, furthermore, that clitoridectomy is evil. Although many of the girls of Ngeca were still being initiated in 1980, it was being done in secret and individually with no attendant ritual. As a consequence, the female age grade system has broken down and there is no longer a set of older girls to instruct the novices in the proper practice of NGWEKO, and premarital pregnancy, which was rare in the traditional system, is now not unusual.

MEDIUM—ENCOURAGED STRATEGY

In this strategy, maidenhood of about 3 years is common; promiscuous premarital sex is encouraged. In this group of societies young women both before and after menarche are encouraged to engage in full sexual intercourse and to change their lovers frequently in order to find a compatible mate. Because of postmenarcheal subfecundity, a maiden in these societies seldom becomes pregnant before she has found a satisfactory mate and married him. The period of license is reported to last for up to 3 or 4 years. If pregnancy should occur during this period, a girl will marry the man of her choice whether or not he is the father of her child.

The Trobriand Islanders of Melanesia (1914) (098). The Trobriand islanders are the classical example of this strategy. Malinowski (1922, p. 53ff) describes the situation as follows:

> Chastity is an unknown virtue among these natives. At an incredibly early age they become initiated into sexual life, and many of the innocent looking plays of children are not as innocuous as they appear. As they grow up, they live in promiscuous free-love, which gradually develops into more permanent attachments, one of which ends in marriage. But before this is reached, unmarried girls are openly supposed to be quite free to do what they like, and there are even ceremonial arrangements by which girls of a village repair in a body to another place, there they publicly arrange themselves for inspection, and each is chosen by a local boy, with whom she spends a night. . . . Again, when a visiting party arrives from another district, food is brought to them by the unmarried girls, who are also expected to satisfy their sexual wants. . . . Marriage is associated with hardly any public or private ceremony. . . . Although the sexual life of the natives are very lax and an unmarried girl can have as many lovers as she likes, a girl is not supposed to become pregnant before she is married.

Using the Tanner scale for judging sexual maturity from breast development (see Buckler, 1979), the authors were able to rate 12 bare-breasted young Trobriand women in a picture published in Malinowski (ibid, Plate XII). The picture was of a group about to leave for a visit to a neighboring village to engage in the sexual behavior described above. Our ratings indicated that the developmental age of the girls ranged from 2 years before menarche to at least 3 years after. This suggests the subfecund period may have been longer among the Trobrianders than the estimate based on the Maasai data. It was this prolonged period of frequent sex without pregnancy that led the Trobrianders to believe that copulation did not cause pregnancy. In any case, postmenarcheal subfecundity apparently permitted a maidenhood of at least 3 years without pregnancy. It may be presumed that the strategies of other societies in this group are also based on this phenomenon.

SHORT—RESTRICTED STRATEGY

A maidenhood of 2 to 3 years is a common characteristic of this category. Multiple standards and complex rules govern premarital sex. Societies with this strategy are ambivalent about chastity during maidenhood. A girl's brothers may favor it and attempt to control the sexual behavior of their sisters and daughters while at the same time they are doing their best to seduce the girls of other clans who are potential spouses. It is not expected that a bride will be virginal, but her value in terms of bride price will be reduced if she becomes pregnant or is openly promiscuous. Other societies in this category provide a maiden with the alternative of being chaste until marriage or being promiscuous. Either alternative is acceptable. These and other complex strategies tend to prolong maidenhood for from 2 to 3 years.

The Kwoma of New Guinea (1937) (095). The Kwoma are a small hill tribe off the Sepik river in New Guinea. They were studied by the senior author in 1937–1938 (see Whiting, 1941, 1970). They were patrilineal, patrilocal, and polygynous. Their subsistence base was yams and taro. They both hunted and raised pigs, and collected the pith of wild sago palms to make flour. They had large ceremonial men's houses and practiced head hunting.

Their maidenhood strategy was complex. Haggling over the amount of the bride price was an important part of the wedding negotiations. Parents of the groom would claim that a potential bride was of little value if she was lazy or promiscuous and in order to reduce the bride price, would try to present evidence that such was the case. Since they would benefit from a high bride price, Kwoma bachelors had a quite different attitude toward the virtue of their sisters whose honor they strove to protect and the maidens of other lineages whose value would be lowered if they could be seduced. The strategy for a young man was to arrange a tryst with an eligible maiden in such a way that her brother would not know about it and at the same time keep careful watch over his own sisters. Kwoma girls, if they liked a suitor would go along with this strategem, and but few of them were virgins by the time they married. Kwoma parents, quite aware of this adolescent game, would arrange for a daughter's marriage soon after her puberty ceremony. Haggling over the bride price usually resulted in some delay and it might be 1 or 2 years before the final arrangements could be made. Premarital pregnancy rarely occurred.

The Papago near Sells Arizona (1910) (151). The Papago are an American Indian tribe in the Southwest. They practice maize agriculture and gather seeds and berries. They also engage in some hunting. The Papago have extended polygynous families with virilocal residence and bilateral descent.

A complex set of rules govern sexual behavior during maidenhood. Underhill (1936, p. 150 ff) describes it as follows:

> In the old days the puberty rite for girls was followed almost immediately by marriage ". . . boys and girls do not associate in unchaperoned groups, for the girls are kept under constant surveillance." . . . There was a class of women who assumed a married woman's privileges of free language and contacts with men, without any of her duties. This same class, which closely resembles that of a prostitute, is found among the Papago and called by a name which means "playful" or light woman. . . . The playful women were always in festal array. . . . So arrayed, the light women would all together go to the girl's puberty dances or to the big drinking ceremonies, where married women appeared only with their husbands and young girls not at all. The playful woman would form a temporary union with some man with whom she would visit several drinking ceremonies or dance through the whole month of puberty dances. Between affairs she would go back to her father's house. Parents made no attempt to control a daughter, if she seemed inclined to this way of life but simply gave up and allowed her to have her way. If she had children, they would take care of them, since no stigma attached to a fatherless child.

VERY SHORT—RESTRICTED STRATEGY

Marriage in this category is delayed for 1 or 2 years after menarche; premarital sex is permitted but not encouraged. The Mbuti and Kwoma maidenhood strategies are similar except that the former has a somewhat shorter maidenhood and premarital sex is less restricted than the latter.

The Efe of Zaire (1980–1981) (011). The Efe are a forest-dwelling group of pigmies situated in Zaire. They are closely related to the Mbuti described by Turnbull (1961) in his "Forest People." The Efe are presently the focus of the Harvard Ituri Project directed by Irven DeVore. The work of Nadine Peacock and Robert Bailey, members of the project, provides this example of the 1.2 maidenhood strategy (N. Peacock and R. Bailey, unpublished fieldnotes, 1982).

The Mbuti subsist from hunting and gathering and from trade with the Lese, a settled horticultural group with whom they exchange labor and forest products for manufactured goods and food. They divide their time between a nomadic life in the forest and the Lese villages. Their descent system is bilateral, but as a consequence of virilocal residence the local groups form weak patriclans. Limited polygny is practiced.

Menarcheal age was estimated from a small sample to be between 15 and 16 and marriage about 2 years later. Girls are not considered nubile until they have first menstruated and even then they are thought to be too young to marry. Early betrothal is not practiced.

Premarital sex is permitted but not encouraged. Incest rules require that a girl's lovers belong to another band. Thus nubile girls meet suitable lovers on visits to other bands to attend dances or to visit with relatives. Unmarried men and women meet when they are living in the Lese villages. Ideally, premarital sex is controlled by a girl's brothers and uncles. A potential lover, might, in fact, approach one of these relatives for permission to have intercourse with a girl. If they agree, the suitor is expected to present a gift of cloth to the girl and arrows to her relatives. Sometimes a girl will leave home and start living with a man who has not asked permission from her relatives. If the latter object, they may forcibly bring her back home. More often than not, however, the girl is permitted to have her own way.

Marriage is based on "sister exchange." Thus if a man decides to become a serious suitor, he is expected to provide one of his potential wife's male patrikin with one of his female patrikin. The couple may or may not live together during these negotiations, but they are not considered to be formally married until they are completed. Furthermore, first affairs and even first marriages are unstable. Peacock estimates that Efe girls go through three trials before they settle down into a stable relationship. This often does not occur until the first child is born. Since fertility is low (35% of a sample of 125 postmenopausal Mbuti women had never had a live birth), marital instability may be prolonged. Thus, the duration of maidenhood has a wide range, but fertile women will usually be married within 2 years after menarche and become pregnant soon thereafter.

ABSENT—PERMITTED STRATEGY

In this strategy marriage occurs before or immediately after menarche; premarital sex is permitted or ignored. Societies using this strategy arrange for their daughters to be married at or before menarche. It generally involves a betrothal arrangement previously made by the parents. The groom may move in with the bride before puberty or he may wait until she first menstruates. In almost all cases initial residence is uxorilocal, i.e., at or near the natal home of the bride.

The !Kung San of Botswana (1967–1969) (002). The !Kung are a gathering and hunting group living in small nomadic bands consisting mostly of closely related cognatic kinsmen. Incest rules require that the husband of a young woman must be found from another band. Since the population density is less than one person per square mile, it is difficult for young women to find a mate without help from her parents. Childhood betrothal is therefore customary and, according to Howell (1979, 178–179), in 65% of the observed cases, her husband moves into the hut of his young bride before she has first menstruated.

A girl's first menses is publicly celebrated. She is oiled, decorated, and secluded in a hut built especially for this purpose. While she remains inside, eating little and hidden from the view of men, other women sing and dance outside. Although the !Kung have no calendar, Howell by using an elaborate and elegant system was able to reconstruct the chronological ages of her sample. The average !Kung San girl will be just over 16 when she first menstruates and will already have been married, perhaps for several years, and perhaps to several different men. It is customary for the groom to come to the bride's camp and live there until after the first child is born or until the marriage breaks up.

Even before marriage, while she is still in her late childhood, she will have engaged in sex play with boys of her age in her band in the nearby bush or in the camp when adults are away. Such play is expected by adults, and unless it is too obtrusive is treated with amused tolerance by them. Although this experience may to some extent prepare a girl for marital intercourse at an early age, she may have an initial negative reaction. Nisa's autobiographical description of her wedding night clearly illustrates this (Shostak, 1981).

The !Kung San are characterized by a low fertility rate (Howell, 1979). This is a consequence of a 4-year interval between pregnancies. Konner and Worthman (1980) show that this long interval is a consequence of a prolonged nursing period combined with frequent nursing bouts. Since the mother sleeps with her infant and carries it in a sling over her hip when she is engaged in gathering food for the family, it is easy for her to nurse her child with little effort and she does so at frequent intervals. It is possible that a short maidenhood is an adjustment to this practice. If !Kung San women did not marry until they were in their middle twenties, they would be limited to four children which, with a high rate of infant mortality, would not be a viable reproductive strategy.

The ease and frequency of divorce before the first child is born defines these early matings as essentially trial marriages. Thus, these early and unsuccessful attempts to find a permanent mate perhaps should be considered as part of a girl's maidenhood even though she is technically married. It may, however, be an effective way for a girl to find a compatible husband. Since these early marriages take place before a young woman is fully fecund, she is not likely to become pregnant for several years and thus have ample time for several childless trials.

ABSENT—PROHIBITED STRATEGY

Brief or no maidenhood is representative of this category. Premarital sex is taboo and virginity highly valued. Societies using this maidenhood strategy also arrange that their daughters are married at or before menarche, in this case, explicitly for the purpose of ensuring premarital virginity. As soon as a girl shows signs of sexual maturity she is expected to obey elaborate rules of modesty which usually includes covering her face and hair with a veil in the presence of men; she is also carefully chaperoned. Most of the societies in this group require the "bloody sheet" test of virginity after the wedding night.

The Egyptians of Silwa (1950) (043). Silwa is a farming village with a population of slightly under 5000 inhabitants. It is situated on the Nile about 40 miles north of the Aswan dam. Preferred marriage was between patrilateral cross-cousins. Since postmarital residence was initially uxorilocal and eventually patrilocal this meant that a girl would usually marry a boy from her own village. Descent was patrilineal and the patriclan was an important political and social entity.

Both boys and girls were legally required to attend school for 5 years between the ages of 7 and 12. Few children continued their education beyond this at the time Ammar carried out his study of the village in 1950. While attending school the sexes were carefully segregated. The boys attended in the morning, while girls attended in the afternoon. As noted by Ammar (1954, pp. 183 and 185):

> In the villagers' view, adolescence (the onset of sexual maturity) and marriage are inextricably connected. It is not unusual for girls to get married by the age of twelve and thirteen. The notion of shame "ar" is a word connoting sex disgrace or sexual infidelity. . . . Boys wear long pants, whereas girls wear a headcloth to cover part of their face and their breasts on passing by men. For both, any conversation about sex is taboo, and they are forbidden to talk about it to their parents or to any grown-up. Chastity as a moral and religious ideal implies the avoidance of any stimulating pleasurable influence from the opposite sex.

Marriage was arranged by the fathers of the bride and groom. Although Ammar does not mention it, the "bloody sheet" test of virginity was probably practiced since it is traditional in Egyptian culture. After marriage a bride "starts her seclusion in the house till she brings forth a child and is never allowed to go out and never seen by a married man, even her husband's father and her married brothers" (ibid, p. 199).

THE CHOICE OF STRATEGIES

A larger and more representative sample would be needed for a fully satisfactory investigation of the reasons for the choice of the maidenhood strategies indicated in Table 15.2. We will, however, present some tentative hypotheses together with some data relevant to testing them.

HISTORICAL INFLUENCES

It is evident that the cases in both samples are not completely independent of one another. In the first sample most of the cases with a maidenhood of over 6.5 and a marriage age over 20 years are closely related. Except for Japan and the Chinese of Hong Kong, they are all European or overseas European cultures. The majority speak an Indo-European language and their religion is Judeo-Christian. There are similar clusters in the ethnographic sample. The Modern strategy is also largely European. The Mbundu and Kikuyu with long—restricted strategies are Bantu-speaking peoples of subsaharan Africa. Four of the cases with a medium—encouraged strategy are Malayo-Polynesian speaking peoples situated in Oceania. Another group of five cases with this strategy are clustered in Southeast Asia. The Amerindians of North and South America for the most part favor the very short or absent—permitted strategies. Finally the absent—forbidden strategy is characteristic of North African and the Middle Eastern Muslim cultures. However, it is also evident that most strategies are distributed over the world in such a way that diffusion and common origins could not entirely explain them, but historical influences should not be neglected if the choice of maidenhood strategies is to be understood.

FAMILY SIZE AND THE DURATION OF MAIDENHOOD

Early marriage and a brief maidenhood makes use of the full female reproductive span and thus should be be preferred by cultures in which large families are valued. Conversely, late marriage and prolonged maidenhood are more compatible with small family preference. These two reproductive strategies should not be confused with the R- and k-strategies of sociobiology. Maidenhood strategies are not transmitted from generation to generation by natural selection but by processes of learning and socialization. Thus theories of social evolution rather than biological evolution are relevant to this investigation. It is the survival of the fittest custom rather than the fittest individual that explains cultural variation. To avoid confusion between these two processes, we have chosen to call investment in large families a "distributive" strategy and in small families, a "selective" strategy.

Societies that value large families and practice a distributive strategy should have maidenhood arrangements that permit women to marry and begin childbearing as soon as they become fecund. Thus the great majority of cases in the ethnographic sample (Table 14.2) had maidenhood practices compatible with a distributive strategy. Only those with a very long—restricted and, to a limited extent, the long—restricted maidenhood strategies prolong marriage beyond the period of subfecundity and thereby limit family size by reducing the length of the female reproductive period.

There are a number of explanations why modern postindustrial societies might choose a selective maidenhood strategy. Increasing population density and decreasing land available for the next generation has been noted by many social scientists (see Goode, 1963; Udry, 1971; Goody 1976; Eekelaar and Katz, 1980) as a reason for limiting family size. Although postmarital family planning accounts for most of the variance in determining family size, late marriage also reduces the possibility of having many children.

In addition, in societies with a social class system of achievable statuses, based on occupational specialization, the success of children can require considerable parental investment. It is usually a better strategy to invest heavily in a few children rather than a little in many.

Our data tend to support both of the above explanations. The more modern societies in the postindustrial sample (see Table 14.1) have maidenhoods that last well beyond the period of subfecundity. They all practice advanced agriculture, have high population densities, occupational specialization, and a social class system of achieved status. Only India, Pakistan, and Bangladesh have brief maidenhood periods.

The ethnographic sample (see Table 14.2) also tends to support this hypothesis. The cases with a very long maidenhood strategy in this sample all have the above characteristics. It should be noted, however, that four of the societies with an absent—forbidden strategy also have an economy based on advanced agriculture, high population density, occupational specialization, and a complex social class system. These cases are Egypt, Turkey, Amhara, and Hausa. As will be discussed below, these societies all have patrilineal descent and thus the certainty of paternity gained by arranging for marriage before fecundity is highly valued. Such is not the case for the complex societies with prolonged maidenhood who all have bilateral descent systems.

It is often adaptive in egalitarian, stateless societies where subsistence is based on horticulture, agriculture, or herding to have as many children as possible. They can help in the fields or with the herds when they are young. Later, sons or sons-in-laws can, as junior warriors, protect the gardens and herds (Whiting and Whiting, 1975; Paige and Paige, 1980).

There were 28 cases in the ethnographic sample that satisfied the above criteria for middle level societies, according to published codes for subsistence type (Murdock and White, 1969) and for social stratification (Murdock and Provost, 1973). Of these, all, save the two cases with a long—restricted maidenhood strategy, make full use of the reproductive lives of their females and thus have a pattern consistent with a distributive reproductive strategy.

Foraging cultures with subsistence economies based on gathering, hunting and/or fishing face quite a different problem in choosing a maidenhood strategy to optimize their reproductive success. They have little property to protect or are young children especially helpful in their economy. Large families are therefore not especially useful. In fact when they are moving camp, as they often do, it is difficult for a mother to carry both an infant and a toddler. Often infanticide is practiced to space children (Whiting, 1964). A long nursing period with frequent bouts of feeding also characterizes many of these societies, particularly those who carry their infants in a sling from which vantage point they have easy access to their mother's breast. As discussed above, Konner and Worthman (1980) have shown that for the !Kung, the exemplar of the absent—permitted strategy, this results in an increased birth spacing and hence a decreased birth rate. The problem for the forager then is not to have a large family but to arrange to start having children as early as possible to compensate for a low birth rate. They also may thus be said to have a distributive maidenhood strategy but one that is quite different from that of the middle-level societies.

The distribution of the cases by maidenhood duration and culture type is shown in Table 14.4.

The above distribution of cases suggests that complex societies are split between maidenhood durations of 5 and 0. It should be noted that all complex cases in the postindustrial sample (Table 14.1) also have prolonged maidenhood and would fall in the top cell of the first column if they were added to this table. Thus complex societies have a stronger preference for a prolonged maidenhood than is indicated in Table 14.4. A brief maidenhood is nevertheless a clear alternative, the possible reasons for which will be discussed below.

Middle-level societies tend to prefer a maidenhood of medium duration, whereas foragers prefer one of brief duration. As it was argued above, both choices are compatible with a distributive strategy. Reasons for the difference may lie in differences in population densities.

TABLE 14.4. The Distribution of the Cases in the
Ethnographic Sample by the Duration
of Maidenhood and Culture Type

Maidenhood duration	Culture type		
	Complex	Midlevel	Foragers
5	4	0	0
4	0	2	0
3	0	11	3
1	0	9	2
0	5	8	10

According to estimates by Murdock and Provost (1973), most middle-level societies in our sample have densities of over 25 persons per square mile whereas most of the foragers have densities of less than one person and none more than five persons per square mile. In denser populations young women can easily meet appropriate partners where this is difficult for the sparsely settled foragers. Marriages are therefore usually arranged by parents at the beginning of puberty for foragers whereas maidens in middle-level societies are given time to make their own choice.

THE AGE OF MARRIAGE

Although chronological age may not be a good basis for estimating reproductive maturity, it does tell us how long a person has lived and learned and thus provides an estimate of socioeconomic competence. To take an extreme example, a precocious girl in the United States, where the median age of menarche is 12.8, may have her first menses at 11 and be fully fecund at 14 or 15. In contrast a late maturing Bundi girl from New Guinea, where the median age of menarche 18 (Malcolm, 1966), would not be equally fecund until she was 23.

Since physical and cognitive growth are positively correlated with reproductive maturity, the American girl in the above example may be above average in size and intelligence if she should become pregnant at 14, but she may still be in junior high school. She would thus be far short of achieving the socioeconomic competence required of an adult female in a society where at least a high school education is needed to compete successfully in the job market. By contrast the 20-year-old Bundi girl will have finished the rudimentary schooling and learned all the economic and social skills expected of adult women in her society.

Unfortunately, as stated above, accurate estimates of the mean chronological ages of menarche and marriage are lacking for most of the cases in the ethnographic sample. They are available only for the following cases: (menarche:marriage) !Kung 16.6:16.5; Kikuyu 15.9:21.8; Maasai 14.9:15.6; Romania 14.2:21.0.

An indirect estimate of the chronological age of marriage may be made on the basis of the 22 "tribal" cases reported in Eveleth and Tanner (1976, Table 15). The mean age of menarche for these cases is 15.4. From these data it can be tentatively assumed that menarcheal age is 2 or 3 years later, on the average, for the ethnographic sample than for the modern societies in the postindustrial sample. The chronological age of marriage for the ethnographic sample can be approximated by adding 15 to the duration of maidenhood. Thus the median age of marriage for the cases coded 0 on the duration of maidenhood scale would fall between 15 and 16 years, for those coded 1 between 16 and 17, and for those coded between 18 and 19.*

Societies with a complex social organization and access to modern medicine have both early menarche and late marriage age. All the cases in Table 14.1 that fit these criteria—from Japan through Czechoslovakia on the list—have a median age of marriage greater than 20 and an age of menarche under 14. This data supports the earlier discussed regularity that the age of marriage is late in postindustrial culture with complex social organization, social stratification with achievable status, universal schooling, and positively valued higher education for women. Maidenhood should therefore be prolonged in order to give a young woman the time and opportunity to learn the skills necessary

---

* Many possible reasons have been suggested for the later occurrence of menarche in preindustrial societies. They include malnutrition, poor health, genetic (racial) factors, climate, female work load, and others. These have been discussed by Eveleth and Tanner (1976). Two other possible reasons should be mentioned. Whiting (1965) and Landauer and Whiting (1981) have shown on a cross-cultural sample similar to the ethnographic sample in this study, that the age of menarche was significantly earlier in societies that had more stressful infant care practices. The use of cribs and cradles that separated the mother from close contact with the infant was one of these stressful practices, the assumption being that close body contact between infant and mother is comforting. Except for the North American Indians who use cradle boards (Chisholm, 1983) nearly all the cases in Table 14.2 are characterized by close mother–infant contact (Whiting, 1981). The second additional reason for late menarche in the third world is suggested in a recent paper by Ellison. He demonstrates that in Scandanavia between 1800 and 1950, the secular decrease in the age of menarche in succeeding generations can be accounted for by a decrease in infant mortality one generation previously. The correlation, adjusted for this lag, was .95. He also reported substantial correlations between infant mortality rates and menarcheal age on two additional data sets, one of them being the Eveleth and Tanner sample. One interpretation of this data might be that female infants genetically programmed to mature early are more at risk in infancy than those programmed for late maturation.

for success in such a cultural milieu. The cases with a very long maidenhood strategy in Table 14.2 also support this hypothesis.

By contrast, in most preindustrial societies with an egalitarian social system, no formal schooling and literacy not a requirement, a young woman should be competent to perform the roles she is expected to play as an adult by her late teens. The frequency of early marriage in the preindustrial sample is thus not maladaptive.

CONTROL OF PREMARITAL PREGNANCY

It is evident that premarital pregnancy can be controlled either by rules governing premarital sex, by marriage before fecundity, by contraception, or by some combination of these. There have been a number of cross-cultural studies of premarital sex restrictions (see Broude, 1980). One of the major findings from these studies are that restrictive premarital sex rules are associated with social complexity as measured by the presence of social stratification (Goethals, 1971), or intensive agriculture as a subsistence base and the belief in high gods (Murdock, 1964). This hypothesis is partially supported by the association is partially supported by the association between sex rules and social complexity in the ethnographic sample used in this study. Premarital sex is either prohibited (0) or restricted (1) in all the complex societies in the sample. By contrast, it is permitted or encouraged in most of the societies with a foraging economy. However, premarital sex is actively encouraged in many of the middle-level societies, a fact that is not consistent with the hypothesis that there is a simple linear relationship between restrictiveness and complexity. The fact that none of the previous studies controlled for the duration of maidenhood may account for the difference in the findings.

The different attitudes toward premarital sexual behavior is, of course, determined by the qualities valued in a bride. Societies that place a high value on a bride's virginity should have a maidenhood strategy that is quite different from those that believe she should be sexually competent. These values often play a part in bride price negotiations. A possible explanation for adopting a strategy of encouraging sex may be related to the reproductive strategy discussed above. In middle-level societies where a distributive strategy is most salient, the sexual competence of a daughter may enhance her value and promiscuous practice is encouraged.

The opposite extreme is represented by those societies that place a high value on a virgin bride, strictly prohibit premarital sex, and arrange for an early marriage for their daughters to make doubly sure that their aim is accomplished. Goethals (1971) argued that the requirement of virginity should be related to patrilineal descent where

the certainty of paternity is more important than in societies where matrilineal or bilateral descent was the rule. If the cases in the ethnographic sample with an absent—prohibited strategy are compared with
those middle-level cases with a medium—encouraged strategy, this
hypothesis is confirmed. The phi value of the association is .606 ($p<.001$).

The certainty of paternity hypothesis may also explain why all the
complex societies with a very long—restricted strategy have bilateral
descent rules while all save one of those with an absent—prohibited
strategy have patrilineal descent. It is worth noting that most of the
former group are Christian while all but one of the latter group are
Muslim.

BACHELORHOOD

An obvious and necessary accompaniment to further research on
maidenhood is an investigation of bachelorhood. In some societies men
and women marry at similar developmental or chronological ages.
More commonly the man is expected to be older than the woman and
this is accomplished by a prolonged bachelorhood during which time
the young man may be a junior warrior, working away, or accumulating enough capital to support a wife. We did not code our sample
for these variables, but this should be done.

DISCUSSION

This chapter describes some of the maidenhood strategies that have
been developed during the course of human social evolution. We have
advanced some hypotheses to account for the choice of particular
strategies in particular contexts and hope that we have successfully
conveyed the more general point that maidenhood strategies are neither arbitrary, nor immutable, but rather are closely attuned to social,
technological, and environmental factors.

There is a need to address what our methods of analysis and findings
might contribute to an understanding of the central concern of this conference: the problem of school-age pregnant girls in the United States.
It appears to us, as we have listened to public debate on this topic,
that the paradigm employed by almost all commentators contains two
central tenets. First, that young girls of school age are too immature
to successfully raise their children. Second, that it is preferrable and
desirable for all young girls to choose a career, complete their education, work, court, marry, possibly work some more, and then, begin
a family. Given these tenets, one can advocate that the ideal American
maidenhood strategy should be followed while limiting sexual activity
(the abstinence approach), or by controlling pregnancy (the planned

parenthood approach). Not infrequently, a compromise plan is advocated: young women should remain chaste until social maturity at 18 or 21 after which sex with contraception is allowed until marriage occurs and the decision to start a family is made.

The first assumption, that teenagers are somehow, prima facie, too young to be mothers, is clearly not supported by the ethnographic record. Through most of human history, young women have married and born their first child within 4 years of menarche while still in their teens. The great difference, of course, between preindustrial societies and the contemporary United States is that in those societies the community was willing and able to support the young mother, both morally and practically. Almost always the young mother could count on the support of her family, and, if married, on the support of her husband's family. In many cases the groom moved in with the bride's family and the couple continued to live there until at least after the first child was born. Alternatively, the young couple set up housekeeping in the groom's parents' residence where his family was available for support. The neolocal residence pattern, common in our society, in which a couple set up a household apart from either family is quite rare in preindustrial societies. From the perspective of a Kwoma or !Kung, the problem of school-age pregnancies is not why are these young women getting pregnant, but why is this society so resentful and unsupportive of them.

The second assumption, that the modern method is somehow prima facie most desirable can also be questioned. Certainly, there is nothing sacrosanct about it. Again, most human societies for most of human history have fared very well without it. The most that can be said for it is that it was well adapted to the historic needs of European and Asian complex societies. However, once the argument is phrased in terms of adaptive fit, then the way is open to question whether it is still an optimal strategy. Clearly, the world has changed from what it was when the "modern" strategy was first developed. In the last 200 years there have been tremendous changes in industry and technology, in education, health care, and contraception, to name but a few. The "modern" maidenhood strategy may no longer be the most appropriate one for most Americans.

Once the above two central tenets are no longer assumed to be self-evident, we are free to explore new and different policy alternatives for teenage girls besides chastity and planned parenthood. We may even look again at some of the patterns used in the preindustrial past and ask whether or not they can be adapted to our needs. In particular, the feasibility of a shorter maidenhood should be explored. For example, some families may want to offer to their daughters the possibility of an early marriage. Using modern contraception, family size would be limited to two or three closely spaced children, and the grandparents would share in their upbringing. By her mid-twenties the young woman would be fully ready to continue her education or enter the work force. She could then concentrate fully on her career and remain continuously employed. By her mid-thirties she has an established career, a completed family, and may even be welcoming grandchildren into her home.

In truth, we need not look very far. Different subcultures within American society are already employing variants of many of the strategies we have discussed in this chapter, and also are developing new ones which meet their psychological and material needs. What we need most is to lose some of our ethnocentric beliefs about what is right and proper, and recognize there are viable alternative maidenhood strategies for young American girls. This alone would be a significant step toward solving the "problem" of teenage pregnancies.

ETHNOGRAPHIC REFERENCES

The references listed below are arranged in order of standard sample identification. The reader is also advised to cross-refer to Table 15.2.

2. *!Kung: The !Kung of Dobe and Nyae Nyae in the 1950's, 1960's and 1970's.*
   Howell, N. *Demography of the Dobe !Kung.* New York: Academic Press, 1979.
   Marshall, L. *The !Kung of Nyae Nyae.* Cambridge, Mass: Harvard University Press, 1976.
   Shostak, M. N. *The life and words of a !Kung woman.* Cambridge, Mass: Harvard University Press, 1981.
5. *MBUNDU: Bailundo subtribe in 1890.*
   Childs, G.M. *Umbundu kinship and character.* London and New York: International Africal Institute and the Witwatersrand University Press, 1949.
11. *KIKUYU: The town of Ngeca in 1900, 1968, and 1980.*
   Kenyatta, J. *Facing Mount Kenya.* New York: Random House, 1939.
   Leakey, L. S. B. *The southern Kikuyu before 1903* (3 vols.). London: Academic Press, 1977.
   Whiting, J., Whiting, B., Herzog, J., and Landauer, T. Unpublished fieldnotes, 1975.
   Worthman, C. *Developmental dysynchrony as normative experience: Kikuyu adolescents.* in this volume, Chapter 6.
   Worthman, C. Unpublished fieldnotes, 1982.
13. *MBUTI: Pygmies of the Ituri region in 1980.*
   Peacock, N. Unpublished fieldnotes, 1982.
21. *WOLOF: The Wolof of Upper and Lower Salum in the Gambia in 1950.*
   Ames, D.W. *Plural marriage among the Wolof in the Gambia, with a consideration of problems of marital adjustment and patterned ways of resolving tensions.* Ann Arbor, Mich: University Microfilms, 4, 145 1, 1953.

23. *TALLENSI: The small Tallensi tribe as a whole in 1934.*
Fortes, M. *The web of kinship among the Tallensi: The second part of an analysis of the social structure of a Trans-Volta tribe.* London: Oxford University Press, 1949.
Fortes, M. *Social and psychological aspects of education in Taleland.* London: Oxford University Press for the International Institute of African Languages and Cultures, 1938.
26. *HAUSA: The Hausa of Province 28 in 1900.*
Smith, M.G. *The Hausa of Northern Nigeria. In* J. L. Gibbs (Ed.), *Peoples of Africa.* New York: Holt, 1965.
Smith, M.G. *The Economy of Hausa Communities of Zaria.* Colonial Office Research Studies 16. London, 1955.
28. *AZANDE: The Azande of the Yambio chiefdom in 1905.*
Evans-Pritchard, E.E. *The dance.* Africa, 1928, *1,* 446–462.
Hutereau, A. *Notes sur la vie familiale et juridique de quelques populations du Congo Belge* (Notes on the family and legal life of some peoples of the Belgian Congo). Bruxelles: Ministre des Colonies, 1909.
34. *MAASAI: The Maasai of Loita Hills, Kenya in 1968–1970.*
Llewelyn-Daves, M. Unpublished fieldnotes, 1972.
36. *SOMALI: The Dolbahanta subtribe in 1900.*
Lewis, I.M. *Peoples of the Horn of Africa.* London: Oxford University Press, 1955.
Lewis, I.M. *A pastoral democracy: A study of pastoralism and politics among the Northern Somali of the Horn of Africa.* London, Oxford University Press, 1961.
37. *AMHARA: The Amhara of the Gondar district in 1953.*
Levine, D.N. *Wax and gold: Tradition and innovation in Ethiopian culture.* Chicago: University of Chicago Press, 1965.
43. *EGYPTIANS: The town and environs of Silwa in 1950.*
Ammar, H. *Growing up in an Egyptian village: Silwa, province of Aswan.* London: Routledge and Kegan Paul, 1954.
Blackman, W.S. *The fellahin of Upper Egypt: Their religious, social and industrial life today with special references to survivals from ancient times.* With a foreward by R. R. Marett. London: Harrap, 1927.
Klunzinger, C.B. *Working days and holidays, days of jubilee and days of mourning. Upper Egypt: Its people and its products.* New York: Scribner, Armstrong, 1878, pp. 158–203.
47. *TURKS: The Turks of the Northern Anatolian plateau in 1950.*
Yasa, Ibrahim. *Hasanoglan: Socio-economic structure of a Turkish village.* Ankara: Yeni Matbaa, 1957.
Stirling, P. Land, marriage and the law in Turkish villages. *International Social Science Bulletin,* 1957.
48. *GHEG: The Mountain Gheg of Northern Albania in 1910.*
Coon, C. S. *The mountains of giants: A racial and cultural study of the North Albanian Ghegs.* Cambridge, Mass.: Peabody Museum, 1950.
Durham, N. E. *Some tribal origins, laws and customs of the Balkans.* London: George, Allen & Unwin, 1928.
000. *ROMANIANS: The Romanians of Baisora in 1981.*
Ratner, M. S. Unpublished fieldnotes, 1981.
51. *RURAL IRISH: The Irish of County Clare in 1932.*
Arensberg, C. M., and Kimbal, S. T. Preface by W. L. Warner. Cambridge, Mass.: Harvard University Press, 1940.

SSIANS: The village of Viratiano in 1955.
ʌnet, S. (Ed.) The village of Viriatino. Garden City, New York: Double Day, 1970.
KURD: The Kurd of the town and environs of Rowanduz in 1951.
Hansen, H. H. The Kurdish woman's life: Field research in a Muslim society. Iraq: Kobenhavn, Nationalmuseet, 1961.
Masters, W. M. Rowanduz: A Kurdish administrative and mercantile center. Ann Arbor, Mich.: University Microfilms, 1954, 358 1. (University Microfilms Publications, no. 7689.) Dissertation, University of Michigan, 1953.

60. GOND: The Hill Maria Gond in 1938.
Elwin, V. The Maria and their ghotul. London: Oxford University Press, 1947.
Grigson, W. V. The Maria Gonds of Bastar. Introduction by J. H. Hutton. Reissued in 1949. London: Oxford University Press, 1949.

61. TODA: The small Toda tribe as a whole in 1900.
Marshall, W. E. A phrenologist amongst the Todas. London: Longmans & Green, 1873.
Rivers, W. H. The Todas. London: New York: Macmillan, 1906.

67. LOLO: The independent and relatively unacculturated Lolo of the Taliang Shan mountains in 1910.
Yueh-hwa, L. Lian-shan I-chia (The Lolo of Liang-shan). Shanghai: Commercial Press, 1947.

68. LEPCHA: The Lepcha in the vicinity of Lingthem in Sikkim in 1937.
Gorer, G. Himalayan village: An account of the Lepchas of Sikkim. Introduction by J. H. Hutton. London: M. Joseph, 1938.
Morris, J. Living with Lepchas: A book about the Sikkim Himalayas. London, Toronto: W. Heineman, 1938.

79. ANDAMANS: The Aka-Bea tribe of South Andaman in 1860.
Man, H. E. On the aboriginal inhabitants of the Andaman Island. London: Royal Anthropological Institute of Great Britain and Ireland, 1932.

89. ALOR: The village complex of Atimelan in North Central Alor in 1938.
DuBois, C. The people of Alor: A social-psychological study of an East Indian island. Minneapolis, Minn: University of Minnesota Press, 1944.

91. ARANDA: The Arunta Mbainda of Alice Springs in 1896.
Spencer, W. B. & Gillen, F. J. The Arunta: A study of a stone-age people (Vol. 2). London: Macmillan, 1927.

94. KAPAUKAU: The village of Botukebo in the Kamu Valley in 1955.
Pospisil, L. J. Kapauka Papuans and their law. New Haven: Yale University Press, 1958.
Pospisil, L. J. Kapauku Papuan political structure. In V.F. Ray (Ed.), Systems of political control and bureaucracy in human societies. Seattle, Washington, 1958.
Pospisil, L. J. Social change and primitive law: Consequences of a Papuan legal case. American Anthropologist, 1958.
Pospisil, L. J. Kapauku Papuan economy. New Haven: Yale University Press, 1963.

95. KWOMA: The Hongwam Sub-tribe of the Kwoma of the upper Sepik River in New Guinea in 1938.
Whiting, J. Becoming a Kwoma, teaching and learning in a New Guinea tribe. New Haven, Conn.: Yale University Press, 1941.

97. NEW IRELAND: The village of Lesu in 1930.
Powdermaker, H. Life in Lesu: The study of a Melanesian society in New Ireland. New York: Norton, 1933.

98. *TROBRIANDS: The island of Kiriwina in 1914.*
Malinowski, B. *Argonauts of the western Pacific: An account of native enterprise and adventure in the archipelagoes of Melanesian New Guinea.* London: George Routledge and Sons, 1922.
Malinowski, B. *The sexual life of savages in northwestern Melanesia: An ethnographic account of courtship, marriage and family life among the natives of the Trobriand Islands, British New Guinea* (Vols. 1 and 2). New York: Horace Liveright, 1929.

105. *MARQUESAS: The Te-i'i chiefdom of southwestern Nuku Hiva Island about 1800.*
Handy, E. W. C. *The native culture of the Marquesas.* Honolulu: Bernice P. Bishop Museum, 1923.
Linton, R. Marquesan culture. In A. Kardiner (Ed.), *The individual and his society: The psychodynamics of primitive social organization.* New York: Columbia University Press, 1939, pp. 138–196.

108. *MARSHALLESE: Marshall Islands, Jaluit Atoll in 1900.*
Endland, A. *Die Marshall-Insulaner: Leben und sitte, sinn und religion eines Sudsee-volkes* (The Marshall Islanders: Life and customs, thought and religion of a South Seas people). Aschendorff, 1914.
Spoehr, A. *Majuro: A village in the Marshall Islands.* Chicago: Chicago Natural History Museum, 1949.
Wedgewood, C. H. Notes on the Marshall Islands. Oceania, 1942–1943.

112. *IFUGAO: The Central and Kiangan Ifugao in 1910.*
Barton, R. F. *The half-way sun: Life among the headhunters of the Philippines.* New York: Brewer and Warren, 1930.
Lembrecht, F. The Mayawya ritual. *Journal of East Asiatic Studies,* 1955 (No. 4), pp. 1–555.

117. *JAPANESE: The village of Suye Mura in 1936.*
Embree, J. F. *A Japanese village.* Chicago: University of Chicago Press, 1939.
Smith, R.J., and Wiswell, E.L. *The women of Suye Mura.* Chicago: University of Chicago Press, 1982.

119. *GILYAK: The Gilyak of Sakhalin Island in 1980.*
Shternberg, L. I. *Giliaki, Grochi, Gol'dy, Negidal'tsy, Ainy: Stat'i i materialy* (The Gilyak, Grochi, Goldi, Negidal, Ainu, articles and materials). IA. P. Al'kor (Ed.), Khabarovsk, Dal'giz, 1933.

120. *YUKAGHIR: The Yukaghir of the Upper Kolyma River.*
Jochelson, W. *The Yukaghir and Yukaghirized Tungus: Memoirs of the American Museum of Natural History,* 1926.

124. *COPPER ESKIMO: The Copper Eskimo of the Arctic mainland in 1915.*
Jenness, D. *The life of the Copper Eskimos.* Ottawa: F. A. Acland, King's Printer, 1922.

126. *MICMAC: The Micmac of the mainland in 1650.*
Le Clercq, C. *New Relations of Gaspesia.* Toronto: Publications of the Champlain Society, 1910.
Denys, N. *The description and natural history of the coasts of Northern America.* Toronto: Publications of the Champlain Society, 1908.

129. *KASKA: The Kaska of the Upper Liard River, reconstructed for 1900.*
Honigmann, J. J. The Kaska Indians: An ethnographic reconstruction. New Haven, Conn.: Yale University Press, 1949.

137. *NORTHERN PAIUTE: The Wadadika or Harney Valley band reconstructed for about 1870.*
Whiting, B. B. *Paiute sorcery.* New York: Viking Fund, 1950.

140. *GROS VENTRE: The Homogeneous Gros Ventre as a whole in 1880.*
     Cooper, J.M. *The Gros Ventres of Montana. Part 2: Religion and ritual.* R. Flannery (Ed.). Washington, D.C.: Catholic University of America, 1956.
     Flannery, R. (Ed.). *The Gros Ventres of Montano. Part 1: Social life.* Washington, D.C.: Catholic University of America, 1953.
147. *COMANCHE: The Comanche as a whole in 1870.*
     Hoebel, E. A. *The political organization and law-ways of the Comanche Indians.* Menasha, Wisconsin; American Anthropological Association, 1940.
150. *HAVASUPAI: The small Havasupai tribe as a whole in 1918.*
     Smithson, C. L. *The Havasupai woman.* Salt Lake City, Utah: University of Utah Press, 1959.
     Spier, L. *Havasupai ethnography.* New York: American Museum of Natural History, 1928.
151. *PAPAGO: The Archie Papago near Sells in 1910.*
     Underhill, R.M. *The autobiography of a Papago woman.* Menesha, Wisconsin: American Anthropological Association, 1936.
158. *CUNA: The Cuna of the San Blas Archipelago in 1927.*
     Nordenskiold, E. *An historical and ethnological survey of the Cuna Indians. In* H. Wassen (Ed.). Eteborg: Guteborg Museum, Ethnographiska Avdelningen, 1938.
     Marshall, D. S. *Cuna folk: A conceptual scheme involving the dynamic factors of culture, as applied to the cuna Indians of Darien.* Unpublished manuscript presented in partial fulfillment of the requirements for the A. B. Degree with honors (Anthropology). Cambridge, Mass: Harvard University Press, 1950.
163. *YANAMAMO: The Shamatari subtribe around the village of Bisaasi-teri in 1965.*
     Chagnon, N.A. *The fierce people.* New York: Holt, Rinehart & Winston, 1968.
164. *CARIB: The Carib along the Barama River in British Guiana in 1932.*
     Gillin, J. *The Barama River Caribs of British Guiana.* Cambridge, Mass: Peabody Museum of American Archaeology and Ethnology, 1936.
169. *JIVARO: The Jivaro proper in 1920.*
     Karsten, R. *The head-hunters of western Amazonas: The life and culture of the Jibaro Indians of eastern Ecuador and Peru.* Helsingfors: Central Trychkeriet, 1935.
     Stirling, M. W. *Historical and ethnographical material on the Jivaro Indians.* Washington, D.C.: Government Printing Office, 1938.
     Simson, A. Notes on the Jivaros and Canelos Indians. Anthropological Institute of Great Britain and Ireland. *Journal,* 1880.
     Up de Graff, F.W. *Head-hunters of the Amazon: Seven years of exploration and adventure,* New York: Duffield, 1923.
173. *SIRIONO: The Siriono in the forests near the Rio Blanco in 1942.*
     Holmberg, A. R. *Nomads of the long bow: The Siriono of eastern Bolivia.*
     Holmberg, A. R. *The Siriono: A study of the effect of hunger frustration on the culture of a semi-nomadic Bolivian Indian society.* New Haven, Conn.: Yale University Press, 294 1. Dissertation (Anthropology), 1946.
176. *TIMBIRA: The Ramcocamercra or Eastern Timbira in 1915.*
     Nimuendaju, C. *The eastern Timbira.* R. H. Lowie (Ed.), Los Angeles, CA: University of California Press, 1946.

177. *TUPINAMBA: The Tupinamba near Rio De Janeiro in 1550.*
   Cardim, F. *A treatise of Brasil and articles touching the dutie of the Kings Majestie our Lord, and to the common good of all the estate of Brasis.* S. Purchas (Ed.). Hakluytus Posthumus or Purchas His Pilgrimes, 1906.
   deSouza, G. S. *Tratado descriptive do Brazil em 1587* (Descriptive treatise on Brazil in 1587). Instituto Historico e Geographico do Brazil, Revista, 1851.
185. *TEHUELCHE: The equestrian Teheulche in 1970.*
   deViedma, A. Description de la costa meridional del sur, llamada vulgarmente Patagonica (Description of the southern shores of that region commonly called Patagonia). In P. De Angelis (Ed.), *Coleccion de Obras y Documentos Relativos a la historia Antigua y Moderna de las Provincias del Rio de la Plata* (Vol. 6). Buenos Aires: Inprenta del Estado, 1837.
   Musters, G. C. On the races of Patagonia. Vol. 1, Anthropological Institute of Great Britain and Ireland, *Journal,* 1872.
186. *YAHGAN: The eastern and central Yahgan reconstructed for 1865.*
   Gusinde, M. *Die Yamana: vom Leben und Denken der Wassernomaden am Kap Hoorn* (The Yahgan: The life and thought of the water nomads of Cape Horn). Modling bei Wien, Anthropos-Bibliothek, 1937.

REFERENCES

Ammar, H. *Growing up in an Egyptian village, Silwa, Province of Aswan.* London: Routledge & Kegan Paul, Ltd., 1954.

Broude, G. J. The cultural management of sexuality. In R. H. Munroe, R. L. Munroe, and B. Whiting (Eds.), *Handbook of cross-cultural human development.* New York: Garland, 1981.

Buckler, J. M. H. *A reference manual of growth and development.* Oxford: Blackwell, 1979.

Chisholm, J. Navajo Infancy. New York: Aldine, 1983.

Dixon, R. B. Explaining cross-cultural variation in age at marriage and proportions never marrying. *Population Studies,* 1971.

Eekelaar, J. M., and Katz, S. N. *Marriage and cohabitation in contemporary societies: areas of legal, social and ethical change.* Toronto: Butterworths, 1980.

Ellison, P. Morbidity, mortality and menarche. *Human Biology,* 1981, 53, 4.

Eveleth, P., and Tanner, J. M. *Worldwide variations in human growth.* Cambridge: Cambridge University Press, 1976.

Goethals, G. W. Factors affecting permissive and nonpermissive rules regarding premarital sex. In J. M. Henslin (Ed.), *Sociology of sex: A book of readings.* New York: Appleton-Century-Croft, 1971.

Goode, W. J. *World revolution and family patterns.* New York: Free Press, 1963.

Goody, J. *Production and reproduction.* New York: Cambridge University Press, 1976.

Howell, N. *Demography of the Dobe !Kung.* New York: Academic Press, 1979.

Kenyatta, J. *Facing Mount Kenya.* New York: Random House, 1939.

Konner, M., and Worthman, C. Nursing frequency, gonadal function and birth spacing among !Kung hunters-gatherers. *Science,* 1980.

Lambert, H. E. *Kikuyu social and political institutions*. London: Oxford University Press, 1956.

Landauer, T. K., and Whiting, J. W. M. Correlates and consequences of stress in infancy. *In* R. H. Munroe, R. L. Munroe, and B. B. Whiting (Eds.), *Handbook of cross-cultural human development*. New York: Garland Press, 1981.

Leakey, L. S. B. *The southern Kikuyu before 1903*. London: Academic Press, 1977 (3 Volumes).

Malcolm, L. A. The age of menarche among the Bundi people of Papua. *Papua New Guinea Medical Journal*, 1966, 9.

Malinowski, B. *The sexual life of savages in northern Melanesia: An ethnographic account of courtship, marriage and family life among the natives of the Trobriand Islands, British New Guinea* (Vols. 1 and 2). New York: Horace Liveright, 1929.

Montague, A. *Reproductive development of the female*. Littleton, Mass.: Wright P.S.G., 1979.

Murdock, G. P. Cultural correlates of the regulation of premarital sex behavior. *In* R. A. Manners (Ed.), *Process and pattern in culture*. Chicago: Aldine, 1964.

Murdock, G. P., and Provost, C. Measurement of cultural complexity. *Ethnology*, 1973, XII, 4.

Murdock, G. P., and White, D. R. Standard cross-cultural sample. *Ethnology*. 1969, *VIII*, 4.

Paige, K. E. and Paige, J. M. *Politics and reproduction rituals*. Berkeley: University of California Press, 1980.

Peacock, N., and Bailey, R. Unpublished fieldnotes, 1982.

Shostak, M. N. *The life and words of a !Kung woman*. Cambridge, Mass.: Harvard University Press, 1981.

Udry, J. R. *The social context of marriage*. Philadelphia: J. B. Lippincott, 1971.

Underhill, R. M. *The autobiography of a Papago woman*. Menasha, Wisconsin: American Anthropological Association, 1936, 2.

Whiting, J. W. M. *Becoming a Kwoma, teaching and learning in a New Guinea tribe*. New Haven, Conn.: Yale University Press, 1941.

Whiting, J. W. M. Effects of climate on certain cultural practices. *In* W. Goodenough (Ed.), *Explorations in cultural anthropology. Essays in honor of George Peter Murdock*. New York: McGraw Hill, 1964.

Whiting, J. W. M. Menarchal age and infant stress in humans. *In* F. A. Beach (Ed.), *Sex and behavior*. New York: Wiley, 1965.

Whiting, J. W. M. *Kwoma journal, HRAFlex Book OJ13-001*. New Haven, Conn.: Human Relations Area Files, 1970.

Whiting, J. W. M. Environmental constraints on infant care practices. *In* R. L. Munroe, R. M. Munroe, and B. B. Whiting (Eds.). *Handbook of cross cultural human development*. New York: Garland, 1981.

Whiting, J. W. M. and Whiting, B. Aloofness and intimacy of husbands and wives. *Ethos*, 1975, *3* (2).

Whiting, J. W. M., Whiting, B., Herzog, J., Landauer, T., Liederman, H. Unpublished fieldnotes, 1973.

Worthman, C. *Developmental dysynchrony as normative experience: Kikuyu adolescents*. Paper delivered at the Social Science Research Council meeting on School-Age Pregnancy and Parenthood, Md., 1982.

15

ADOLESCENT SEXUALITY, PREGNANCY, AND CHILDBEARING IN EARLY AMERICA: SOME PRELIMINARY SPECULATIONS*

Maris A. Vinovskis

While adolescent sexuality, pregnancy, and childbearing in the United States today are suddenly receiving an extraordinary amount of attention, there is almost no research available from the past on these issues. On the one hand, historians of human sexuality and fertility usually do not distinguish between the behavior of adolescents and adults (Vinovskis, 1981b; Wells, 1975). On the other hand, most of the historical studies of teenagers do not include an analysis of adolescent sexuality and childbearing (Kett, 1977). As a result of this lack of historical scholarship, this chapter will of necessity only provide an exploratory and cursory overview. Yet by bringing together the available scattered pieces of information, it will at least delineate some of the basic issues as well as provide some tentative answers. Although the chapter will try to present comparative data whenever possible, its focus and evidence are mainly from New England in the seventeenth, eighteenth, and nineteenth centuries.†

*Revision of paper presented at the Social Science Research Council Conference on "School-Age Pregnancies and Parenthood" at the Belmont Conference Center, Baltimore, Maryland, May 23–26, 1982. This research was made possible by a fellowship from the John Simon Guggenheim Memorial Foundation.

†In the past, people were more likely to use the term "youth" rather than "adolescent" or "teenager" and it encompassed individuals roughly from age 15 to 21 or 24. For purposes of this chapter, however, the terms "adolescent" and "teenager" will be used interchangeably and will refer to children from 13 through 19.

AGE AT MENARCHE AND MARRIAGE

One explanation for the lack of attention to adolescent sexuality, pregnancy, and childbearing in the past may be that they were not important factors in the lives of those individuals. If the age of sexual maturity in the past, for example, was much higher than today, then most teenagers would not have been concerned about becoming pregnant or bearing children. We should not assume that our forebears matured sexually at the same ages as we do today—especially since there is considerable evidence of a secular decline in the age of menarche (Wyshak and Frisch, 1982; Tanner, 1965; Brundtland and Walloe, 1976).

The age at menarche is particularly important for understanding family life in early America because the puritans did not consider marriage valid unless both partners were sexually mature and the marriage had been consummated. In fact, the inability to have sexual intercourse was considered grounds for annulling a "marriage" (Laslett, 1971). Therefore, the age at menarche set the lower limits for the ages at which girls could marry in colonial America.

Information on the age at menarche in the past is quite limited and of varying quality, although enough data has survived to allow some general observations. While girls today experience menarche at about 12.8 years, their American and European counterparts 100 years ago had to wait several more years. Grace Wyshak and Rose Frisch (1982) recently reviewed 218 reports on the age of menarche in Europe from 1875 to 1981 (including 220,037 individuals). They found that in the early nineteenth century the age of menarche may have been as high as 17 or 18 years old. In Europe the age at menarche declined by two or three months per decade in the century and a half, the greatest decline occurring in the Scandinavian countries and the smallest occurring in France.

The age at menarche appears to be associated with many different factors, such as, fatness in adolescence, physique, health status, genetics, and socioeconomic status (Johnston, 1974). The best-established factor, however, is nutrition with severe malnutrition delaying menarche (Frisch and McArthur, 1974).

Since age at menarche appears to be closely linked with the environmental conditions under which children develop, any attempt to extrapolate directly from the age at menarche in Europe to colonial America is highly questionable. In fact, when information on the ages at menarche are available for the United States in the late nineteenth and twentieth centuries, those figures are consistently lower than the European averages. Data from the United States indicates a secular decline in age at menarche from 14.75 years in Bowditch's study of

1877, to about 14 years at the turn of the century, and to 12.8 years in 1947. Since that time, the age at menarche in the United States seems to have leveled off (Wyshak and Frisch, 1982).

Although we have reasonable estimates of the age at menarche in the United States in the last quarter of the nineteenth century, we do not have comparable data for the seventeenth and eighteenth centuries. There are, however, some estimates of the age of menarche among slaves for the antebellum period.

A recent analysis by Fogel and Engerman (1974) of antebellum slavery argued that plantation owners did not try to maximize their profits by deliberately breeding their slaves. As proof, they cited the relatively late age at first birth among slaves compared to their lower age of menarche. Critics of Fogel and Engerman quickly challenged many of their assumptions including their discussion of the age at menarche (Gutman and Sutch, 1976). As a result, Trussell and Steckel (1978) recalculated the ages at menarche and first birth for antebellum slaves using probate and plantation records. Based on an estimate of the caloric intake of slaves as well as on an analysis of spurts in their heights, Trussell and Steckel concluded that menarche occurred at least by age 15 and probably somewhat earlier.

Another indirect indicator of the age at menarche among the white population in the United States in the nineteenth century is provided by the debates over the advisability of older girls attending colleges or universities. Many nineteenth-century physicians such as Horatio Storer described menstruation as "periodic infirmity . . . temporary insanity" (cited in Walsh, 1977, p. 111). Similarly, Dr. Edward Clarke warned against educating women the same way as men since the uterus was connected to the central nervous system. Energy expended on intellectual pursuits would necessarily arrest the normal but sudden spurt of reproductive development at the time of puberty. The results of female education under these circumstances would be "monstrous brains and puny bodies; abnormally active cerebration and abnormally weak digestion; flowing thought and constipated bowels" (Clarke, 1873, p. 41). Although the advice of doctors such as Storer and Clarke were challenged by others, the debates implied that girls experienced menarche at about age 14 or 15—quite close to the figure suggested by the Bowditch study as well as the estimate of menarche among antebellum slaves.

If the age at menarche in the United States in the nineteenth century was around 14 or 15, is it possible to make any inferences about the seventeenth and eighteenth centuries? Unfortunately, we do not have any detailed studies of the age at menarche for that period, but the investigations of nutrition and wealth suggest that American colonists fared better than their European counterparts (Jones, 1980). Furthermore, since the height of individuals is considered to be a reasonable proxy of their nutritional background, the fact that the average height of army enlistees in the United States from 1799 to 1894 remained fairly constant (Soltow and Stevens, 1981) reinforces the idea that little change in nutrition had occurred between the late eighteenth and nineteenth centuries. Therefore, one might speculate that the age at menarche in colonial America was around 15 or 16, although no substantial direct evidence on this has thus far been uncovered.

One additional point should be made about the age at menarche. While menarche signified to early Americans the sexual maturity of girls, it does not mean that they were all immediately capable of child-bearing. There is a period of adolescent subfertility, which considerably reduces fecundability (Talwar, 1965; Trussell and Steckel, 1978). Furthermore, there are some indications that adolescent subfertility and age at menarche may be related so that the period of reduced fecundability is shortened as the age at menarche declines (Frisch, 1975). Therefore, even if adolescents in early America experienced menarche by age 15 or 16, we should not expect most of them to bear children at those ages even if they were already sexually active.

Having speculated about the age at menarche, we should now turn to the age at marriage as another potentially important factor affecting the lives of adolescents in the past. If teenagers married soon after puberty, then many of the problems currently associated with adolescent sexuality, pregnancy, and childbearing (Card and Wise, 1978; Furstenberg, 1976; Moore and Caldwell, 1977) would not have been historically present.

In many societies marriage signifies the transition from being dependent upon one's own family to establishing a separate household. At least by the sixteenth and seventeenth centuries, individuals in Western Europe were expected to enter into matrimony only if they were economically able to create and maintain their own home. Under these circumstances, an early marriage was usually considered desirable as it signified relative independence from others and the start of one's own family (Stone, 1977).

The requirement of being able to maintain an independent home meant that many individuals were forced to postpone their marriages or to remain single throughout their lives. J. Hagnal (1965) characterized this as the "European marriage pattern" with men marrying in their late twenties and women in their early or mid-twenties. As a result, it was common for adolescents to go through their teenage years without experiencing sexual intercourse or bearing a child (Stone, 1977).

Whereas economic scarcity generally precluded early marriages in Western Europe in the seventeenth and eighteenth centuries, it should not have been a major deterent in the New World where economic opportunities were more plentiful (Walton and Shepherd, 1979; Jones, 1980). Indeed, early historians of the American family such as Earle (1895) and Calhoun (1960) simply assumed that girls married at a very young age.

> The early Puritans married young . . . . Girls often married at sixteen or under. Old maids were ridiculed or even despised. A woman became an "antient maid" at twenty-five (p. 67).

While present-day analyses of adolescents almost uniformly point to the problems caused by early marriages and childbearing, these studies suggest just the opposite—those women in colonial America who did not marry as young teenagers were the ones who were considered to be unfortunate and disadvantaged.

The early historians of the family relied almost exclusively on literary evidence for estimating age at first marriage in colonial America. However, in the late 1960s demographic historians such as Demos (1970), Greven (1970), and Lockridge (1970) tried to determine empirically the age at first marriage by reconstituting the lives of the early settlers from the local town and church records in New England. They discovered (to everyone's surprise) that few New England girls married as early as age fifteen or sixteen.

The general contours of the age at first marriage in colonial New England are now fairly clear. Compared to their counterparts in England, men and women married at younger ages. Overall, women married in their very early twenties and men married during their late twenties. There was a gradual increase in the ages at which women married from the seventeenth to the eighteenth centuries while there was a corresponding decrease in the age at which men married (Vinovskis, 1981b). Although the data on the ages at first marriage for the nineteenth century are more scarce than for the colonial period, they suggest a slight increase. Thus, the mean age at first marriage in Massachusetts from 1845 to 1860 was about 26 for males and 24 for females. The relative insignificance of marriage among teenagers in the nineteenth century is illustrated by the fact that only 3.6% of native-born women, ages 14–19, were married and 4.7% of foreign-born adolescents (Massachusetts, 1887). The important point is that at no time during the colonial or early national period were large numbers of very young adolescents marrying in New England.*

---

*The situation in the South may be somewhat different than in the North since women may have married at earlier ages in the first years of settlement. As new studies of the demographic history of the South become available, we should be able to undertake a broader and more comparative analysis of this topic.

While there has been no comprehensive examination of the trends in the ages at marriage in New England, some tentative explanations can be offered. Settlers to the New World brought with them the cultural expectations of a late age at first marriage. However, favorable economic conditions allowed them to marry sooner than in the Old World. In addition, the relative scarcity of women in the early decades of settlement may have encouraged men to marry younger women. As the eighteenth century progressed and the sexual imbalance was corrected, it was no longer as essential to take a young wife (Vinovskis, 1981b; Jones, 1981; Norton, 1981). While some Americans had praised the virtues of very early marriages, few of them personally followed that advice. Indeed, in the nineteenth century there was a growing feeling among many women that they should enjoy their youthful independence as long as possible before settling down to the responsibilities of married life (Degler, 1980; Rothman, 1981).

The ages at menarche and first marriage in early America suggest that most adolescents experienced puberty several years before they married. If they did not encounter some of the same problems associated with adolescent sexuality, pregnancy, or childbearing that are present today, it was not because they did not experience a period of time between sexual maturity and marriage. In fact, since the age at first marriage rose from the seventeenth to the nineteenth centuries for women and the age of menarche probably somewhat declined, the amount of time adolescents spent in this transition phase increased.

ADOLESCENT PREMARITAL SEXUAL ACTIVITY

During the 1970s adolescent premarital sexual activity had increased dramatically. Zelnik and Kantner (1980) estimate that the percentage of never-married metropolitan area females ages 15–19 who have engaged in sexual intercourse increased from 27.6% in 1971 to 46.0% in 1979. While some policymakers have reluctantly accepted such high rates of sexual activity as given and mainly focus their energies on ways of improving contraceptive use among teenagers, others like Senator Jeremiah Denton are trying to reverse the trend in adolescent sexual activity. A related issue of considerable interest is whether sexual activity among adolescents has varied in the past and the causes of those fluctuations in behavior among different societies over time.

It is virtually impossible to directly measure sexual activity in the past. We can, however, estimate trends in sexual behavior prior to marriage in societies without modern contraceptives by calculating the percentage of births born 6 or 8½ months after marriage. Naturally, only a small proportion of premarital sexual activity results in the birth of a child, but the overall trends provided by this index of premarital pregnancies can be useful for approximating shifts in premarital sexual activity in early America (Stone, 1977, pp. 607–609).

Smith and Hindus (1975) assembled premarital pregnancy data from 5665 marriages in the United States in the seventeenth, eighteenth, and nineteenth centuries (see Fig. 15.1). The sample is heavily biased toward rural New England and one-third of the cases come from Hingham, Massachusetts. Nevertheless, this series provides us with the most comprehensive and systematic information that is currently available on premarital pregnancies in early America.

The series on premarital pregnancies indicates wide fluctuations over time—from a low proportion of premarital pregnancies in the seventeenth century (under 10% of first births) to a high percentage in the second half of the eighteenth century (nearly 30%). Although fecundability, pregnancy wastage, contraceptives, abortions, and illegitimacy may have affected the extent of premarital pregnancies, it is unlikely that these factors can account for the dramatic trends over time (Smith and Hindus, 1975).

The cycle of premarital pregnancies in America is very similar to the ones found in England and France. The American pattern, however, differs in that it reveals a sharp decline in the early nineteenth century whereas the European data indicate that decline a half century later (Laslett et al., 1980).

To consider the trends in adolescent premarital pregnancies over time, we need to separate the data by the age at marriage of the woman. Unfortunately, we only have such historical data from two Massachusetts communities—Andover and Hingham (see Figs. 15.2A and B) (Smith and Hindus, 1975).

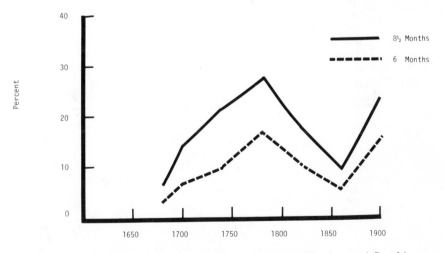

Figure 15.1. Premarital pregnancies in America (Hindus and Smith).

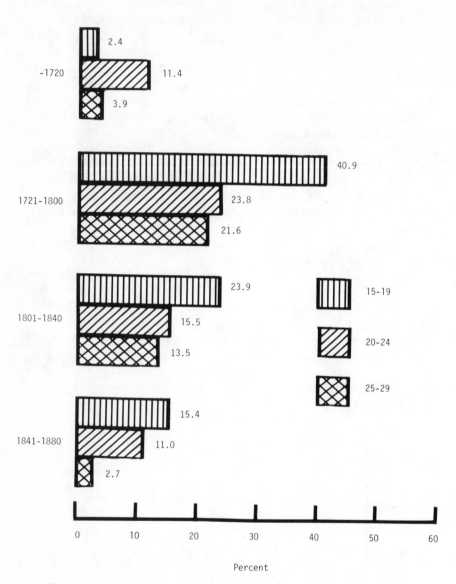

Figure 15.2. (A) Premarital pregnancies in Hingham by age (%).

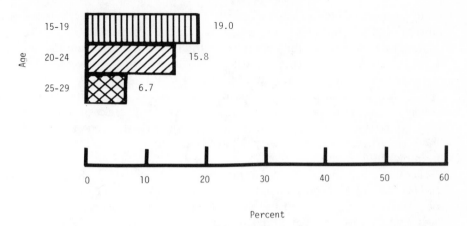

Figure 15.2. (B) Premarital pregnancies in Andover by age (%).

The age-specific pattern in those communities roughly corresponds to the trend in total premarital pregnancies. Interestingly, during most of this time period, the rate of teenage premarital pregnancies is significantly higher for women marrying later—perhaps reflecting a desire among women to postpone their marriages unless they are forced into an earlier one by an unintended pregnancy. The relatively low rate of adolescent premarital pregnancies in Hingham before 1720 may, in part, reflect teenage subfecundity—particularly if the age of menarche in seventeenth-century Hingham was higher than in the eighteenth or nineteenth centuries (Smith and Hindus, 1975). It may also reflect, however, tighter controls on adolescent rather than adult sexual behavior by the Puritans during the seventeenth century.[*]

The low rate of premarital pregnancies in the seventeenth century does not seem very surprising since we have always assumed that Puritans were strongly opposed to premarital or extramarital sex. New England Puritans were not hostile to sex, in fact, they regarded it as an essential and welcome part of matrimony. However, they placed great stress on the need for self-control and self-denial in sexual matters for those who were not married (Morgan, 1966).

New England Puritans in the seventeenth century demanded that the entire community conform to the exemplary moral codes drawn up by the first settlers. Sexual offenders were quickly and publicly chastized by the civil magistrates or the ministers. As late as the 1670s it is estimated that well over one-half of the guilty couples involved in pre-

---

[*]Parents in seventeenth-century New England probably exercised more control over sexual and marital behavior of their children than in the eighteenth or nineteenth centuries (Smith, 1973).

marital pregnancies in Essex County (Massachusetts) were convicted and punished (Smith and Hindus, 1975). Whereas sexual activity prior to marriage had been quite common in the fifteenth and sixteenth centuries in England, Puritans in England and the New World succeeded in greatly reducing that behavior (Stone, 1977).

Perhaps the most surprising finding from the data by Smith and Hindus (1975) is the rapid rise and the peak of premarital pregnancies in the late seventeenth and eighteenth centuries. By the second half of the eighteenth century, nearly 30% of first births occurred within 8½ months of the marriage.

The rise in premarital pregnancies was not peculiar to the United States. In England the loosening of popular convention about sexual behavior quickly followed the restoration of the monarchy in 1660 as secularization replaced Puritanism (Stone, 1977). In New England there was a steady and quite visible erosion of church and civil opposition to premarital sexual activities. In Essex County, for example, the number of civil prosecutions for fornication dropped and the severity of the penalties for them were reduced from corporal punishment to the payment of a fine (Smith and Hindus, 1975). When prominent church leaders such as Jonathan Edwards in the eighteenth century tried to enforce the lax moral standards of their parishioners, they no longer could count on the support of their congregation or the rest of the community (Tracy, 1979). Simultaneous with the unwillingness of civil or church authorities to punish cases of bridal pregnancies, parents gradually lost their ability to "persuade" their children whom and when they should marry (Smith, 1973).*

In the absence of concerted communal or familial efforts to curb premarital sexual activity, there was a general loosening of sexual behavior among early Americans. Sexual intimacy returned as a normal part of courtship behavior and practices such as bundling became more common (Stiles, 1934). The promise to marry rather than the marriage ceremony itself often led to sexual intercourse among couples. As long as the community was assured that they would not be saddled with the financial burden of any out-of-wedlock births, they were quite willing to tolerate premarital pregnancies. The result was less of a breakdown in sexual mores in the early Republic than a shift in the definition of appropriate behavior between individuals in love with each other (Ulrich, 1982).

While there is some consensus on the low level of premarital pregnancies in the seventeenth century and the increase during the eighteenth century, there is considerable disagreement over their pattern in the nineteenth century. Shorter (1975, p. 334), looking at Western

*For a review of the relationship between religion and the family, see Moran and Vinovskis (1982).

Europe and the United States, rejects the Smith and Hindus (1975) data as overrepresenting the experience of a few New England towns and dismisses their argument that premarital intercourse declined in the nineteenth century. Instead, Shorter (1975) concludes that:

> The central fact in the history of courtship over the last two centuries has been the enormous increase in sexual activity before marriage. Before 1800 it was unlikely that the typical young woman would have coitus with her partner—certainly not before an engagement had been sealed, and probably not as a fiancee either. But after 1800 the percentage of young women who slept with their boyfriends or fiancees rose steadily, until in our own times it has become a majority. (p. 80)

But others have challenged both Shorter's portrayal of the trends in premarital pregnancies and out-of-wedlock births as well as his interpretation of them. Shorter sees the rise in premarital sexual activity in the late eighteenth and nineteenth centuries as an entirely new phenomenon, but other scholars suggest that it was already quite high in the fifteenth and sixteenth centuries (Laslett et al., 1980). In addition, although Shorter dismisses the work of Smith and Hindus (1975) as unrepresentative and incorrect, he does not produce any evidence to counter it. Therefore, we have no reason at this time to doubt that the rise and decline in premarital pregnancies in the United States did not occur about a half century earlier than in Western Europe.* Finally, whereas Shorter explains much of the rise in sexual activity as the result of changes in the lives of young women fostered by urban and industrial development, others have questioned both his interpretation of the lives of those women as well as pointing to the fact that similar shifts in sexual activity were occurring in agricultural and rural areas (Tilly and Scott, 1978).

Assuming that Smith and Hindus (1975) are correct in dating the decrease in premarital pregnancies in America in the early nineteenth century, how can we account for this change? The answer probably lies in the development of a nineteenth-century attitude toward sex which accepted it within marriage, but strongly condemned it outside of marriage.

In the early nineteenth century, reformers in America stressed the importance of individuals controlling their own lives and avoiding

---

*Part of the decline in the Smith and Hindus (1975) index of premarital pregnancies in rural areas, such as Hingham, Massachusetts in the nineteenth century, may be the result of women from those communities going to Boston as unwed mothers because of the increased stigma attached to out-of-wedlock births (Hobson, 1980). While this factor may account for some of that decline, it is doubtful that it will explain most of it as it is unlikely that very large numbers of unwed women from rural Massachusetts went to Boston for that purpose.

committing any sins. Whereas colonial Americans placed great stress on the public censure of deviants, the early nineteenth-century reformers devoted more of their efforts to instilling the values of self-control and self-discipline.*

The waves of religious revivals that swept across America in the early nineteenth century involved teenagers as well as adults and preached the gospel of sexual abstinence before marriage.† Whereas religion did not appear to be a major factor in preventing premarital pregnancies in the eighteenth century, it now assumed a much more important role.‡

The aversion to sex prior to marriage was reinforced by medical writings which warned adolescents of the dangers of dissipating their strength and vitality through sexual involvement with another or by masturbation (Bullough and Voight, 1973). Even married couples were warned to practice moderation in their sexual relations lest they damage themselves by excessive indulgence. Some writers specifically warned against early marriages because they would injure both the parents, who were still maturing, as well as their offspring. An anonymous clergyman (*Physiology of Marriage*, 1856, p. 22) in Massachusetts cited an eminent British writer in condemning the dangers of an early marriage:

> Dr. Johnson proceeds to say that for every year the female marries below the full age of twenty-one, "there will be, on an average, three years of premature decay of the corporeal fabric, and a considerable abbreviation of the usual range of human existence." Thus, if she marries at eighteen, instead of twenty-one, there will be, according to this estimate, which he insists is "a fair one," nine years of premature decay; and, if she marries at sixteen, instead of twenty-one, her physical decline will be hastened no less than fifteen years!

Perhaps, most important of all, prohibitions against sex prior to marriage became part of a broader ideology of what constituted respectability for women in the nineteenth century. Anyone who transgressed was punished by social ostracization. The notion of a "fallen" woman became prevalent so that any sexual experience prior to marriage was now deemed to make any woman a less desirable marriage partner (Berg, 1978). In addition, female delinquency became associated with sexual impropriety and thus reinforced the link between early sexual activity and deviance (Sedlack, 1980; Schlossman and Wallach, 1980; Brenzel, 1975, 1980).

*On reform efforts in the antebellum period, see Rothman (1971).
†On the role of religious revivals, see McLoughlin (1978).
‡Smith and Hindus (1975) found that after controlling for wealth, religion did not predict whether someone would become premaritally pregnant in Hingham, Massachusetts in 1767.

Of course, not everyone was able to live up to the new expectations of sexual abstinence prior to marriage and many engaged couples still became sexually intimate with each other. The penalties for such behavior, however, seemed much more severe than in the eighteenth century (Parkes, 1932; Erikson, 1966). While the diffusion of contraceptive information in the early nineteenth century may have made premarital sex less likely to be exposed, the pressures against premarital pregnancies probably led to even more induced abortions among single women (Mohr, 1978). Furthermore, as the nineteenth century progressed and the value of sexual abstinence became routinely accepted, there probably was a real decline in premarital sexual activity rather than just an increase in the effectiveness of contraceptives or the use of abortions (Smith and Hindus, 1975).

ADOLESCENTS AND THE CHANGES IN SEXUAL ACTIVITY AND PREGNANCY

We have established thus far that most adolescent girls probably were sexually mature by the ages of 15 or 16, but that they usually did not marry until age twenty. We have also detected wide fluctuations in premarital sexual activity for both adolescents and adults, although the explanations for these changes are still quite sketchy. Now we must turn to the issue of whether Americans in the seventeenth, eighteenth, or nineteenth centuries perceived and dealt with adolescents as a special category of individuals as they are currently dealt with.

Aries (1962) has argued that children were treated as miniature adults in the past so that no special distinctions would have been made for adolescents. This notion was accepted by colonial historians such as Demos (1974, p. 428):

> Colonial society barely recognized childhood as we know and understand it today. Consider, for example, the matter of dress; in virtually all seventeenth-century portraiture, children appear in the same sort of clothing that was normal for adults. In fact, this accords nicely with what we know of other aspects of the child's life. His work, much of his recreation, and his closest personal contacts were encompassed within the world of adults. From the age of six or seven he was set to a regular round of tasks about the house or farm (or, in the case of a craftsman's family, the shop or store). When the family went to church, or when they went visiting, he went along. In short, from his earliest years he was expected to be—or try to be—a miniature adult.

If Demos is correct about childhood in early America, then the notion of adolescents as separate or apart from adults was simply missing in that society. Yet while Demos is correct in saying that the Puritans did not treat their children the same as we do today, he was incorrect in suggesting that New Englanders did not distinguish between adolescents and adults. In fact, Puritans commonly referred to children roughly in the age group 15 to 21 or 24 as youths and treated them somewhat differently, depending upon the issue, from older adults (Stannard, 1975; Kaestle and Vinovskis, 1978).

Early Americans did differentiate between youths and adults, but that distinction was a general one rather than being closely linked to exact chronological age. Colonial Americans did not pay much attention to age, but focused on other attributes of individuals. It is only in the second half of the nineteenth century when age-grading in schools became prevalent that chronological age and developmental attributes began to be tied together.

Historians are still debating whether adolescence as a phase of life as we know it today existed in the past. Many scholars of the family argue that adolescence is a late nineteenth and early twentieth-century development. According to them, while the concept of youth as a general period of semidependency existed in the first three quarters of the nineteenth century, nothing fully resembling adolescence today had emerged. Yet the transformation of America from an agricultural to an urban-industrial society during these years created sharp discontinuities in the lives of children and fostered an environment in which adolescence as a stage of life was to develop (Demos and Demos, 1969). Others have challenged this interpretation by pointing out that in the early eighteenth century youths experienced many of the same emotional impulses and tensions that we associate with adolescence today (Hiner, 1975). At the present time there is no way to resolve this debate, but we can conclude that in the seventeenth, eighteenth, and nineteenth centuries the teenage years were loosely defined by contemporaries and based more on economic and social status rather than chronological age.

Did adolescents in the past who married early suffer from any adverse consequences? Were their early marriages regarded as undesirable by contemporaries? Most of the studies today (Card and Wise, 1978; Furstenberg, 1976; Moore and Caldwell, 1977) suggest that early marriage and childbearing are detrimental to the parents—especially the mother.

In the seventeenth and eighteenth centuries there does not appear to have been any strong bias against early marriages or childbearing as long as the individuals involved were both sexually mature, capable of supporting an independent household, and had the approval of their parents. There was a tendency to postpone marriage until the woman was about 20 years old, but individuals who married earlier were not frowned upon or penalized.

In the nineteenth century, however, there was a growing feeling that children should not marry too early. Physicians cautioned young men and women against engaging in sex while their bodies were still growing since they assumed that sexual activity drained the body of vital energy necessary for normal growth (Walsh, 1977; Bullough and Voight, 1973). In addition, the emphasis on receiving a common school education, especially for males, made early marriages less desirable from an educational perspective.* Finally, there was a growing feeling among women that they should postpone their marriages in order to enjoy their youthful independence and to earn money in the textile mills or teaching profession. While most unmarried women only worked for a few years before finally getting married and having a family, it was a period of time that was cherished even by girls from middle-class backgrounds who did not need to work in order to support their parents or put aside money for their own dowries (Mason et al., 1978).

If early marriage and childbearing did not evoke cries of social disapproval in the past, did it handicap those individuals later in life? Although we do not have any longitudinal information on the effects of early marriage and childbearing from the seventeenth, eighteenth, or nineteenth centuries, we can speculate on what such data might reveal by considering whether education was really necessary or useful for success. Certainly educators like Horace Mann felt that the completion of a common school education was an important factor in getting ahead in nineteenth-century America and most educational historians have agreed with him (Vinovskis, 1970). Thus, children of foreign-born parents who did not receive as much education as those of native-born parents are seen to have suffered when they attempted to advance in their careers (Thernstrom, 1964). Yet Graff (1979) has recently challenged this idea by arguing that the acquisition of literacy in early America was not essential or even especially helpful for achieving material success.

Again, there is no way that we can settle the debate over the economic productivity of education in the past, but I suspect that education had more value than suggested by Graff. Nevertheless, education, beyond the ability to read and write, probably was much less important then than today so that anyone denied that opportunity because of early marriage and childbearing would not be as disadvantaged as their contemporary counterparts. Furthermore, since most women did not continue employment outside their own households after marriage in the nineteenth century, any disadvantages caused by early withdrawal from school probably were minimal. Certainly there was no effort by common school reformers in the mid-nineteenth century to encourage or even to allow pregnant teenagers to continue their ed-

---

*On the development of common schools, see Kaestle and Vinovskis (1980).

ucation for fear that their lack of access to that schooling would hand-icap them later.

If early Americans did not express disapproval of early marriages or childbearing, did they oppose sexual intercourse among adolescents beyond condemnation of premarital sex in general? In other words, were teenagers who engaged in premarital sex singled out for attack more than adults when magistrates or ministers commented on such practices?

Although ministers in the early nineteenth century frequently ad-dressed teenagers in regard to the sins of premarital sexual behavior, it appears to have been done more as a way of reaching this audience rather than considering this particular activity to be especially sinful and harmful among the young. Thus, the general societal attitudes toward premarital sex were more important in determining how young people would be treated rather than any special view of adolescents.

One interesting perspective on whether sexual activity was viewed any differently among adolescents than adults is in the public reactions to prostitution in nineteenth-century America. As reformers denounced the evils of prostitution and sought to eradicate it, did they pay particular attention to teenage prostitutes? And, in appealing to the sympathy of the public and the magistrates, did they evoke the image of the par-ticular vulnerability of the young prostitute?

According to the recent work of Hobson (1981) on prostitutes in an-tebellum Boston, juvenile prostitution was not a focal point of discourse among reformers. Moral reformers, administrators in public and private agencies, and police and court personnel who voiced concern about prostitution emphasized women's vulnerability and passivity to sexual exploitation due to their dependency on males without any particular emphasis on the age of the woman, nor were the early anti-prostitution laws age-specific. At what period juvenile prostitutes were singled out for pity and attention more than adult prostitutes is not clear, but it may have occurred only in the late nineteenth and early twentieth centuries. Thus, the evidence from religious leaders as well as anti-prostitution activists supports the notion that premarital sexual inter-course among adolescents was not seen as especially problematic compared to the same behavior among adults prior to the mid-nine-teenth century.

CONCLUSION

Adolescent sexuality, pregnancy, and childbearing were not seen as particularly important problems and issues in early America. Even though adolescent girls were sexually mature by age 15 or 16, most of them postponed marriage until they were at least 20 years old. Those that did marry early and started their families as teenagers did not seem to suffer either in the eyes of the public or in their subsequent lives. While premarital sexual activity was strongly opposed in the seventeenth and nineteenth centuries, adolescents do not appear to have been singled out from other adults when this behavior was denounced.

Part of the explanation for the lack of attention to adolescent sexuality, pregnancy, and childbearing in the past is that it occurred so infrequently compared to the current situation. Contrary to the popular image of the past, few girls married or had children as young teenagers in early New England. Furthermore, although the Puritans did distinguish between youths and adults, they did not focus on that distinction when judging the suitability or advisability of sexual activity, marriage, or childbearing.

If our contemporary problems of adolescent pregnancy were not perceived or treated the same as in the past, it does not imply that we cannot benefit from an historical perspective on this issue today. For example, during the debates in the U.S. Congress over adolescent pregnancy in 1978 and 1981, there was considerable disagreement over whether it is really possible to reverse the recent increases in sexual activity among teenagers (Vinovskis, 1981a). A glance at the fluctuations in the rates of premarital pregnancy in America during the past 350 years should be enough to convince anyone that such increases can be reversed. However, whether the mechanisms of social control used in the early nineteenth century would be deemed acceptable by most Americans today is questionable. Yet an understanding of the relationships between broader societal changes and more specific aspects of life such as adolescent premarital behavior may help us to see our own problems within a more appropriate framework an context than many people today have been willing to acknowledge.

REFERENCES

Aries, P. *Centuries of childhood: A social history of family life.* (Trans. R. Baldick.) New York: Vintage, 1962.

Berg, B.J. *The remembered gate: Origins of American feminism: The woman and the city, 1800–1860.* New York: Oxford University Press, 1978.

Brenzel, B. Lancaster industrial school for girls: A social portrait of a nineteenth-century reform school for girls. *Feminist Studies*, 1975, *3*, 40–53.

Brenzel, B. Domestication as reform: A study of the socialization of wayward girls, 1856–1905. *Harvard Educational Review*, 1980, *50*, 196–213.

Brundtland, G.H., and Walloe, L. Menarchal age in Norway in the 19th century: A reevaluation of historical sources. *Annals of Human Biology*, 1976, *3*, 363–374.

Bullough, V., and Voight, M. Women, menstruation, and nineteenth century medicine. *Bulletin of the History of Medicine*, 1973, *47*, 66–82.

Calhoun, A. *A social history of the American family* (3 Vols., Reprint). New York: Barnes & Noble, 1960.

Card, J. J., and Wise, L.L. Teenage mothers and teenage fathers: The impact of early childbearing on the parent's personal and professional lives. *Family Planning Perspectives*, 1978, *10*, 199–205.

Clarke, E.H. *Sex education; Or, a fair chance for the girls*. Boston: J.R. Osgood, 1873.

Degler, C. *At odds: Women and the family in America from the revolution to the present*. New York: Oxford University Press, 1980.

Demos, J. *A little commonwealth: Family life in Plymouth Colony*. New York: Oxford University Press, 1970.

Demos, J. The American family in past times. *American Scholar*, 1974, *43*, 428.

Demos, J., and Demos, V. Adolescence in historical perspective. *Journal of Marriage and the Family*, 1969, *31*, 632–638.

Earle, A.M. *Colonial dames and goodwives*. Boston: MacMillan, 1895.

Erikson, K.T. *Wayward Puritans: A study in the sociology of deviance*. New York: Wiley, 1966.

Fogel, R., and Engerman, S. *Time on the cross: The economics of American negro slavery* (2 Vols.). Boston: Little Brown, 1974.

Frisch, R.E. Demographic implications of the biological determinants of female fecundity. *Social Biology*, 1975, *22*, 17–22.

Frisch, R., and McArthur, J.W. Menstrual cycles: Fatness as a determinant of minimum weight necessary for their maintenance or onset. *Science*, 1974, *435*, 949–951.

Furstenberg, F. F. *Unplanned parenthood: The social consequences of teenage childbearing*. New York: Free Press, 1976.

Graff, H.J. *The literacy myth: Literacy and social structure in the nineteenth-century city*. New York: Academic Press, 1979.

Greven, P.J., Jr. *Four generations: Population, land, and family in colonial Andover, Massachusetts*. Ithaca, NY: Cornell University Press, 1970.

Gutman, H., and Sutch, R. The slave family: Protected agent of capitalist masters or victim of the slave trade? *In* P.A. David *et al.* (Eds.), *Reckoning with slavery*. New York: Oxford University Press, 1976, pp. 94–162.

Hajnal, J. European marriage patterns in perspective. *In* D. V. Glass and D.E.C. Eversley (Eds.), *Population in history: Essays in historical demography*. Chicago: Aldine, 1965, pp. 101–143.

Hiner, N.R. Adolescence in eighteenth-century America. *History of Childhood Quarterly*, 1975, *3*, 253–280.

Hobson, B. A wolf in gentleman's garb: Sources of a parable of seduction and betrayal. Unpublished paper, 1980.

Hobson, B. Sex and the marketplace: Prostitution in an American city, Boston, 1820–1880. Unpublished Ph.D. thesis, Boston University, 1981.

Johnston, F.E. Control of age at menarche. *Human Biology*, 1974, *46*, 159–171.

Jones, A.H. *Wealth of a nation to be: The American colonies on the eve of the Revolution*. New York: Columbia University Press, 1980.

Jones, D.L. *Village and seaport: Migration and society in eighteenth-century Massachusetts*. Hanover, NH: New England Press, 1981.

Kaestle, C., and Vinovskis, M.A. From apron strings to abcs: Parents, children, and schooling in nineteenth-century Massachusetts. *In* J. Demos and S. Boocock (Eds.), *Turning points: Historical and sociological essays on the family*. Chicago: University of Chicago Press, 1978, pp. S539–S580.

Kaestle, C.F., and Vinovskis, M.A. *Education and social change in nineteenth-century Massachusetts*. Cambridge, England: Cambridge University Press, 1980.

Kett, J.F. *Rites of passage: Adolescence in America, 1790 to the present.* New York: Basic Books, 1977.

Laslett, P. Age at menarche in Europe since the eighteenth century. *Journal of Interdisciplinary History,* 1971, *2,* 221–236.

Laslett, P., Oosterveen, K., and Smith, R.M. (Eds). *Bastardy and its comparative history.* Cambridge, Mass.: Harvard University Press, 1980.

Lockridge, K.A. *A New England town, the first hundred years: Dedham, Massachusetts,* New York: Norton, 1970.

McLoughlin, W.G. *Revivals, awakenings, and reform.* Chicago: University of Chicago Press, 1978.

Mason, K., Vinovskis, M.A., and Hareven, T.K. Women's work and the life course in Essex County, Massachusetts, 1880. *In* T.K. Hareven (Ed.), *Transitions: The family and the life course in historical perspective.* New York: Academic Press, 1978, pp. 187–216.

Massachusetts. *Census of Massachusetts, 1885* (4 Vols). Boston: Wright and Potter, 1887.

Mohr, J.C. *Abortion in America: The origins and evolution of national policy, 1800–1900.* New York: Oxford University Press, 1978.

Moran, G.F., and Vinovskis, M.A. The Puritan family and religion: A critical reappraisal. *William and Mary Quarterly* (3rd Series), 1982, *39,* 29–63.

Morgan, E.S. *The Puritan family: Religion and domestic relations in seventeenth-century New England.* New York: Harper & Row, 1966.

Moore, K.A., and Caldwell, S.B. Early childbearing and educational attainment. *Family Planning Perspectives,* 1977, *9,* 220–225.

Norton, S.L. Age at marriage and marital migration in three Massachusetts towns, 1600–1850. Unpublished Ph.D. thesis, University of Michigan, 1981.

Parkes, H.B. Morals and law enforcement in colonial New England. *New England Quarterly,* 1932, *5,* 431–435.

Physiology of marriage. Boston: John P. Jewett, 1856.

Rothman, D.J. *The discovery of the asylum: Social order and disorder in the new republic.* Boston: Little Brown, 1971.

Rothman, E.K. Intimate acquaintance: Courtship and the transition to marriage in America, 1770–1900. Unpublished Ph.D. thesis, Brandeis, 1981.

Schlossman, S., and Wallach, S. The crime of precocious sexuality: Female juvenile delinquency in the progressive era. *Harvard Educational Review,* 1980, *48,* 65–94.

Sedlack, M.W. *The education of girls with special needs, 1865–1972.* Unpublished paper presented at Teachers College conference on History of Urban Education, December 1980.

Shorter, E. *The making of the modern family.* New York: Basic Books, 1975.

Smith, D.S. Parental power and marriage patterns: An analysis of historical trends in Hingham, Massachusetts. *Journal of Marriage and the Family,* 1973, *35,* 406–418.

Smith, D.S., and Hindus, M.S. Premarital pregnancy in America, 1640–1971: An overview and interpretation. *Journal of Interdisciplinary History,* 1975, *5,* 537–570.

Soltow, L., and Stevens, E. *The rise of literacy and the common school in the United States: A socioeconomic analysis to 1870.* Chicago: University of Chicago Press, 1981.

Stannard, D.E. Death and the Puritan child. *In* D.E. Stannard (Ed.), *Death in America.* Philadelphia: University of Pennsylvania Press, 1975, pp. 9–29.

Stiles, H.R. *Bundling: Its origin, progress, and decline in America.* New York: Book Collectors Association, 1934.

Stone, L. *The family, sex and marriage in England, 1500–1800.* New York: Harper & Row, 1977.

Talwar, P.P. Adolescent sterility in an Indian population. *Human Biology,* 1965, *37,* 256–261.

Tanner, J.M. The trend toward earlier physical maturation. *In* A.S. Parker and J.D. Meade (Eds.), *Biological aspects of social problems.* New York: Plenum Press, 1965, pp. 40–65.

Thernstrom, S. *Poverty and progress: Social mobility in a nineteenth-century city.* Cambridge, Massachusetts: Harvard University Press, 1964.

Tilly, L.A., and Scott, S.W. *Women, work, and family.* New York: Holt, Rinehart, & Winston, 1978.

Tracy, P.J. *Jonathan Edwards, pastor: Religion and society in eighteenth-century Northampton.* New York: Hill & Wang, 1979.

Trussell, J., and Steckel, R. The age of slaves at menarche and their first birth. *Journal of Interdisciplinary History,* 1978, *8,* 477–505.

Ulrich, L.T. *Good wives: Images and reality in northern New England, 1650–1750.* New York: Alfred Knopf, 1982.

Vinovskis, M.A. Horace Mann on the economic productivity of education. *New England Quarterly,* 1970, *43,* 550–571.

Vinovskis, M.A. An epidemic of adolescent pregnancy? Some historical considerations. *Journal of Family History,* 1981, *6,* 205–230.(a)

Vinovskis, M.A. *Fertility in Massachusetts from the Revolution to the Civil War.* New York: Academic Press, 1981. (b)

Walsh, M.R. *Doctors wanted, no women need apply: Sexual barriers in the medical profession, 1835–1975.* New Haven, Conn.: Yale University Press, 1977.

Walton, G.M., and Shepherd, J.F. *The economic rise of early America.* Cambridge, England: Cambridge University Press, 1979.

Wells, R.V. *The population of the British colonies in America before 1776: A survey of census data.* Princeton, NJ: Princeton University Press, 1975.

Wyshak, G., and Frisch, R.E. Evidence for a secular trend in age of menarche. *New England Journal of Medicine,* 1982, *306,* 1033–1035.

Zelnik, M., and Kantner, J. Sexual activity, contraceptive use and pregnancy among metropolitan-area teenagers, 1971–1979. *Family Planning Perspectives,* 1980, *12,* 230–237.

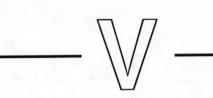

THE MODERN WORLD

16

ADOLESCENT PREGNANCY AND CHILDBEARING: AN ANTHROPOLOGICAL PERSPECTIVE

Melvin Konner
Majorie Shostak

INTRODUCTION

In the minds of some who consider the problem of school-age pregnancy and childbearing, there is an implicit assumption that it is somehow a return to a more primitive form of reproductive life cycle. That is, the basic human condition is viewed as one in which reproductive activity begins early, fertility is poorly controlled, and childbearing, the main business of life, preoccupies young women and girls from the earliest possible age. Only when (so this thinking runs) higher-level civilizations, with their need for prolonged education and maturation, began to impose strictures on adolescent sexual activity, did the teenage years become free from childbearing activity.

Our experience with the !Kung San ("Bushmen") of the Kalahari Desert in Botswana, an African hunting and gathering people, led us to question the validity of this viewpoint. Further, systematic review of the cross-cultural and historical evidence suggested that in fact the opposite might be the case; that is, that the most primitive human condition may be one in which the teenage years are relatively free, and the early and middle teenage years completely free, of pregnancy and childbearing, and that this freedom might be the result of primarily biological rather than primarily cultural causes. While it would be unfortunate to replace one oversimplification with another, our working hypothesis at present is the one just stated, and the purpose of this chapter is to review very briefly the justification for this position.

EPIDEMIOLOGY OF ADOLESCENT PREGNANCY

It is difficult to obtain reliable estimates of the incidence of pregnancy, but the number of reported pregnancies to teenagers (individuals under 20 years of age) has for a decade been increasing from about one million annually to about 10% above that figure. For 1974, or about the time that adolescent pregnancy began to be a matter of widespread public concern, the Alan Guttmacher Institute reported on the characteristics of these pregnancies (Guttmacher Institute, 1976). About 600,000 were completed, the others ending in early termination either spontaneously or therapeutically. About 250,000 were to girls 17 and younger, and about 13,000 to girls 14 and younger. In the early 1970's the birth rate for all women, and for women 20–24 years old, declined markedly, while births for 14–17 year olds stayed at about 30 per thousand. Out-of-wedlock births, a subcategory of total births, rose in the younger age group during the same period, as they had been doing since 1960.

By 1975 (National Center of Health Statistics, 1977; Klerman and Stekel, 1978), a trend toward stabilization of births to teenagers was noted, However, since this was 2 years after the Supreme Court abortion decision and 2 years before the withdrawal of Medicaid funding for abortions, it was not clear that it reflected a stabilization in pregnancies, or that it could be projected forward. Further, since birth rates for all women were dropping, and since teenagers were not participating in the downward trend but only stabilizing, it seemed that the proportion of all children who would have teenagers as mothers would continue to rise.

By 1978 (Guttmacher Institute, 1981) and certainly by 1979 (Baldwin, 1983), it was clear that the teenage birthrate was declining, and that all ages were now participating in the decline. However, this was due to a marked (approximately two-thirds) increase in the number of therapeutic abortions to teenagers, and the overall rate of pregnancy was estimated to have increased by 10–15% since 5 years earlier. Also, it was noted at this time that the percentage of births to teenagers that occurred out-of-wedlock had continued to rise steadily. Of births to 17 year olds in 1970, 35% were out-of-wedlock, whereas 53% of births to 17 year olds in 1979 were out-of-wedlock, and comparable increases were seen for other ages under 20 (Baldwin, 1983). In 1979, 1.3 million children were living with teenage mothers, about one-half of whom were unmarried (Guttmacher Institute, 1981).

It must be noted that aggregating the data for whites and blacks, as is done above (and in many policy statements and news reports) obscures important differences in the trends for the two groups (Baldwin, 1983). In 1979 the black:white ratio of birth rates ranged from 1.8:1

at age 19 to 4.8:1 at age 14, indicating a marked difference in the development of adolescent fertility. Between 1970 and 1979 the number of births per thousand in the 15–19 year age group in blacks changed from high 90's to the low 90's, while the same age group in whites increased its birthrate from 10.9 to 14.9 per thousand, a numerically much more significant change at the national level. Finally, the increase in nonmarital births during this time period was largely accounted for by whites.

In 1981, the last year for which there are national data at this writing, there were 537,024 births to women under 20, 37% of which were to girls or women under 18. Births to teenagers continued to decline both in rates and in absolute numbers, and this decline had occurred for all ages under 20 between 1970 and 1981 (National Center for Health Statistics, 1983, 1984). The proportion of births to teenagers which were nonmarital continued to be high; one-half of all births to teenagers in 1981 were out-of-wedlock. Trends distinguishing blacks and whites, as reported by previous observers, were reconfirmed.

In summary, it can be said that the levels and trends reported in the mid-1970's have improved in some respects but not in others. Births to teenagers, although they continue to represent a significant proportion of all births, have been declining steadily in relative and absolute numbers. However, pregnancies to teenagers appear to have increased, and therapeutic abortions to teenagers have increased even more markedly. Thus the decline in teenage childbearing is owed primarily to an increase in the utilization of therapeutic abortion and not to the comparatively minor increase in the use of effective methods for prevention of conception (Baldwin, 1983). There is no reason to believe that abstinence has played a role in the decline of births during the late 1970's; on the contrary all methods of estimating sexual activity showed it to be increasing among teenagers during this period (Guttmacher, 1981). Finally, the proportion of births to teenage mothers that have occurred nonmaritally has risen steadily.

All these generalizations apply to young teenagers (those under 17) as well as to all teenagers, although there are some age differences in the magnitude of some of the trends. Black-white differences are very marked; although the incidence statistics have always been in conventional terms "worse" for blacks (higher rates of birth, pregnancy, abortion, and nonmarital birth), the trends are "worse" for whites. In all likelihood there are many more ethnic and subcultural variations that are obscured by the lumping of all teenagers into two racial groups. Interestingly, studies in the United Kingdom (Russell, 1982) and various European countries (Deschamps and Valentin, 1978) show that with the exception of France the phenomena of increasing rates of teenage and early teenage pregnancy, and of nonmarital pregnancy in the same age groups, are cross-national ones, although the proportion of completed pregnancies varies greatly with social context and with the availability of therapeutic abortion.

It is, of course, not possible to project these forward. Even the current situation may be different from that in 1981, the last year for which we have data, because of increasing consciousness of the existence of nationally endemic venereal herpes simplex, or because of decreasing availability of funds for therapeutic abortion for indigent teenagers. Within the next decade there are likely to be marked changes in one direction or another due to improvements in contraceptive technology, favorable or unfavorable changes in contraceptive education, changing venereal disease patterns, and the possible development of vaccines against genital herpes simplex and/or gonorrhea—not to mention unpredictably changing standards of sexual morality. It is further likely that increasing public consciousness about adolescent pregnancy has affected and will continue to affect the situation, through the development of social, educational, medical, and health programs.

CONSEQUENCES OF ADOLESCENT PREGNANCY AND CHILDBEARING

Two opposing kinds of conventional wisdom exist with regard to the consequences of adolescent pregnancy and childbearing. One, associated especially with educators, psychologists, and psychiatrists, although also subscribed to by many pediatricians and obstetricians, holds that the teenage years, particularly the early teenage years, are no time for pregnancy, childbirth, or parenthood (Duenhoelter et al., 1975; Guttmacher Institute, 1976, 1981; Lobl et al., 1971; Russell, 1982). The other, in a sense both older and newer, associated with some pediatric and obstetrical tradition as well as with the folk wisdom of some ethnic groups, holds that the younger a woman is when she bears a child the better off she (and her child) are, youth being synonymous with resilience, health, and strength (Baird, 1967; Morris, 1981; Rothenberg and Varga, 1981).

As with many long-standing controversies, both viewpoints have some validity. Part of the fruit of this controversy has been an increasing consciousness of the need to separate the teenage years into two or even three separate groups for analysis. For example, risk of both fatal and nonfatal pregnancy complications is only slightly higher in 18 and 19 year olds than in 20–24 year olds, but these risks increase steadily as maternal age drops below 18. To girls under 15, the risk of infant mortality and the risk of low birth weight infants is more than twice what it is for women 20–24 years old (Shapiro et al., 1968; Guttmacher Institute, 1976, 1981). The risks to the mother under 20 have been shown to be higher for—in various studies—toxemia of pregnancy, anemia, hemorrhage, spontaneous abortion, postnatal complications, and maternal death (including suicide), as have the risks to the child for low birth weight, prematurity, congenital anomalies, low postnatal gain in length and weight, impaired cognitive development, and abuse and neglect; most of these risks have also been found in various studies to become significantly higher as maternal age drops through the teenage years (e.g., Battaglia et al., 1963; Lobl et al., 1971; Duenholter et al., 1975; Dott and Fort, 1976; see Rothenberg and Varga, 1981; Russell, 1982 for reviews).

However, most such studies, especially those analyzing population statistics, have been justly criticized for failure to control adequately for factors other than maternal age. The younger mothers have tended to have poorer nutrition and poorer health care prenatally, and have differed significantly from older mothers in a variety of socioeconomic background variables relevant to the natal and postnatal outcomes of their children. Studies in which such variables have been well controlled (as well as some studies in which they have not) have failed to confirm many of the above-mentioned disadvantages (e.g., Briggs et al., 1962; Isreal and Wouterz, 1963; Morris, 1981; Rothenberg and Varga, 1981; Osbourne et al., 1981; Horon et al., 1983).

Such studies have led to a newly emerging view—in effect, a new "conventional wisdom"—which holds that adolescent pregnancy is biologically advantageous although socially disadvantageous (Morris, 1981). Three qualifications are helpful with regard to this view. First, while it is now generally agreed that ages 17, 18, and 19 are biologically desirable times for most young women to have pregnancies (whether completed or not) there remains doubt as to the biological suitability of younger teenagers for pregnancy and delivery. Second, research is only in its earliest stages regarding some fundamental biological problems that may be uniquely faced by young teenagers, such as exaggerated maternal–fetal nutrient competition (Naeye, 1981; Frisancho et al., 1983) and immaturity of the pelvis with size limitation of the birth canal (Moerman, 1982); thus a final conclusion about the biological adequacy (in the sense of "biological" that excludes psychological factors) of young teenage mothers is probably premature. Third, studies that control all background variables other than age (socioeconomic status, prenatal care, education, marital status, nutrition, etc.) may show that in abstract terms there are no basic biological reasons for young teenagers to avoid motherhood. In practical terms, however, young teenagers have a much higher incidence of other risk factors. They seek prenatal care later, have poorer nutrition, stay unmarried at higher rates, and decline in socioeconomic status and education with respect to their age-mates who avoid pregnancy and motherhood.

The fact that these risk factors could theoretically be removed does not change the risk to which adolescent mothers and their children are exposed in the world as it is. Stated another way, maintaining poor standards of nutrition, prenatal care, childbirth preparation, and post-natal care is to some extent inherent in being a teenager. To do research in which the control group of older mothers is equally poor in these areas may be to eliminate the phenomenon we need to be studying, and may be valuable for scientific interpretation but only indirectly relevant to policy. In practical terms, the cost/benefit analysis of coun-terbalancing these disadvantages of adolescent pregnancy with ag-gressive policies and programs—as opposed to trying to prevent young adolescents from becoming parents—may not be a favorable one.

That the social and psychological risks incurred by the young teen-ager who becomes a mother are great is almost generally agreed. Of women who first give birth during their twenties, 96% have high school diplomas, while about one-half of women who first gave birth before age 18 have completed or will complete high school. The mean annual income of white mothers who gave birth before age 16 is slightly more than one-half that of mothers who first gave birth in their late twenties. Marriage disruption, if marriage occurs, is three times more likely for mothers under age 17 than for mothers over age 20 (Guttmacher In-stitute, 1981). Thus the picture is one of impaired educational, economic, and marital status for women who have become mothers during their early teens, and this impairment exists despite mitigation by Aid to Families with Dependent Children (AFDC) and other social welfare programs.

There is also the question of psychiatric risk, which is more difficult to study. It has been repeatedly shown that for fully adult mothers the postpartum period is one of particular psychiatric vulnerability, when a greatly disporportionate incidence of onset, or exacerbation, of mental illness takes place (Pugh et al., 1963; Paffenbarger, 1964; Hamburg et al., 1968). This vulnerability may result from hormonal, psychological, or social changes that accompany delivery, and most likely results from some combination of those causes. While postpartum psychiatric vul-nerability in young teenagers specifically has not been adequately studied, it does not seem likely that their risk would be lower than that for the general population of parturient women. Studies of suicide have shown a high relative risk during pregnancy, and this applies to teen-agers as well as to older women (Pretzel and Cline, 1978). Although it is not clear that therapeutic termination of pregnancy resolves the added risk, either abstinence or effective contraception would presum-ably do so.

Finally, it must be considered that there are individual adolescents, families, and perhaps even subcultures, for whom early pregnancy and motherhood are not undesirable outcomes, even psychosocially, and even at the younger ages. Some girls correctly perceive early motherhood as a route to social and economic independence. This independence may be meager compared with national standards, but may be markedly superior to the particular adolescent's situation in her family of origin. Or, childbearing may greatly improve her status within that family, which may in turn cheerfully provide adequate psychosocial or even economic support for her and her child. Some young women in their late twenties or early thirties have completed not only the childbearing but the child-rearing phase of their lives and are prepared to enter the labor force or to advance their educations. As in all areas of medical practice and social policy implementation, there is a need for clinical judgment that will take into account individual situation and subcultural variation, and will sometimes depart from generally agreed upon guidelines, This is another lesson of the anthropological perspective on this or indeed almost any social problem.

THE CULTURAL HYPOTHESIS OF INCREASING ADOLESCENT PREGNANCY

Why has this relative increase in adolescent pregnancy occurred? The explanation most frequently advanced relates to the liberalization of sexual mores that has affected American society during the past two decades. It is easy to document that such a change has taken place (Chilman, 1979; see also this volume) and it is obvious to anyone who has lived through that period as an adult. Today's adolescents have been exposed to a much more liberal set of sexual mores than was the case for the adolescents of 20 years ago, whether the measures involve transmission of knowledge, adult models, peer pressure, or rules and restrictions governing their own behavior. It seems logical to account for the increasing proportion of adolescent pregnancies mainly by reference to this cultural change.

But this logic runs aground against at least some ethnological experience, which suggests that liberal premarital sexual mores, however new they may be for us, are not new for a large proportion of the cultures of the ethnological record, and that, contrary to what may seem obvious, liberal sexual mores and even active sexual lives among adolescents are not necessarily associated with pregnancies among young teenagers. Using the Standard Cross-Cultural Sample of 186 societies—chosen for their representativeness of the ethnological universe, their geographic independence of one another, and the quality of the data available for them—Broude and Greene (1976) rated twenty sexual practices and attitudes toward sex, including premarital sex. It was possible to rate 107 societies on frequency of premarital sex for males, and, of these, premarital sex was rated as universal or almost universal in 59.8%, moderate or not uncommon in 17.8%, occasional in 10.3%, and uncommon in 12.1%. For females ($n = 114$ societies) the corresponding percentages are 49.1, 16.7, 14.0, and 20.2%.

It was also possible to rate 141 societies on attitudes toward premarital sex, as explicitly expressed in the cultural norms. Premarital sex is rated as "expected, approved; virginity has no value" in 24.1%; "tolerated; accepted if discreet" in 20.6%; and "mildly disapproved; pressure toward chastity but transgressions are not punished and nonvirginity ignored" in 17.0%. The cumulative percentage of these three more lenient categories is 61.7%, with the stricter, more disapproving categories distributed as follows: "moderately disapproved; virginity valued and token or slight punishment for nonvirginity," 8.5%; "premarital sex disallowed except with bridegroom," 4.3%; and "premarital sex strongly disapproved; virginity required or stated as required (virginity tests, severe reprisals for nonvirginity, e.g., divorce, loss of bride price)," 25.5% (Broude and Greene, 1976, pp. 414-415).

Since most of these societies do not place much emphasis on chronological age, many not even keeping track of it, it is not possible to separate premarital sex or attitudes toward it with regard to age. However, it is clear from much of the ethnographic material that teenagers are among the main targets of these strictures, or the lack therof.

It thus appears that our much discussed liberal shift in mores regarding premarital sex during the past 25 years has put the more liberal sector of our population in a category that includes at least 60% of the traditional societies in the ethnological record. Yet there is no widespread occurrence of early teenage pregnancies in these societies, as there is in ours at present. For example, the cultural atmosphere with regard to sex among the traditional !Kung San was at least as open and liberal as that in the United States during the past few years, yet early teenage pregnancy was unknown and at most about one-half of all women who had children had their first child before age nineteen. For this and other reasons, it seems worthwhile to summarize briefly this apparently paradoxical case. (For an account of adolescence in another, quite different African society, the Kikuyu, who also have late menarche compared with our own, see Worthman, this volume, Chapter 6.)

THE !KUNG HUNTER–GATHERER MODEL

The !Kung are the most extensively studied hunting-gathering population to date, and are thought to provide evidence regarding human adaptation during the vast majority of the course of human evolution (Lee and DeVore, 1968, 1976). There have been excellent studies of ogy (Lee, 1979), and demography (Howell, 1979). In addition one of us (Shostak, 1981) has worked extensively on the life cycle of women, while the other (Konner, 1976; Konner and Worthman, 1980) has focused on infant growth and development, infant care, and the relationship between nursing and reproductive function. The following discussion is drawn from these observations, as well as from those of Draper (1975, 1976), Marshall (1976), Lee (1979), and Howell (1979).

The demographic facts are, briefly, as follows (Howell, 1979). Prospective study of the age at menarche, which is easy to determine accurately for reasons of ritual, gives a mean of 16.6 and a median of 17.1 years, respectively, with the majority of girls passing this milestone between age 16 and 18 years (Howell, ibid, p. 178). About one-half of all girls are married by the time they reach menarche. Careful retrospective study of women who were 45 years old or older in 1968 yielded an estimate of the timing of first birth reflected by a mean of 18.8 and a median of 19.2 years, with all but a handful of mothers having had their first births between ages 17 and 22 (ibid, p. 128). Prospective study of women having their first births in the period 1963–1973 yielded higher estimates, with a mean of 21.4 and a median of 19.6 years (ibid, p. 141). Completed fertility determined retrospectively gave an estimate of 4.7 live births per woman, with the average age of last birth being in the middle thirties. Of 179 births occurring in the study population during the decade 1963–1973, only 16 occurred before age 20 (15 of these were first births), and only one occurred before age 17.

These demographic data must be understood in relation to the ethnographic context, which is as follows. Experimentation with sex starts quite early for the !Kung, beginning in early childhood and continuing through middle childhood without the interruption familiar in our society (and in psychoanalytic theory) as the "latency period." Children do not assume responsibility for subsistence until late in their teens, and their play groups are frequently out of sight of adults; sexual awareness and curiosity are allowed to flourish in the unrestricted time that comprises most of their day. Adults do not actually approve of sexual play among children and adolescents, and when it becomes obvious they make some effort to discourage it. But these efforts are half-hearted— of the order of verbal chastisements with no real or threatened consequences—and do little to ensure that the infractions will not recur. Interviews with adults reveal that they consider sexual experimentation in childhood and adolescence to be inevitable and even healthy. Certainly for adults sexual activity is considered essential for mental health, and they often referred to mentally ill people (for example, a woman who ate grass) as having suffered derangement because of sexual deprivation.

For the growing child among the !Kung, as opposed to among ourselves, the effect seems to be one of making sex seem less taboo, less frightening, and less unknown. It is not likely that a !Kung girl would engage in sex without understanding what is involved or what the consequences can be; she knows too much to allow herself naively to be "taken advantage of."

However, despite childhood sexual experimentation, the transition from the playful sex of childhood to the real sex of adulthood can be difficult, especially for girls. The main explanation for this is the early age at first marriage in the traditional system, in which one half of all girls were married before the time of their first menstruation (age 16½). However, they were typically married to men about 10 years older than themselves. Thus a teenage girl was confronted with the sexual advances of an adult man after having had prior experience only with boys her own age. Although in principle these advances would be delayed until her menarche, the transition from casual sex play with age mates to adult sex with a husband was stressful for many.

Contraception does not play a significant role in !Kung reproductive life. Some individuals claim to be vaguely aware of herbal medicines used by neighboring Bantu cultures, but few women of any age claim to have taken them at any time in their lives, and, in any case, they are of unknown effectiveness. The !Kung carry out their reproductive lives under the misconception that conception results from the mixing of menstrual blood, late in the menstrual flow, with semen; thus nothing resembling a conscious rhythm method could be operating. Children are highly desired by almost all women, regardless of age.

Nisa, a woman from whom an extended life history was collected by one of us (Shostak), described a more or less continual experience with childhood sexuality, all in the course of play with other children. In her early-to-mid-teens she had two unsuccessful arranged marriages to older men. Both were soon dissolved—the first because her husband had sex with a woman his own age in the marriage hut, while the much younger Nisa was presumed to be sleeping; the second because the young man proved unlikable to Nisa's father. Dissolution of these relationships was easily achieved. Both involved her in resistance to her husbands' sexual advances; despite extensive sex play in childhood, reportedly including sexual intercourse with penetration, these first experiences with adult men were awkward and essentially unwelcome. She was married for the third time through yet another arrangement by her parents, about 1 year before her first menstruation. She ran away from her husband many times before she settled down to married life with him. She finally agreed to have sex with him once, but subsequently refused due to the pain this had caused her. It took years before their relationship actually assumed an adult cast. As she explained, "We lived and lived, the two of us together, and after a while I started to really like him, and then to love him. I had finally grown up and learned how to love. I thought, 'A man has sex with you. Yes, that's what a man does. I had thought that perhaps he didn't'. . . I thought that, and gave myself to him, gave and gave. We lay with each other and my breasts were very large. I was becoming a woman."

The years from age 16½, when first menstruation occurs, to age 19, the mean age at first birth—a delay due mainly to adolescent subfertility—are important ones for the young !Kung woman. It is as though time were temporarily suspended; she is sexually mature but has no significant responsibility for taking care of a family or for contributing to subsistence. She can ease gradually into adult roles and adult sexuality without having to deal with the consequences of early pregnancy. She has years—some before menarche, some after—to determine whether she is compatible with her husband. As long as she has not yet become pregnant, divorce is possible. Whether she is married or not, the primary responsibility for feeding herself and her husband is deferred, while being borne by her mother and father. Even after her first birth, her need to remain near her mother is recognized, and it is not until the second child that she may be expected to move, with her family, to her husband's parents' village-camp. At that time—when she is 23 or 24 years old—she is essentially on her own, with the full psychological and social responsibilities pertaining to motherhood. Still, she is never quite "on her own" in the sense that many young American mothers are; she remains in a social and economic context dense with her own and/or her husband's relatives, and it is very rare for a marriage to be dissolved after it has produced living children.

Thus, this example of a very primitive society that is representative of the basic human social and demographic adaptation presents a picture of adolescent sexuality quite different from conventional assumptions about such societies. They indeed have active sexual lives from an early age, and restrictions on sexual relations are few. However, they have a late age of first menstruation, a presumed period of adolescent subfertility, and some contribution from pregnancy wastage that result in a mean age at first live birth of just under 20. Even then, the context of the kinship system is such as to limit responsibility and provide extensive economic and psychological support, diminishing only gradually as the young woman reaches her mid-20's and her family grows.

THE SECULAR TREND IN GROWTH AND MATURATION

A broader cross-cultural and historical view may now be invoked to present the spectrum of variation against which we must assess the

American and the !Kung models. In general it may be summarized as showing that whether compared with current underdeveloped populations or with European and American populations prior to the twentieth century, the ratio of births in the 15- to 19-year-cohort to those in the subsequent 5-year cohort is high in the current American population. Observed from the perspective of the child, the cohort of children born in the United States this year will include a proportion with mothers under age 20 that is higher than the comparable proportion for current populations in the underdeveloped world or for European and American populations at various times in the past, a circumstance due both to the current teenage birthrate and to the limitation of total family size.

Evidence that the age at first menstruation, or menarche, has been dropping in the United States and Europe for more than a century, has been repeatedly summarized (Tanner, 1962, 1968, 1973; Tanner and Eveleth, 1975; Wyshak and Frisch, 1982; Eveleth, see this volume). There is disagreement (e.g., Bullough, 1981) about the magnitude of this phenomenon, about its cross-national variability, and about whether and where it may be continuing, but there is general agreement that the phenomenon is real. A very conservative estimate would be that the age of menarche has declined 2 years since the early nineteenth century, and estimates as high as between 4 and 5 years have been presented.

This secular trend in growth has been well documented not only for age at menarche but for general growth rate (height and weight) as well as for maximum body size attained (Meredith, 1967, 1976). It is noteworthy that such measures lead to an estimate of the rate of acceleration of growth that confirms the estimate derived from studies of menarche. For example, the age of the peak of growth velocity in the pubertal height spurt, as indicated by changing height-for-age curves, has decreased at about the same rate as the age at menarche, namely 4 months per decade. This is of particular interest since studies of age at menarche are subject to methodological challenges that do not apply to studies of height growth.

The secular trend appears to have stopped in some populations, notably Oslo, Norway, where the earliest historical data come from (Brundtland and Walloe, 1973), London, England (Tanner, 1973), Newton, Massachusetts (Zacharias et al., 1976), and among old Americans at Harvard and Eastern women's colleges (Damon, 1974). The trend is reported to be continuing in some other populations (Guarniere et al., 1978), especially in the underdeveloped world (Eveleth and Tanner, 1976). In northern Europe, it appears to have stabilized at just about 13 years (Tanner, 1973) and in New England at a slightly younger age. Zacharias and her colleagues (Zacharias et al., 1970; Zacharias, et al., 1976) found that a large sample of girls in Newton, Massachusetts menstruated for the first time at 12.65 years, no earlier than the menarcheal age of their mothers. In the wealthiest New England families, the secular acceleration of growth apparently ended early in the twentieth century (Damon, 1974). It now seems possible, despite some exceptions, that the mean age at menarche may not drop much below 12½ to 13 years anywhere in the world, and that this may be a basic biological lower limit for this milestone in our species. But the youngest estimates for the United States place the mean at about 14 years during the early twentieth century. Norway, Germany, Finland, and Sweden, for which the data are much better, show a steady decline beginning in the middle of the nineteenth century, when the average age at menarche for various populations was 15, 16, or perhaps even 17 years. Conservative estimates thus leave room for a 2- or 3-year decline in northern Europe over a period of 150 years.

There is considerable variation in the age at menarche within populations, with the 95% confidence interval being bracketed by an 8-year period with the mean in the center (Eveleth, this volume, Chapter 3). Thus reports of menarche at age 12 and pregnancy at age 13 in some girls must be expected even with the highest estimated mean menarcheal ages ever presented. In our population menarche at age 8 or 9 and pregnancy at age 10 or 11 can no longer be considered to reflect endocrine pathology, as they certainly would have been at the turn of the century.

As previously noted, one can be skeptical about historical data on age at menarche, but the average age at which a given height is reached as also been dropping at about 4 months per decade (Meredith, 1976); this too has stopped in populations with higher socioeconomic status.

The reasons for the growth acceleration are not agreed upon. Frisch (1984) has accumulated evidence that nutritional improvements have led to increases in fatness at each age, which, in turn, lead to earlier menarche through the production of physiologically potent estrogens in fat cells. An effect of intense and prolonged exercise training is now well demonstrated in studies of young dancers and athletes (e.g., Frisch et al., 1980), and this effect may be obtained through the reduction of body fat or through endocrinological stress responses unfavorable to reproductive function. Other hypotheses of variation in age at menarche have been advanced, including improved public health and medical care in controlling chronic diseases of childhood (Tanner, 1968), changes in environmental lighting (Zacharias and Wurtman, 1964, 1969), increased consumption of refined carbohydrates (Schaefer, 1970), increased stimulation during infancy (Whiting, 1965), and genetic changes resulting from outbreeding or natural selection (Cavalli-Sforza and Bodmer, 1971). Urban living is definitely associated with earlier maturation, an effect that has been shown throughout the world (Eveleth and Tanner, 1976), but the meaning of this association is difficult to determine, since urbanization is accompanied by changes in most or all of the other, more specific, proposed causes. It is likely that the specification of determinants of the secular trend will await a better understanding of the neuroendocrine control of the onset of puberty, a rapidly advancing field, but one with many unexpected and puzzling findings (Sizonenko, 1978a,b; Grumbach, 1980; Reiter, Chapter 4, this volume).

It is necessary as well to consider the phenomenon of "adolescent sterility," more properly called adolescent subfertility, which has recently been extensively reviewed (Montagu, 1979). The erratic quality of menstrual cycles during the first year or more after menarche has been repeatedly documented, as has the existence of a high proportion of anovulatory cycles. Thus it is not surprising that first fecundity lags behind menarche by one or more years in many populations, and that this phenomenon is greater in underdeveloped countries. In view of the effect of nutrition and exercise on fecundity it is possible that this infertile period has decreased in length in recent generations, in parallel with the decrease in age at menarche. if so, then the mean age at first fecundity (or first consistent ovulation) would have dropped more markedly and rapidly than the mean age at menarche. However, this notion is at present still in the realm of speculation.

EVIDENCE FROM HISTORICAL DEMOGRAPHY

Historical demographers have provided a body of evidence on adolescent fertility (and, indirectly, fecundity) that is independent of the above-mentioned studies, and that also takes into account changing patterns of marriage and mores. Through the study of church, family, and other records, the lateness of first childbearing in Europe, England, and the United States during the sixteenth to nineteenth centuries has been shown (Laslett, 1965, Chapter 4; 1977, Chapter 6). The frequently cited case of Shakespeare's Juliet, whose nurse chides her for not marrying and becoming pregnant by age thirteen (as Juliet's mother allegedly had done) is carefully considered by Laslett. His discussion shows the nurse to have been a poor historical demographer, since such a case would have been exceedingly rare in either Juliet's Italy or Shakespeare's England. (Actually, as Laslett also shows, Juliet's age in Shakespeare's source for the play was eighteen. The change probably gives the play much of its urgency and poignancy, but it makes the nurse's impatience quite unrealistic.)

For the United States, Cutright (1972a,b) has reviewed the history of illegitimacy during the twentieth century, specifically addressing the relationship of earlier maturation to adolescent childbearing. He shows that there have been increases in the rate of teenage childbearing at least since 1940, and attempts to explain these increases in part by reference to the secular trend toward earlier menarche. He refers specifically to "the myth of an abstinent past," the thrust of which is to assume that because teenagers at the turn of the century had few pregnancies they must have obeyed their society's much greater strictures against sex. He presents the contrasting view that they were in fact more active sexually than we imagine them to have been, but did not become pregnant because they were reproductively immature. Vinovskis (see this volume, Chapter 15) reviews literature that carries this discussion back to the colonial period, arguing that premarital pregnancies not resulting in out-of-wedlock births have fluctuated rather than steadily increasing, and appear to have declined during the early nineteenth century due to an increasing stringency of sexual mores. However, this discussion does not change the basic assessment of pregnancy and childbearing in the early United States. Pregnancies in the late teens were incorporated decisively into a framework of marriage and family, while pregnancies in the early teens were virtually unknown.

DISCUSSION

A careful consideration of the ethnological literature, and of the experience of the !Kung San, hunter-gatherers of northwestern Botswana, in particular, leads to a revision of the common notion that in primitive societies young people enter the childbearing phase of the reproductive life cycle in the early teenage years. Although this may be true of some primitive societies, the majority appear to avoid this transition until later. Despite commonly nonrestrictive mores with regard to adolescent sexuality, and despite apparent high levels of adolescent sexual activity, pregnancy and childbearing usually do not occur. One explanation for this is probably that most such societies have puberty that is late compared with ours, and have, in addition, a significant period of adolescent infertility and/or subfertility.

It is against this broad ethnographic and evolutionary background that historical patterns of adolescent development in our own society must be seen. One hundred fifty years ago, a young woman menstruating at age 15 and becoming a mother by age 18 could take her place as an adult in a relatively simple society designed to support her in every way through firm institutions of marriage and family. Today, a girl menstruating at age 12 and becoming a mother by age 15, often unmarried and likely to remain so, is only a school-child at sea in a grown-up world that is much more complex and unforgiving. Even if all systems of physical maturation have accelerated, so that today's 15 year old has the body and even the brain of the 18 year old of the past, there is no way for her to compensate for the three years of lost experience, or to struggle successfully in a complex society in which maturity, education, and experience are increasingly valued.

Whatever the causes, it seems reasonable to judge the secular trend in human maturation to be one of the most profound changes in the biology of the species in recorded history, with what would seem to be important implications for adolescent psychology, education, and law. It is not our intention to argue that recent changes in rates of adolescent pregnancy are the simple result of longer-term changes in rates of human growth. Many other factors have intervened, and in fact the increase in the rate of maturation in the United States may have been largely completed before the beginning of the most recent change in adolescent sexual activity that has brought the current high incidence of pregnancy in this growth phase. However, it is clear that no rise in early teenage pregnancies could have occurred in a historical period when it was physiologically impossible. One does not have to postulate or discover a tight historical coupling between the secular trend and the adolescent pregnancy rate in order for them to have been causally related. The sexual activity of adolescents—and, even more so, our mores with regard to that activity—could be expected to resist change against the background of the long-term biological transformation, and then perhaps to change quite rapidly as the illogic of continued resistance became widely apparent.

Many expect moral restraint from teenagers, reasoning, not illogically, that loose morals explain teenage pregnancy. The expectation of moral restraint, characteristic of Europe and the United States in recent centuries, arose for complex reasons that are poorly understood and that are beyond the scope of this discussion. It must be seen against the background of the ethnological record, which shows that most societies have not traditionally had such expectations. Equally important, it must be seen in the context of a quite different biological reality, one that is now part of the past—a reality in which the late maturation of mature sexual impulses and the lateness of first fertility combined to prevent teenage pregnancy (and certainly early teenage pregnancy) with or without active moral restraint.

We may be tempted to blame changes in adult sexual mores for the rise in teenage pregnancy, imagining that if by legal or religious fiat exposure of teenagers to sexual ideas and stimuli could be drastically reduced, teenage sexual activity would revert to the patterns of 30 years ago. It is likely that this hypothesis has some validity. But the direction of causality may be much more complex, and indeed may be interactive, if not weighted in the other direction. Teenagers, especially the older ones in college, appear to have actually played a role in *producing* the changing sexual mores of recent decades, rather than being passive recipients of adult liberalization. If so, it is plausible that it is exactly accelerated sexual maturation that has led them to strive for earlier sexual freedom, and that this striving may have affected adult mores as much or more than it was affected by them. In other words, the secular trend seems to us a viable hypothesis for partial explanation of the change in mores itself.

Infancy and adolescence are probably two of the most sensitive periods of human growth. An early teenage pregnancy brought to term thus affects two growing children, one in each of the sensitive periods. Fetuses and infants are resilient, but only within limits, and it is doubtful whether a young teenager could provide the environment necessary for optimal development, even under conditions of optimal support and care for the mother.

Young teenage mothers, for their part, are completing the most rapid period of growth they have experienced since their own infancy, and are in the midst of a hormonal, psychological, and social turmoil centering around their own approach to adulthood. To bring a baby into this turmoil is often to pit two children against each other, children with needs that may be incompatible.

It is doubtful that we can turn back the clock on teenage sexual activity. Although this kind of reversal may have occurred before in our history, we are now in a different circumstance—not merely culturally but also biologically. Current high levels of teenage sexual activity are probably partly the product of television and magazine influences, but against the background of biological changes in the pace of maturation that have been going on for more than a century. To expect today's teenagers to live up to moral standards inherited from centuries past is not only to give them conflicting cultural and ethical messages but also to fail to recognize that the teenagers themselves are different— psychologically, physiologically, and anatomically.

Under the circumstances it is perhaps not too strong to say that to withhold information about contraception from a young teenager who may be sexually active, and then to deny her the possibility of therapeutic termination of her pregnancy, may in itself be a form of child abuse. Whatever our opinions of the complex moral issues of contraception and therapeutic abortion, our decisions could be made with a larger measure of compassion for the plight of today's teenager, caught between a mature body and immature, inexperienced emotions. The same logic we apply to protect young delinquents from adult punishment in juvenile court would presumably apply *a fortiori* to the protection of young teenagers from the consequences of their own sexual indiscretions. The practice, invoked by some authorities, of referring to even the youngest teenagers as women and men, rather than as girls and boys, simply *because* they have managed to achieve sexual intercourse, conception or even parenthood, contributes to the forces tending to rob them of their childhood.

Numerous other changes have taken place in the behavior of young teenagers in parallel with the increase in their sexual activity. These include a rise in school-age suicide (Petzel and Cline, 1978), school-age alcoholism (Hartford, 1976), and school-age substance abuse (Hein *et al.*, 1979). Despite the undoubted great complexity and obscurity of the causation of these trends, they must be understood against the background of the prior secular change in the organization of maturation. The ultimate and perhaps very general implications of this change, for adolescence specifically and for recent changes in our culture more widely, are only beginning to be explored.

REFERENCES

Baird, D. Prerequisites for successful childbearing. *Medical Services Journal (Canada)*, 19 23; 490–499, 1967.

Baldwin, W., Trends in adolescent contraception, pregnancy and childbearing. *In* E. R. McAnarney, (Ed.), *Premature adolescent pregnancy and parenthood*. New York: Grune and Stratton, 1983.

Battaglia, F., Frazier, T., and Hellegars, A. Obstetric and pediatric complications of juvenile pregnancy. *Pediatrics*, 1963, *32*, 902.

Briggs, R. R., Herren, R. R., and Thompson, W. B. Pregnancy in the young adolescent. *American Journal of Gynecology*, 1962, *84*, 436–441.

Broude, G. J., and Greene, S. J. Cross-cultural codes on twenty sexual attitudes and practices. *Ethnology*, 1976, *15*, 409–429.

Brundtland, G. H., and Walloe, L. Menarchal age in Norway: Halt in the trend towards earlier maturation. *Nature (London)*, 1973, *241*, 478–479.

Bullough, V. L. Age at menarche: A misunderstanding. *Science*, 1981, *213*, 365–366.

Cavalli-Sforze, L. and Bodmer, W. *The genetics of human populations*. San Francisco: Freeman, 1971.

Chilman, C. *Adolescent sexuality in a changing American society: Social and psychological perspectives*. Washington, D.C.: U.S. Government Printing Office, 1979.

Cutright, P. Illegitimacy in the United States: 1920–1968. *In* C. Westoff and R. Parke (Eds.), *Commission on population growth and the American future. Vol. I: Demographic and social aspects of population growth*. Washington, D.C.: Government Printing Office, 1972. (a)

Cutright, R. The teenage sexual revolution and the myth of an abstinent past. *Family Planning Perspectives*, 1972, *4(1)*, 24–31. (b)

Damon, A. Larger body size and earlier menarche: The end may be in sight. *Social Biology*, 1974, *21*, 8–11.

Deschamps, J. B., and Valentin, G. Pregnancy in adolescence. Incidence and outcome in European Countries. *Journal of Biosocial Science Suppl.*, 1978, *5*, 117–126.

Dott, A. B., and Fort, A. T. Medical and social factors affecting early teenage pregnancy. *American Journal of Obstetrics and Gynecology*, 1976, *125(4)*, 532–536.

Draper, P. !Kung women: Contrasts in sexual egalitarianism in the foraging and sedentary contexts. In R. Reiter (Ed.), *Toward an anthropology of women*. New York: Monthly Review, 1975.

Draper, P. Social and economic constraints on child life among the !Kung. In R. Lee and I. DeVore (Eds.), *Kalahari hunter-gatherers*. Cambridge, Mass.: Harvard University, 1976.

Duenhoelter, J. H., Jimenez, J. M., and Bauman, G. Pregnancy performance of patients under fifteen years of age. *Obstetrics and Gynecology*, 1975, *46(1)*, 49–52.

Eveleth, P. E., and Tanner, J. M. *Worldwide variation in human growth. International biological programme* Vol. 8. Cambridge, England: Cambridge University, 1976.

Frisancho, A. R., Matos, J., and Flegel, P. Maternal nutritional status and adolescent pregnancy outcome. *American Journal of Clinical Nutrition*, 1983, *38(5)*, 739–746.

Frisch, R. Body fat, puberty and fertility. *Biological Review*, *1984, 59*, 161–188.

Frisch, R., and Revelle, R. Height and weight at menarche and a hypothesis of menarche. *Archives of Disease in Childhood*, 1971, *46(249)*, 695–701.

Frisch, R., Wyshak, G., and Vincent, L. Delayed menarche and amenorrhea in ballet dancers. *New England Journal of Medicine*, 1980, *303*, 17–19.

Grumbach, M. M. The neuroendocrinology of puberty. *Hospital Practice*, 1980, *15*, 51–60.

Guarniere, J., Ferlazzo, G., and Amagliani, G. L'eta del menarca nella popolazione scolastica di Messina. *Acta Medica Auxologica*, 1978, *10*, 209–215.

Guttmacher Institute, *11 Million teenagers: What can be done about the epidemic of adolescent pregnancies in the United States*. New York: Alan F. Guttmacher Institute, 1976.

Guttmacher Institute, *Teenage pregnancy: The problem that hasn't gone away.* New York: Alan F. Guttmacher Institute, 1981.

Hamburg, D., Moos, R., and Yalom, I. Studies of distress in the menstrual cycle and the postpartum period. In R. Michael (Ed.), *Endocrinology and human behavior*. London: Oxford, 1968.

Hartford, T. C., Teenage alcohol use. *Postgraduate Medicine*, 1976, *80*, 73.

Hein, K., Cohen, M. I., and Litt, I. F. Illicit drug use among urban adolescents. A decade in retrospect. *American Journal of Diseases of Children*, 1979, *133*, 38.

Horon, I. L., Strobino, D. M., and MacDonald, H. M. Birth weights among infants born to adolescent and young adult women. *American Journal of Obstetrics and Gynecology*, 1983, *146(4)*, 444–449.

Howell, N., *Demography of the dobe !Kung*. New York: Academic Press, 1979.

Isreal, S. L., and Wouterz, T. B. Teenage Obstetrics. *American Journal of Obstetrics and Gynecology*, 1963, *85*, 659.

Klerman, L. V., and Stekel, J. F. Teenage pregnancy. *Science*, 1978, *199 (4336)*, 1390.

Konner, M. J. Maternal care, infant behavior and development among the Kung. In R. Lee, and I. Devore (Eds.), *Kalahari hunter-gatherers*. Cambridge, Mass.: Harvard University, 1976.

Konner, M. J., and Worthman, C. M. Nursing frequency, gonadal function and birth spacing among !Kung hunter-gatherers. *Science*, 1980, *207*, 788-791.

Laslett, P. *The world we have lost: England before the industrial age.* New York: Scribner's, 1965.

Laslett, P. *Family life and illicit love in earlier generations.* Cambridge, England: Cambridge University, 1977.

Lee, R. *The !Kung San: Men, women and work in a foraging society.* New York: Cambridge University, 1979.

Lee, R., and DeVore, I. *Man the hunter.* New York: Aldine, 1968.

Lee, R., and DeVore, I. *Kalahari hunter-gatherers.* Cambridge, Mass.: Harvard University, 1976.

Lobl, M., Welcher, D., and Mellitts, E. Maternal age and intellectual functioning of offspring. *Johns Hopkins Medical Journal,* 1971, *128,* 347, 1971.

Marshall, L. *The !Kung of Nyae Nyae.* Cambridge, Mass.: Harvard University, 1976.

Meredith, H. A synopsis of puberal changes in youth. *The Journal of School Health,* 1967. *37,* 210–215.

Meredith, H. Findings from Asia, Australia, Europe, and North America on secular change in mean height of children, youths and young adults. *American Journal of Physical Anthropology,* 1976, *44,* 315–326.

Moerman, M. L. Growth of the birth canal in adolescent girls. *American Journal of Obstetrics and Gynecology,* 1982, *143(5),* 528–532.

Montagu, M. F. A. *The reproductive development of the female: A study in the comparative physiology of the adolescent organism* (3rd ed.). Littleton, Mass.: Wright PSG, 1979.

Morris, N. M. The biological advantages and social disadvantages of teenage pregnancy. *American Journal of Public Health,* 1981, *71,* 810–817.

National Center for Health Statistics, *Monthly Vital Statistics Report,* 1977, *26* (5, Suppl.).

National Center for Health Statistics. Advance report of final natality statistics, 1981. *Monthly Vital Statistics Report,* 1983, *32* (9, Suppl.), 14–40 (Dec. 29).

National Center for Health Statistics. Trends in teenage childbearing, United States, 1970–81. *Vital and Health Statistics, Series,* 1984, *21, No. 41.* Hyattsville, Md.: U.S. Public Health Service (September).

Naeye, R. L. Teenaged and pre-teenaged pregnancies: consequences of the fetal-maternal competition for nutrients. *Pediatrics,* 1981, *67(1),* 146–50.

Osbourne, G. K., Howat R. C., and Jordan, M M. The obstetric outcome of teenage pregnancy. *British Journal of Obstetrics and Gynaecology,* 1981, *88(3),* 215–221.

Paffenbarger, R. S. Epidemiological aspects of post-partum mental illness. *British Journal of Preventive and Social Medicine,* 1964, *18,* 189.

Petzel, S. V., and Cline, D. W. Adolescent suicide: Epidemiological and biological aspects. *Adolescent Psychiatry,* 1978, *6,* 239–266.

Pugh, T., Jerath, B., Schmidt, W., and Reed, R. Rates of mental diseases related to childbearing. *New England Journal of Medicine,* 1963, *268,* 1224.

Rothenberg, P. B., and Varga, P. E., The relationship between age of mother and child health and development. *American Journal of Public Health,* 1981, *71,* 810–817.

Russell, J. K. *Early teenage pregnancy.* New York: Churchill Livingstone, 1982.

Schaefer, O. Pre- and post-natal growth acceleration and increased sugar consumption in Canadian Eskimos. *Canadian Medical Association Journal,* 1970, *103,* 1059.

Shapiro, S., Schlesinger, E., and Nesbitt, R. Jr., *Infant, perinatal, maternal and childhood mortality in the United States: A vital and health statistics monograph of the American Public Health Association.* Cambridge, Mass.: Harvard University, 1968.

Shostak, M. *Nisa: The life and words of a !Kung woman.* Cambridge, Mass.: Harvard University, 1981.

Sizonenko, P. C. Endocrinology in preadolescents and adolescents. I. Hormonal changes during normal puberty. *American Journal of Diseases of Children,* 1978, *132,* 704–712. (a)

Sizonenko, P. C., Preadolescent and adolescent endocrinology: Physiology and physiopathology. II. Hormonal changes during abnormal pubertal development. *American Journal of Diseases of Children,* 1978, *132,* 797–805. (b)

Tanner, J. M. *Growth at adolescence* (2nd ed.). Oxford: Blackwell, 1962.

Tanner, J. M. Earlier maturation in man. *Scientific American,* 1968, *218(1),* 21–27.

Tanner, J. M. Trend towards earlier menarche in London, Oslo, Copenhagen, the Netherlands and Hungary. *Nature (London),* 1973, *243,* 95–96.

Tanner, J. M., and Eveleth, P. B. Variability between populations in growth and development at puberty. *In* S. R. Berenberg (Ed.), *Puberty: Biologic and psychosocial components.* Leiden: Stenfert Kroese, 1975.

Whiting, J. Menarcheal age and infant stress in humans. *In* F. Beach (Ed.), *Sex and behavior.* New York: Wiley, 1965.

Wyshak, G., and Frisch, R. Evidence for a secular trend in age of menarche. *New England Journal of Medicine,* 1982, *306,* 1033–1035.

Zacharias, Z., and Wurtman, R. J. Blindness: Its relation to age of menarche. *Science,* 1964, *144,* 1154–1155.

Zacharias, L., and Wurtman, R. J. Age at menarche: Genetic and environmental influences. *New England Journal of Medicine,* 1969, *280,* 868–875.

Zacharias, L., Wurtman, R. J., and Schatzoff, M. Sexual maturation in contemporary American girls. *American Journal of Obstetrics and Gynecology,* 1970, *108,* 833–846.

Zacharias, L., Rand, W. M., and Wurtman, R. J. A prospective study of sexual development and growth in American girls: The statistics of menarche. *Obstetrical and Gynecological Survey,* 1976, *31,* 325–337.

17

SCHOOL-AGE PARENTS AND CHILD ABUSE

Richard J. Gelles

Are school-age parents at greater risk of abusing their children? The answer, according to both those who study the consequences of teen-aged childbearing and those who are concerned with the etiology of child abuse, is, YES. Students of teenaged childbearing report consistent and compelling deleterious effects of what is referred to as "premature parenthood" on the mother, child, and family (Crawford and Fursten-berg, 1982; Furstenberg, 1976; Klerman and Jeckel, 1973; Menken, 1978; Moore and Caldwell, 1977; Moore and Waite, 1977). The death rate for children born to teenage mothers is more than double the death rate for infants born to older mothers (Thornburg, 1978). Premature or low birth weight babies, and the medical problems correlated with this condition, including death, asphyxia, birth injuries, neurological prob-lems, epilepsy, cerebral palsy, and retardation are also more common among teenage mothers (National Center for Health Statistics, 1978; Pasamanick and Lilienfeld, 1956; Newcombe and Tarendale, 1964; Menken, 1972). Included among the other deficits disproportionately experienced by children of teenaged mothers are deafness and blind-ness (Goldberg et al., 1967) and motor and intellectual development problems (Clifford, 1964; Drillien, 1969; Eaves et al., 1970; Weiner, 1970).

Noting the health problems of adolescent mothers and their offspring, as well as the social and psychological correlates of teenage child-bearing, child abuse researchers have proposed that since these same factors are correlated with abuse of children, then teenage parenthood is probably causally linked to the abuse of children (Bolton, 1980: Bolton et al., 1980).

The actual empirical evidence to support the hypothesized corre-lation between teenaged childbearing and increased risk of child abuse is considerably more ambiguous than one would expect based on reviewing the literature concerned with teenaged parenthood and child abuse.

METHODOLOGICAL DIFFICULTIES IN ASSESSING THE RELATIONSHIP BETWEEN SCHOOL-AGED PARENTHOOD AND CHILD ABUSE

Kinard and Klerman (1980) have identified three important methodological problems with research that attempts to assess the relationship between teenaged parenthood and child abuse: (1) how to measure the age of the parent; (2) which parent's age should be measured, and (3) selection of appropriate comparison groups.

AGE OF PARENT

Kinard and Klerman (1980) identify three possible ways the age of the parent can be measured in a study of teenage parenthood and child abuse: (1) age at time of the abuse incident; (2) age at time of the birth of abused child; and (3) age at time of the birth of the first child. One obvious problem arises when there are three possible means of measuring age—that of noncomparability of various studies if they each use a different measure of age of the parent. The weakest measure of age, especially if child abuse is operationalized as a reported and validated case of child abuse, is age of parent at time of the abuse. If this measure is used, it can underestimate the relationship between age and abuse, since the time at which the abuse is reported is not necessarily the time at which the abuse began. Thus, a teenager may have a child, and even commence mistreating the child, but the abuse might not come to public attention until the parent is 20 or 25 years of age. Kinard and Klerman (1980) also note problems with the second measure, since the parent may have begun his or her career as a parent when a teenager, but might be abusing a child born after he or she had turned 20. The preferred measure of age for Kinard and Klerman is age at time of birth of first child.

WHICH PARENT'S AGE TO MEASURE

In their discussion of which age to measure, Kinard and Klerman discuss "mother's age." However, as the literature on child maltreatment clearly points out (e.g., Straus et al., 1980), mothers are only slightly more likely than fathers to be the offenders in acts of abuse. Thus, measuring the age of the mother (at time of abuse, at time of birth of abused child, and at time of birth of first child), might not capture the true relationship between age and abuse. Clearly, children can, and are, abused by caretakers other than their mothers.

COMPARISON GROUPS

A fatal flaw in a considerable number of child abuse studies is that the research designs do not include comparison groups. The lack of a comparison groups means that the investigator can not determine whether or not there is a relationship between abuse and an independent variable. Of course, an investigator could assess the proportion of a sample of abusers who are teenage parents and compare that to national or regional natality statistics. However, this is far less satisfactory than designing a study which includes some kind of matched comparison group (Kinard and Klerman, 1980).

ADDITIONAL METHODOLOGICAL PROBLEMS

There are additional methodological problems in studying school-age parenthood and child abuse which were not identified by Kinard and Klerman. One of the most important problems is the confounding of the factors which cause child abuse with those factors which lead persons or families to be identified as child abusers. Most child abuse and neglect researchers draw their samples of abused children from publicly identified and validated cases of abuse (Gelles, 1975). Physicians, social workers, and other clinicians tend to consider factors which are believed to be associated with child abuse when they assess children and families who are suspected of being involved in abuse. *Thus, socioeconomic status, race, and age, because they are thought to be strongly associated with abuse, can become significant factors in the diagnosis of child abuse* (Gelles, 1975). Researchers have noted a preferential susceptibility of blacks and lower socioeconomic status families to be labeled "child abusers" (Newberger et al., 1977; Turbett and O'Toole, 1980). In short, a belief that teenage parents are likely to abuse their children may cause clinicians to preferentially identify (correctly and falsely) young parents as abusers. This, in turn, would mean that a researcher would find a disproportionate number of teenaged parents among official cases of abuse. A more valid measure of the relationship between age and child abuse would require a research design which does not confound causal factors with factors which lead individuals to be identified as abusers and abused.

Another methodological difficulty with research on school-age parenthood and child abuse (and for that matter, a problem with most research on school-age parenthood—Crawford and Furstenberg, 1982) is that few studies employ careful statistical controls for race, income, class, or other social factors that might be confounded with school-age childbearing. The inability to rule out spuriousness in the analysis of the relationship between school-age parenthood and child abuse is a major problem, and one which is not easily overcome. Irrespective of the research design, it is difficult to gather a sufficient number of cases and controls to prepare a complete analysis. This is due to both child abuse and school-age parenthood being essentially low base-rate phenomena. Estimates of the national incidence of child abuse run from a conservative 1% to as high as 3.8% (Burgdorf, 1980; Gelles, 1978). Teenagers (14–17 years of age) constitute 7% of the national population (Bureau of the Census, 1979). While much is made of teenage pregnancy rates and their recent increase (Baldwin, 1976), estimates are that of the 40% of teenagers who become pregnant, only 20% will give birth (Tietze, 1978). Thus, teenagers who become parents make up only 1% of the national population. In short, few studies have sufficient numbers of teenage abusive parents to run the normal tests for spuriousness.

EVIDENCE ON THE LINK BETWEEN SCHOOL-AGE PARENTHOOD AND CHILD ABUSE

Kinard and Klerman (1980) reviewed four studies of child abuse which provide evidence on the hypothesized relationship between school-age parenthood and child abuse. In addition, there are two other bodies of data which can be examined to shed light on the possible relationship between these two important social issues.

The oldest and best known body of data is David Gil's 1967 nationwide epidemiological study of reported and validated cases of child abuse (1970). Gil's data provide measures of whether the mother was under 20 years of age at the time of the reported abuse, and her age at the time of the birth of the abused child (see Table 17.1 for summary). According to Kinard and Klerman's reanalysis of the Gil data, teenage mothers at the time of the reported abuse were overrepresented in the Gil sample. However, mothers under age 20 at the time of the birth of the abused child were no more likely to be abusers than mothers who were older than 20 years of age when they gave birth to the abused child (Kinard and Klerman, 1980).

A second national sample of abuse cases comes from the American Humane Association (see Table 17.1 for summary). The American Humane Association operates a national clearing house for child abuse and neglect reports. Kinard and Klerman analyzed 36,822 validated cases of abuse and neglect reported to AHA by 38 states in 1976. The data provide information only on the mother's age at the time of the birth of her first child. From these data, Kinard and Klerman (1980) find that teenage mothers are overrepresented as child abusers.

A third set of data are 2436 confirmed reports of child abuse or sexual

TABLE 17.1. Teenage Childbearing in Relationship to Child Abuse[a]

Study	N	Mothers less than age 20 (%)		
		At time of abusive incident	At birth of abused child	At birth first child
Kinard (1978)	30	3.45	34.5	51.7
Gil (1970)	1,104	9.29	37.9	—
AHA (1978)	36,822	—	—	39.3
McCarthy (1978)	1,903	8.00	34.8	51.7
Bolton et al. (1978)	4,851	6.40	—	36.5

[a]Adapted from Kinard and Klerman (1980) and Elster et al. (1981).

abuse received by the Georgia Child Abuse Registry between June, 1975 and July, 1978 (McCarthy, 1980). The McCarthy data (see Table 17.1) include all three measures of age of mother. The Kinard/Klerman (1980) analysis of the McCarthy data suggests that teenage mothers are more likely than older mothers to be perpetrators of abuse.

Finally, Kinard and Klerman review Kinard's own research (Kinard, 1978). While the number of abuse cases is small (N = 30), all three measures of age are available as is a matched comparison group (N = 30). When Kinard compared the percentage of abusive mothers who were teenagers when they gave birth to their first child to a matched control group, she found that a higher percentage of the control group mothers were teenagers at first birth. However, the percentage of mothers in both groups who started childbearing when they were younger than 20 years of age was higher than the general population.

In the end, Kinard and Klerman (1980) conclude that the findings from the four studies indicate that teenage mothers are more likely than older mothers to be perpetrators of maltreatment.

Table 17.1 reviews the findings from the four studies reviewed by Kinard and Klerman and includes a fifth study, an analysis of a large random sample of reported child maltreatment incidents in Arizona (Bolton et al., 1980). Compared to Kinard and Klerman's data on the national percentage of first births to mothers under 20 years of age between 1965 to 1971, it would appear that teenage mothers are not overrepresented as abusers in the Bolton et al. data.

DATA FROM A NATIONAL SURVEY OF FAMILY VIOLENCE

A final source of data on the relationship between school-age parenthood and child abuse is the national survey of family violence carried out by Straus et al. (1980). This was a national survey carried out in 1976 of 2143 households. The survey examined violence between husband and wife, violence between parent and child, and violence between children. To be eligible for inclusion in the sample, a household had to have a man and a woman living together in a relationship.

To be part of the analysis of parent and child violence, there had to be at least one child living in the household who was between the ages of 3 and 17 years.*

Violence was nominally defined as an act carried out with the intention, or perceived intention, of causing pain or injury to the other person (Straus et al., 1980). Abusive violence was nominally defined as violence which included the high potential of injuring the person being hit. Violence was operationalized through the use of the Conflict Tactics Scales (Straus et al., 1980; Straus, 1979). The Conflict Tactics Scales were designed to measure intrafamily conflict in the sense of the means used to resolve conflicts of interests. Three different tactics are measured: (1) reasoning: the use of rational discussion and argument (Items a–d, Fig. 17.1); (2) verbal aggression: the use of verbal and symbolic means of hurting, such as insults or threats to hurt the other (items e–j); (3) violence: the actual use of physical force (items k–r); and (4) abusive violence (items n–r).

The operationalization of abusive violence in this study was quite different than the typical operationalization of child abuse. First, and most importantly, this definition of abuse does not limit child abuse to actions which injure a child. Thus, it is a broader definition of abuse than is typically found in the literature. Second, the operationalization is based on a parent's self-report, rather than the official report and validation of abuse. On the one hand, this means that this definition of abuse is not confounded with factors which lead a person to be publicly labeled a child abuser. On the other hand, the definition is confounded with factors which lead an individual to admit or not admit violence toward a child to an interviewer.†

Of the 2143 households surveyed, 1146 included children between 3 and 17 years of age. Of these families, 623 mothers and 523 fathers were interviewed. Subjects were asked to report their own use of conflict tactics with their children, so that the data on mother's violence is reported by mothers, and father's violence is reported by fathers.

Assessing age during the year of reported violence, Straus and his colleagues (1980) found an inverse relationship between parent's age and abusive violence. However, since the lower limit of age of respondents was 18, no data on school-age parents are available from this study.

Age of the parent at the time of the birth of the child was available. Table 17.2 provides a summary of all forms of conflict resolution by the age and gender of the parent.

*The rationale for setting the age limit between 3 and 17 years of age was the result of the goal of measuring the extent of sibling violence. In order to arrive at a meaningful measure, a lower limit of 3 years of age was set—so as to exclude the hitting and throwing of objects carried out by infants and toddlers.

†For a complete discussion of the methodology, see Straus et al., 1980.

TABLE 17.2. Age at Birth of Child By Gender, By Conflict Tactics in Previous Year

Age	Reasoning		Verbal aggression		Violence		Severe violence	
	Mothers	Fathers	Mothers	Fathers	Mothers	Fathers	Mothers	Fathers
Under 17	96	100	80	50	78	58	30	0
	(23)[a]	(11)	(20)	(12)	(23)	(12)	(23)	(12)
18–21	97	92	70	63	75	77	21	13
	(126)	(53)	(129)	(51)	(129)	(32)	(130)	(53)
22–25	96	97	65	63	71	66	21	9
	(165)	(98)	(167)	(103)	(167)	(100)	(167)	(101)
26–30	97	99	67	61	70	67	18	14
	(128)	(128)	(129)	(132)	(129)	(131)	(130)	(132)
31–40	98	93	55	50	57	47	11	8
	(118)	(162)	(116)	(163)	(122)	(163)	(122)	(163)
Over 40	83	87	48	36	48	29	0	3
	(30)	(38)	(31)	(36)	(31)	(38)	(31)	(38)
	$p \leq .05$	$p \leq .05$	$p \leq .05$	$p \leq .05$	$p \leq .01$	$p \leq .001$	$p \leq .01$	NS

[a]Numbers in parentheses are cell sizes.

Mothers who were 17 years of age or less at the time they gave birth to the child who was discussed during the interview (when mothers had more than one child aged 3–17 living at home, a single "referent child" was selected using a table of random numbers), were most likely to use violence and abusive violence toward that child. Interestingly, the same relationship was not found for fathers. Men who were 18–21 or 26–30 years of age at the time of the birth of the child, reported the highest levels of abusive and general violence.

Women who were teenagers at the time of the "referent child's" birth were also the most likely to use some form of verbal aggression in dealing with their children. Again, fathers who were teenagers at the time of the child's birth were not the most likely to be verbally aggressive.

Parents who were teenagers at the time of the birth of their children were not significantly different from other parents (with the exception of those who were over 40 years of age when they became parents of the referent children) in terms of the use of reasoning as a means of settling conflicts of interest.

EXPLAINING THE RELATIONSHIP BETWEEN SCHOOL-AGED PREGNANCY AND CHILD ABUSE

The dominant model used to explain the hypothesized relationship between commencing child rearing as a teenager and child abuse is a "stress and coping" model.

57. Parents and children use many different ways of trying to settle differences between them. I'm going to read a list of some things that you and (CHILD) might have done when you had a dispute. Still using Card A, I would like you to tell me how often you did it with (CHILD) in the last year.

	Q.57 RESPONDENT								Q.58 EVER HAPPENED			Q.59 CHILD								
	Never	Once	Twice	3-5 Times	6-10 Times	11-20 Times	More than 20 Times	Don't Know	Yes	No	Don't Know	Never	Once	Twice	3-5 Times	6-10 Times	11-20 Times	More than 20 Times	Don't Know	
a. Discussed the issue calmly	0	1	2	3	4	5	6	X	1	2	X	0	1	2	3	4	5	6	X	421-23
b. Got information to back up (your/ his or her) side of things	0	1	2	3	4	5	6	X	1	2	X	0	1	2	3	4	5	6	X	424-26
c. Brought in or tried to bring in someone to help settle things	0	1	2	3	4	5	6	X	1	2	X	0	1	2	3	4	5	6	X	427-29
d. Insulted or swore at the other one	0	1	2	3	4	5	6	X	1	2	X	0	1	2	3	4	5	6	X	430-32
e. Sulked and/or refused to talk about it	0	1	2	3	4	5	6	X	1	2	X	0	1	2	3	4	5	6	X	433-35
f. Stomped out of the room or house (or yard)	0	1	2	3	4	5	6	X	1	2	X	0	1	2	3	4	5	6	X	436-38
g. Cried	0	1	2	3	4	5	6	X	1	2	X	0	1	2	3	4	5	6	X	439-41
h. Did or said something to spite the other one	0	1	2	3	4	5	6	X	1	2	X	0	1	2	3	4	5	6	X	442-44

i. Threatened to hit or throw something at the other one	0	1	2	3	4	5	6	X	1	2	X	0	1	2	3	4	5	6	X	445-47
j. Threw or smashed or hit or kicked something	0	1	2	3	4	5	6	X	1	2	X	0	1	2	3	4	5	6	X	448-50
k. Threw something at the other one	0	1	2	3	4	5	6	X	1	2	X	0	1	2	3	4	5	6	X	451-53
l. Pushed, grabbed, or shoved the other one	0	1	2	3	4	5	6	X	1	2	X	0	1	2	3	4	5	6	X	454-56
m. Slapped or spanked the other one	0	1	2	3	4	5	6	X	1	2	X	0	1	2	3	4	5	6	X	457-59
n. Kicked, bit, or hit with a fist	0	1	2	3	4	5	6	X	1	2	X	0	1	2	3	4	5	6	X	460-62
o. Hit or tried to hit with something	0	1	2	3	4	5	6	X	1	2	X	0	1	2	3	4	5	6	X	463-65
p. Beat up the other one	0	1	2	3	4	5	6	X	1	2	X	0	1	2	3	4	5	6	X	466-68
q. Threatened with a knife or gun	0	1	2	3	4	5	6	X	1	2	X	0	1	2	3	4	5	6	X	469-71
r. Used a knife or gun	0	1	2	3	4	5	6	X	1	2	X	0	1	2	3	4	5	6	X	472-74
s. Other (PROBE): _____	0	1	2	3	4	5	6	X	1	2	X	0	1	2	3	4	5	6	X	475-77

FOR EACH ITEM CIRCLED AS "NEVER" OR "DON'T KNOW" ON Q. 57, ASK:
58. When you and (CHILD) have had a disagreement, have you ever (ITEM)?

ASK EVERYONE:
59. Now, let's talk about (CHILD). Tell me how often in the past year when you had a disagreement (he/she) (FIRST ITEM CIRCLED). (RECORD ABOVE) _____

TAKE BACK CARD A

Figure 17.1. Example of Conflict Tactics Scales: reasoning.

355

In their discussion of teenage fathers, Elster and Lamb (1983) note that high stress and reduced ability to manage stress are linked to child-rearing failure. Among the variables which Elster and Lamb find correlated with both young fathers and child abuse are: low education, low vocational success, and high marital disorganization. The psychological immaturity of adolescent fathers not only contributes to the stress they are believed to experience, but also their ability to manage this stress, thus raising their risk of child maltreatment (Elster and Lamb, 1983).

Kinard and Klerman (1980) explain that poverty can contribute to both early parenthood and child abuse.

Bolton et al. (1980), while finding little differences in comparing the dynamics of families where there are adolescent pregnancies and families where there are no adolescent pregnancies, agree that stress and coping ability are means of explaining the hypothesized higher risk of child maltreatment among teenaged parents. Bolton (1980), following the same logic as Elster and Lamb, compares the factors related to both abuse and teenage pregnancy, and finds indicators of social stress and coping ability are means of explaining the hypothesized higher risk of child maltreatment among teenage parents.

DISCUSSION AND SUMMARY

The strong feeling that school-age parents are at greater risk than other parents for abusing their children is shared by many students of school-age parenthood and child maltreatment. the data supporting such a claim are often contradictory and suspect on numerous methodological grounds.

Among the major problems with research and theory on the possible relationship between school-age parenthood and child abuse are that most investigations cannot separate out the factors related to school-age parenthood from the factors related to the likelihood of being reported for child abuse. Even more importantly, the widespread belief that school-age parents are at risk for child abuse may mean that a disproportionate number of these parents to be both correctly and falsely identified as abusers, thus overestimating the true relationship.

Even if the problem of confounding of causal factors with identification factors was resolved or not present, the current research still suffers from the problem of trying to find a link between two phenomena with low base rates. No study to date has a sufficient sample which would allow for even the crudest control for factors such as race, income, education, or social support. Thus, it can not be determined whether school-age parenthood is the prime factor leading to abuse, or whether social class is related both to the risk of abuse and early childbearing.

The current theoretical explanations for the proposed link between abuse and early parenthood are social-structural and social psychological in nature. *Although few, if any, studies include direct measures of stress and coping, the assumption is that early childbearing is highly stressful, and in and of itself lowers the ability of young parents to cope with stress.* The most popular dynamic applied to the study of school-age parents and abuse is that poverty and social class are related to early (immature) childbearing. Poverty is stressful, as is early childbearing, so that school-age parents are thought to suffer from excessive stress. Unable to cope with this stress, they are at risk of battering their children. In addition, early childbearing is thought to produce physical and psychological stress for the mother, as well as increasing the probability of problems for the child, including prematurity, low birthrate, mental retardation, reduction in intelligence, and other problems which add to the stress of early childbearing.

Although alluded to in some discussions of school-age parenthood and child maltreatment, biosocial parameters are rarely investigated. The physiological impact of school-age parenthood on both the mother and the child are rarely measured or included in a theoretical discussion of child abuse.

In conclusion, it would be fair to say that the proposed risk of child abuse among school-age parents is neither adequately demonstrated nor explained in the available literature. Even if a consistent correlation between the two events is found, numerous plausible rival hypotheses for the relationship need to be considered. Should there actually be a direct and nonspurious relationship found, the current thinking on explaining such a relationship ought to be broadened to include a variety of factors beyond simply stress and coping.

ACKNOWLEDGMENT

A revised version of a paper presented at the Conference on School-Aged Pregnancies and Parenthood. Sponsored by the Society for Social Sciences Research, Baltimore, Maryland, May, 1982.

This research was partially sponsored by a Grant from the National Institute of Mental Health (MH 27557).

REFERENCES

Baldwin, W. Adolescent pregnancy and childbearing—Growing concerns for Americans. *Population Bulletin*, 1976, *31*, 3–21.

Bolton, F. G., Jr. *The pregnant adolescent*. Beverly Hills, Ca.: Sage Publications, 1980.

Bolton, R. G., Jr., Laner, R. H., and Kane, S. P. Child maltreatment risk among adolescent mothers: A study of reported cases. *American Journal of Orthopsychiatry*, 1980, *50*, 469–504.

Bureau of the Census. *Statistical Abstract of the United States*, 100th Edition. Washington, D.C.: Government Printing Office, 1979.

Burgdorf, K. *Recognition and reporting of child maltreatment*. Rockville, Maryland: Westat, Inc., 1980.

Clifford, S. H. High risk pregnancy: I. Prevention of pregnancy the "sin qua non" for reduction of mental retardation and other neurological disorders. *New England Journal of Medicine*, 1964, 271, 243.

Crawford, A. G., and Furstenberg, F. F., Jr. *Teenage sexuality, pregnancy, and child welfare*. Unpublished manuscript, 1982.

Drillien, C. M. School disposal and performance for children of differential birth weight born 1953–1960. *Archives of Diseases of Childhood*, 1969, 44, 562.

Eaves, L. C., Nuttall, J. C., Klonoff, H., and Dunn, H. G. Developmental and psychological test scores in children of low birth weight. *Pediatrics*, 1970, 45, 9.

Elster, A. B., and Lamb, M. E. Adolescent fathers: a Group potentially at risk for parenting failure. *Infant Mental Health Journal*, 1983, 3, 148–155.

Elster, A. B., McAnarey, E. R., and Lamb, M. E. *Adolescents and their children: Pediatric challenges*. Unpublished manuscript, 1981.

Furstenberg, F. F., Jr. *Unplanned parenthood: The social consequences of teenage childbearing*. New York: The Free Press, 1976.

Gelles, R. J. The social construction of child abuse. *American Journal of Orthopsychiatry*, 1975, 43, 363–371.

Gelles, R. J. Violence towards children in the United States. *American Journal of Orthopsychiatry*, 1978, 48, 580–592.

Gil, D. *Violence against children*. Cambridge, Mass.: Harvard University Press, 1970.

Goldberg, I. D., Goldstein, H., Quade, D., and Rogot, E. Association of perinatal factors with blindness in children. *Public Health Reports*, 1967, 82, 519.

Kinard, E. M. Emotional development in physically abused children: A study of self-concept and aggression. Doctoral dissertation, Brandeis University, 1978. University Microfilms, Ann Arbor, Michigan.

Kinard, E. M., and Klerman, L. V. Teenage parenting and child abuse: are they related? *American Journal of Orthopsychiatry*, 1980, 50, 481–488.

Klerman, L. V., and Jekel, J. *School-Age mothers: Problems, programs, and policy*. Hamden, Conn.: Linnet Books, 1973.

McCarthy, B. Unpublished data, Centers for Disease Control, DHEW, Atlanta, 1978. (As cited in Kinard, E. M., and Klerman, L. V. Teenage parenting and child abuse: Are they related? *American Journal of Orthopsychiatry*, 1980, 50, 481–488.)

Menken, J. Teenage childbearing: Its medical aspects and implications for the U.S. population. In C. Westoff and R. Parks (Eds.), *Demographic and social aspects of population growth*. Washington, D.C.: Government Printing Office, 1972.

Menken, J. Health and demographic consequences of adolescent pregnancy and childbearing. In C.Chilman (Ed.), *Teenage childbearing: Recent research on determinants and on consequences*. Washington, D.C.: Government Printing Office, 1978.

Moore, K. A., and Caldwell, S. B. The effects of government policies on out-of-wedlock sex and pregnancy. *Family Planning Perspectives*, 1977, 9 (4), 164–168.

Moore, K. A., and Waite, L. Early childbearing and educational attainment. *Family Planning Perspectives*, 1977, 9(5), 220–225.

Newcombe, H. B., and Tarendale, O. G. Maternal age and birth order correlations. *Mutation Research* 1964, *1*, 446.

Newberger, E. H., Reed, R. B., Daniel, J. H., Hyde, J. N., Jr., and Kotelchuck, M. Pediatric social illness: Toward an etiologic classification. *Pediatrics*, 1977, *60*, 178–185.

National Center for Health Statistics. Final natality statistics, 1978. *Monthly Vital Statistics Report 26* (No. 12), Washington, D.C.: National Center for Health Statistics, U.S. Department of Health and Human Services, 1978.

Pasamanick, B., and Lilienfeld, A. The association of maternal and fetal factors with the development of mental deficiency: II. Relationship to maternal age, birth order, previous reproductive loss, and degree of mental deficiency. *American Journal of Mental Deficiency*, 1956, *60*, 557–569.

Straus, M. A. Measuring intrafamily conflict and violence: the conflict tactics (CT) scales. *Journal of Marriage and the Family*, 1979, *41*, 75–88.

Straus, M. A., Gelles, R. J., and Steinmetz, S. K. *Behind closed doors, violence in the American family.* Garden City, NY: Anchor/Doubleday, 1980.

Teitze, C. Teenage pregnancy: Looking ahead to 1984. *Family Planning Perspectives*, 1978, *10*, 205–207.

Thornberg, H. *Teenage pregnancy: Have they reached epidemic proportions?* Phoenix: Arizona Governor's Council on Children, Youth and Families, 1978.

Turbett, J. P., and O'Toole, R. *Physician's recognition of child abuse.* Paper presented at the meetings of the American Sociological Association, New York, August, 1980.

Weiner, G. The relationship of birth weight and length of gestation to intellectual development at ages 8 to 10 years. *Journal of Pediatrics*, 1970, *76*, 694.

18

THE ECONOMIC IMPACT OF SCHOOL-AGE CHILD REARING

Lorraine V. Klerman

Pregnancy, childbearing, and child rearing among young women who have not yet finished school has many negative consequences. This chapter will examine the literature on these consequences with particular emphasis on the economic ones. It will also review the policies and programs that are attempting to minimize the negative effects of school-age parenthood.

HEALTH AND SOCIAL CONSEQUENCES

School-age or adolescent pregnancy has become a source of professional concern only in the last two decades. Prior to that time attention focused on marital status, rather than age. Out-of-wedlock births were believed to place prospective mother and child at increased health and social risk. It was not until the 1960s and the War on Poverty that interest shifted to the consequences of being or having a school-age mother. Since that time both research and programs have expanded rapidly.

SHORT-TERM EFFECTS FOR MOTHERS AND CHILDREN

Early studies focused on young mothers' medical, educational, marital, fertility, and economic problems during pregnancy and in the first year or two following delivery. They also examined the health of the infant at birth and during the first year of life. Studies by Sarrel (1967), Osofsky (1968), Klerman and Jekel (1973), Presser (1975), Furstenberg (1976), and others documented high rates of maternal morbidity, non-completion of school, illegitimacy and marital instability, inability to control subsequent fertility, and low birth weight or otherwise less than healthy infants. The tendency for young mothers to come from welfare families and to themselves become beneficiaries of the Aid to Families with Dependent Children (AFDC) program was also noted. The Alan Guttmacher Institute (AGI) booklet, *11 Million Teenagers: What Can Be Done About the Epidemic of Adolescent Pregnancies* (1976), brought the facts about this problem to the attention of the American public and to policymakers in a very dramatic way. Its charts were captioned, "Babies of Young Teens Two to Three Times More Likely to Die in First Year," "Maternal Death Risk 60 Percent Higher for Young Teenagers," "Twice as Many Teenage Mothers Drop Out of School," "Teen Mothers Face Greater Risk of Unemployment, Welfare Dependency," "Teen Marriages Two to Three Times More Likely to Break Up," "Young Mothers Will Have 1.3 Times More Children," and so on.

Although some of the earliest studies in this area were funded by the Children's Bureau, the focus of research activity in the federal government soon shifted to the Center for Population Research of the National Institute of Child Health and Human Development (NICHD). Under NICHD's guidance, research interest expanded to explore the consequences of adolescent sexuality beyond the pregnancy and early postpartum period in time, and beyond the mother–infant unit in extent. In addition, since the cause and effect link joining early childbearing and negative outcomes was being challenged, more sophisticated studies of larger samples over longer periods of time were supported. These projects attempted to determine whether maternal age was independently a risk factor, aside from its association with other risk factors such as poverty, low educational attainment, and race.

LONG-TERM CONSEQUENCES FOR CHILDREN

This second generation of studies also focused on the longer-term consequences for the child of being born to an adolescent mother. Baldwin and Cain (1980) reviewed those studies and concluded that the increased risk of low birth weight infants and perinatal mortality was the result of inadequate prenatal care rather than of maternal age. In addition, they stated that the evidence on the impact of young parents on the social-emotional development of their children was inconclusive, suggesting some negative effect as the child reached school age. The problems, however, seemed related to the mothers' educational and economic deficits and marital and household status rather than to age directly. The claim frequently made by clinicians that adolescent mothers were overrepresented among child abusers was challenged as possibly being due not to the age of the mother but the fact that both child abusers and adolescent parents were likely to be from families of low socioeconomic status (Kinard and Klerman, 1980). Studies of the intellectual status of the children of young mothers also were questioned on the same grounds (Kinard and Klerman, 1983), and research in both areas continues (Leventhal, 1981).

ECONOMIC CONSEQUENCES

Three types of economic consequences have been studied: the economic effects of early childbearing on the young mother herself; the impact on her male partner and on the larger family unit; and the costs to society. At the 1975 NICHD/AGI Conference on Consequences of Adolescent Pregnancy and Childbearing, Trussel (1980) clarified the problems involved in studying these issues. Bacon (1974), Presser (1973), and others had already reported higher levels of poverty, unemployment, and welfare dependency for women who began child rearing before age 20. Research was needed, and subsequently conducted, which would separate the effect of early child rearing from preexisting poverty and low aspirations and would reveal the links between the early pregnancy and later economic well being.

CONSEQUENCES FOR YOUNG MOTHERS

Teenage childbearing appears to influence economic status through its direct effect on education, family size, and marital status and the impact of these factors on labor force participation, employment, and wages.

Education. Although it is clear that low scholastic attainment and dropping out of school are not always a result of pregnancy, but rather precede it in many cases, research has shown that women who have their first child before age 18 are less likely to complete high school or to continue their schooling than their peers who delay childbearing. For example, Moore and Waite (1977) using the National Longitudinal Survey of the Education and Labor Market Experience of Young Women, found that "young women who had a first birth at 15 or younger completed about 1.4 fewer years of schooling by age 24 than did their classmates who delayed motherhood until 16 or 17, and 1.9 fewer years than those who waited until 18 to bear their first child." These differences were significant even if race, family background, parental attitudes, and individual motivation were controlled.

Card and Wise (1978), on the basis of TALENT data, investigated the relationship between early childbearing and the probability of receiving a high school or college degree, using samples matched on race, socioeconomic status, academic aptitude, and educational expectation.

They found that approximately one-fifth of young women who experienced a first birth before age 18 received their high school diplomas at age 18 compared to nearly three-quarters of those who delayed childbearing until 18 or 19 and to almost nine-tenths of those who delayed until age 20 or later. By age 29 one-half of the earliest childbearers had achieved this milestone as compared to over four-fifths of the middle age group, and almost all of the oldest age group. There were also differences among the males, although of lesser magnitude. Similar findings were reported for college degrees. Very few of the early mothers and fathers graduated college: 1.6% of mothers and 10.9% of fathers under 18 at birth of first child as compared to 7.9% of mothers and 17.5% of fathers who had their first child at 20–24 and 22.4% of mothers and 29.2% of fathers with no children at 24.

Trussell and Abowd (1979) reported that level of schooling had a significant indirect effect on labor force participation in this population. Mott and Maxwell (1981) showed that young mothers who drop out of school are even less likely than other adolescent mothers to enter the labor force, and, if they do, are more likely to be unemployed. They also noted, however, on the basis of two national surveys, that the percentage of pregnant adolescents remaining in school before and after they give birth had risen in recent years. The proportion of pregnant students stating that they were in high school 5 months before delivery in 1968 was 17% for whites and 43% for blacks compared to 37% for whites and 60% for blacks in 1978. At 9 months postpartum the percentage still enrolled went from 4 to 14% among whites and from 13 to 31% among blacks. McCarthy and Radish (1982) using the June 1980 Current Population Survey also found that the amount of education obtained by women who gave birth before age 20 had increased over time, perhaps as a result of the Title IX legislation or special education programs. They noted, however, that when the mean number of completed years of education was considered, women who gave birth at later ages and childless women had also made gains and that, in fact, younger mothers had not gained more than older ones so that they were still at a disadvantage.

Family Size. Another factor which has been found to have a significant impact on economic well being is family size. Younger mothers are more likely to have large families. Their difficulties with family planning have been described by many authors (Jekel *et al.*, 1979; Cartoof, 1979). Fortunately, the magnitude of the disparity in family size between younger and older mothers is beginning to decline (Millman and Hendershot, 1980; Koenig and Zelnik, 1982), but a discrepancy still remains. Large family size makes it more difficult to seek employment and to hold a job once it is obtained. Also it means that less money is available per individual.

Marital Status. The influence of marital status on economic well being is both direct and indirect and positive and negative. Young mothers who, before or after childbirth, marry men who are employed at reasonable wages usually have higher family incomes than those who do not marry (Furstenberg and Crawford, 1978). Early marriage, however, often leads to large family size and to leaving school, both of which have negative economic impacts. In addition, the high rate of separation, divorce, and widowhood among women who marry as teenagers makes marriage a poor solution to the economic problems of early childbearing (Moore et al., 1978).

In summary, early childbearing affects educational attainment and family size which influence the ability to enter the labor market, the potential to find employment, and the amount of money earned. Early childbearing also may be caused by or result in an early marriage which impacts on welfare dependency and avoidance of poverty through its negative effects on educational attainment and its positive impact on family size (Hofferth and Moore, 1979).

IMPACT ON MALE PARTNER AND FAMILY UNIT

Project TALENT, a large prospective nationwide study of high school boys and girls, was analyzed by Card and Wise (1978) who found that in the years after the date of their expected high school graduation, males who fathered a child at age 18 or under were significantly overrepresented in blue collar jobs and underrepresented in professions, compared to males who had waited until after 18 to become fathers.

Moore and Hofferth (1978) using data from a 1975 AFDC survey showed that approximately half of households receiving AFDC included at least one woman who had borne her first child when she was less than 20. More recent studies by Wertheimer and Moore (1982) and Scheirer et al. (1982) confirm the fact that teenage mothers are overrepresented among welfare families.

PUBLIC SECTOR COSTS

Another group of studies has translated some of these economic consequences for individuals and families into societal costs, or at least public sector costs. The first major project in this area was commissioned by the Select Committee on Population, U.S. House of Representatives. Moore (1978), using the March 1976 Current Population Survey, reported that in 1975, $4.65 billion of the $9.4 billion disbursed by AFDC went to households that contained one or more women who had borne their first children before the age of 20. This figure included only direct AFDC payments to households. It excluded administrative costs, Medicaid, food stamps, and other payments and services linked to poverty. The magnitude of the AFDC figure was due not only to the greater likelihood of teenage, as compared to older mothers, receiving AFDC, but also to the larger size of families started by teenagers.

More recent analyses by Wertheimer and Moore (1982) place the AFDC total at $5 billion or 53% of the AFDC budget. Moreover, public sector costs are not limited to AFDC. AFDC families are automatically eligible for Medicaid. The same researchers estimated that in 1975 Medicaid paid $1.17 billion of medical expenses for teenage mothers, including charges for prenatal care and delivery and $.93 billion of medical expenses for their children. Food stamps are estimated to have added another $1.45 billion. Thus, the dollar expenditures in 1975 for AFDC households in which the mother was a teenager when her first child was born were estimated at over $8 billion, including AFDC.

On the basis of his analyses of the 1977 and 1978 welfare files in Monroe County, New York, Block (1981) challenged the assumption that teenage mothers place a disproportionate burden on welfare rolls. His overall findings were similar to those just described: 57% of public assistance cases were women who conceived their first child as a teenager and these cases absorbed 60% of total public assistance costs. When these data were disaggregated by age, however, an interesting reversal occurred. In 1978 among women under 30 those who conceived their first child as a teenager (TAP's) comprised 80% of the public assistance cases and 83% of the costs, while those who conceived after their teenage years (N-TAP's) comprised 20% of the cases and 17% of the costs. Over age 30, however, TAP's were 36% of cases and 40% of costs and N-TAP's were 64% of the cases and 60% of the costs. The author explained this as follows:

> . . .women who conceived as teenagers enter the welfare system at a more rapid rate than N-TAP's. . .Subsequently TAP's at a family age* of 13 to 16 years, when they are approximately 30 years old, leave the welfare system. N-TAP's on the other hand, enter at a slower rate and tend to remain . . .a reasonable explanation. . .is that women who conceived as teenagers have grown children when they are still young enough to consider other income opportunities. N-TAP's, on the other hand, tend to enter later in the family age cycle, and are therefore older but have younger children, forcing them to stay for longer periods of time. As a group, N-TAP's are older when they are able to consider other income possibilities. (p.84)

*Family age is defined as number of years after birth of first child.

SRI International (1979) approached the same problem from a somewhat different perspective. Instead of looking at current AFDC costs for households with a teenage mother, the investigators projected the total health and welfare costs over a 20-year period for the estimated 442 thousand first births to teenagers in 1979. Separate cost estimates were made for those under 15, 15–17, and 18 and 19, and then these estimates were combined. All costs were calculated in constant 1979 dollars. Medical costs for the combined three cohorts were estimated at $485 million in 1979 and $695 million from 1980 to 1988, for a total of $1.18 billion. Welfare costs, which included AFDC, food stamps, other nutrition programs, subsidized public housing, and social services were estimated at $275 million in 1979, $4.815 million from 1980 to 1988, and $2.02 million from 1989 to 1998 for a total of $7.11 billion. Thus the estimated 20-year total was $8.29 billion or $18,710 per first teenage birth with a range from $23,450 for the youngest group to $14,426 for the oldest.

Walentik (1983) used a similar procedure to estimate the economic costs of teenage pregnancy to the St. Louis Standard Metropolitan Statistical Area (SMSA). He based his figures on the 11,400 teenage pregnancies in that SMSA in 1981, excluding the costs of almost four thousand abortions. The total of $81.8 million included Medicaid-financed medical costs associated with delivery ($5.3 million) and the value of welfare that federal, state, and local governments might expect to pay in welfare payments and other social services by the time the almost six thousand children* reached maturity—$14,041 for the average child.

It should be noted that not all these costs would be prevented if births were postponed until 20 or older. Some percentage of these women would also have required assistance from the AFDC, Medicaid, food stamps, and other programs, even if they delivered their first children at a later date. The estimates of what could be saved by delay of childbearing or other changes will be reviewed later in this chapter.

ATTEMPTS AT SOLUTIONS

Since the early 1960's, the health, education, and welfare fields have responded to the information about the negative consequences of early childbearing by creating programs which attempt to prevent these occurrences. Two approaches to prevention have been tried: programs that seek to delay the birth of the first or subsequent child (primary prevention) and programs that assist the pregnant adolescent, young mother, and significant others.

---

*Walentik estimated that 1600 of the pregnancies ended in miscarriages or stillbirths and that 100 infants died in the first year.

PRIMARY PREVENTION

In the primary prevention area, little was done until the mid-1970's when family planning clinics began, with federal encouragement, to reach out to adolescent clients. The Roe vs. Wade decision of the United States Supreme Court and the use of Medicaid funds made abortions more available for a time, and despite the decrease in public funds and a variety of restrictive state laws, abortions remain an important way to avoid first and subsequent births to young mothers (Klerman, 1981; Vinovskis, 1981). Sex education programs are also on the increase (Orr, 1982) and although the education does not appear to influence whether the teenager engages in sexual activity, it may have a positive effect on contraceptive use (Zelnik and Kim, 1982).

It is generally believed that the stabilization and gradual decline in the adolescent birth rate is attributable largely to the availability of abortions, with family planning programs having limited success in some areas. The St. Paul, Minnesota school program is one of the few that can document significant changes in adolescent births (Edwards et al., 1980).

PROGRAMS FOR PREGNANT WOMEN AND PARENTS

Much attention and money has also gone into programs for reducing the negative consequences for women who become pregnant, complete their pregnancies, and raise their children. Through provision of health, educational, and counseling services, supplemented by welfare and other economic supports, day care, parenting classes, and other services, these programs hope to prevent the detrimental negative economic consequences, as well as the health and social ones described earlier. Evaluations of programs developed in the 1970s indicated that they had a positive effect, at least over a short period of time (Klerman, 1979). The number of comprehensive programs relative to the need, however, is still relatively small (JRB Associates, 1981; Wallace et al., 1982). Also, although favorable cost/benefit ratios have been demonstrated (Hardy and Flagle, undated; JRB Associates, 1981; Zellman, 1981), the per patient costs are high enough to make local communities reluctant to develop such programs. While the federal government has passed two laws* that provide funds for such programs, the level of appropriations has made possible only the support of demonstration programs scattered across the country rather than a network capable of responding to all areas in need. Fortunately, local programs have been able to find other sources of support such as federal Title X (family planning) and Title XX (social services) funds, state health, education,

*Title VI of P.L. 95-626 and Title XX of P.L. 97-35.

and welfare agencies, United Ways, and private foundations (Weatherley et al., 1985).

Two recent reports, however, suggest that even the best of these programs have a limited effect on economic problems. The Urban Institute (Burt et al., 1984) evaluated twenty-three of the projects funded by the federal Office of Adolescent Pregnancy Programs (OAPP). Twelve months after the last child's birth, 61% of the mothers were receiving welfare support and 12 months later that figure was slightly reduced for those who delivered while in the program ("delivered clients"—52%) but increased for those who entered as mothers ("entry mothers"—67%). Thirteen percent of delivered clients were working 20 or more hours per week at 12 months and 21% at 24 months. Among entry mothers the figures were 10% at both 12 and 24 months. Perhaps the program's impact will be experienced later since almost two-thirds of the study population was in or had completed school at 24 months. Only 12% of the delivered clients and 21% of the entry mothers, however, were in or had completed a job training program. The authors comment:

> . . .independence from welfare appears to be an unrealistic goal for clients of these projects at 12 months postpartum. . . It may be that support from welfare enables project clients. . .to continue with their schooling and develop the motivation to avoid subsequent pregnancies. In the long run, completion of schooling will contribute more to self-sufficiency than what is perhaps premature insistence on independence from welfare as an outcome variable. (p. 126)

The authors also attempted to determine the cost-effectiveness of the OAPP programs using a success index. A client was scored as a success if she had a positive outcome at 12 months in two of the three outcome variables: no subsequent pregnancy, not on welfare, and in school or graduated. The eight projects analyzed had success rates ranging from 22 to 92% and the cost of services per successful client ranged from $1823 to $6739.

Project Redirection, a multi-site demonstration project supported by the Ford Foundation, listed among its objectives: acquisition of employability and job skills. This was reflected in the services offered to the participants including individual vocational counseling, group workshops on possible careers, techniques for obtaining and keeping a job, and job placement assistance. About 70% of the enrollees received these services. Yet at 24 months after enrollment only 15% of both the Redirection participants and of a comparison group were employed. A greater percentage of Redirection than comparison subjects, however, had ever been employed and the number of jobs held was higher for Redirection participants. Those teenagers who obtained jobs or employability training through Redirection and who spent more time in the program were more likely to show positive impacts on employment. In both groups approximately three-fifths of the adolescents were receiving their own AFDC grants at 24 months postpartum (Polit et al., 1985; Quint and Riccio, 1985).

ALTERNATIVE APPROACHES

Many believe that school-age pregnancy and its negative consequences can be only minimally affected by programs serving thousands, primarily young women, and costing millions. Significant changes may occur only as a result of modifications of much larger and more expensive federal and state programs and policies, such as AFDC, Medicaid, the minimum wage, and preschool and secondary education. A few examples of the studies in these areas and their implications are reviewed in the following sections.

AFDC. The research of Ellwood and Bane (1984) indicated that the size of the welfare benefit does not influence childbearing decisions, but does modify the living arrangements as well as divorce and separation rates among young single mothers. Using information from the Survey of Income and Education, the Census, and vital statistics, they concluded that in states with low AFDC benefits, young women not living with a husband were likely to live at home, while in high benefit states, such women were likely to live independently. Moreover, among women who married before age 20 and who had a child, divorce and separation rates increased with the size of the AFDC benefit. No one would suggest that young mothers living with abusive or nonsupportive parents or spouses should be forced to stay with them in order to obtain benefits adequate for healthy living, nevertheless, the consequences of high benefit levels should be examined. Several studies have found that living in the parental home increases the probability that a young mother will continue or complete her education and delay a subsequent birth (Furstenberg and Crawford, 1978; Goldstein, 1984). Similarly, marriage is probably the most usual way of obtaining support for a young mother, or any mother. In fact, Bane and Ellwood (1983) have shown that one-third of the women who leave the AFDC rolls do so because of marriage or reconciliation.

It is not only welfare benefits but also the practices of welfare workers at the local level that need to be examined. The availability of benefit levels high enough to permit independent living should not be used to encourage it, when other and possibly more supportive arrangements are possible. Teenage mothers, in common with most adolescents, usually want to leave home and become independent. Convincing the young mother and her family that this may not be the best arrangement may be difficult and time-consuming, and welfare workers without recourse to social services, visiting nurses, or other resources may make the easier decision (Klerman, 1982).

Minimum Wage. Wise (1984) and others have shown that the minimum wage significantly reduces the employment of adolescents, with women, blacks, and those in school particularly impacted. Increasing employment opportunities would be expected to affect the economic consequences of school-age pregnancy in several ways. It might reduce the number of pregnancies and births as young men and women found other outlets for their energies, alternative ways to prove their adult status, and activities which would be hindered by pregnancy and childbearing. In addition, a rise in adolescent and young adult employment might increase the rate of marriage among young people, especially non-whites. The drop in marriage rates in this population has been associated with the decline in employment, suggesting that young mothers realize that marriage to men who cannot support them and their children may have fewer benefits than being on welfare. An increase in marriages to working husbands would reduce welfare dependency among young mothers. The potential for exploitation of young workers and for repercussions throughout the labor market would have to be carefully considered before any changes in the minimum wage were instituted.

Medicaid. The present policies regarding health benefits also contribute to welfare dependency. Medicaid eligibility is usually tied to AFDC and AFDC is only available to women with no male in the household. If they could be assured of free or low-cost medical care for themselves and their children, many women would seek employment and leave the AFDC rolls.

Education. Evidence is mounting of the effectiveness of certain types of compensatory educational programs. The 20-year follow-up of children who participated in a high-quality preschool education has revealed that teenage pregnancy was less prevalent in this group than in a control population (Berrueta-Clement *et al.*, 1984). Another example is the Basic Educational Opportunity Grant program. Recent research by Manski and Wise (1983) has shown that the program has had a substantial positive impact on low-income students' attendance at junior colleges and vocational schools. Moreover, Wise (1984) found that young women who attended such secondary institutions earned approximately 9% more 7 years after high school graduation than did similar women who did not attend.

POTENTIAL IMPACT ON DIFFERENT APPROACHES

A recent study by Moore and Wertheimer (1984) provides new insights into the effectiveness of some of these approaches to reducing the societal costs of early childbearing. Using a microsimulation computer model they attempted to determine, under seven different "scenarios," the public sector costs associated with different patterns of teenage childbearing as well as the effects of those scenarios on related sociodemographic factors.

The first or baseline analysis showed what might be expected if trends as measured in 1980 were continued unchanged through 1990. Under this assumption teenage mothers would continue "to have lower educational attainment, lower participation in the work force, lower personal and family earnings, larger families and greater welfare dependency than women who bear their children at older ages." Moreover, 79% of 20- to 24-year-old women and 52% of 25- to 29-year-old women would have had their first birth before age 20; and the costs of three transfer programs, AFDC, Medicaid, and food stamps, would be $5.83 billion for AFDC families of women aged 20–29.

The greatest decrease in expenditures for these three programs, to $4.40 billion, would occur with a 50% reduction in fertility under age 20. Reductions were also predicted if average family size of teenage childbearers was reduced so that it was not greater than that of women who gave birth at age 20 or later ($4.86 billion); if births to unmarried women under age 18 were eliminated ($4.93 billion); if the probability of marriage among unmarried mothers was raised by one-half the difference between 100% and the marriage probability for all women in each age, race, and parity subgroup ($5.06 billion); if there was a 50% reduction in the age- and race-specific probabilities of birth among married and unmarried women under age 18 ($5.11 billion); and if the annual probability of dropping out of school was no higher for teenage mothers than for other teenagers of the same age, race, and sex ($5.61 billion).

The minor impact of the educational scenario is disappointing since so much current effort is directed at keeping pregnant students and young mothers in school. Yet reduction of dropouts did not affect family size, percentage of women married, women's labor force participation, personal earnings, or family earnings. The authors believe this is because labor participation rates, hours worked, and wage rates are lower for women than for men.

These analyses suggest that the best approach to reducing public sector costs is the prevention of first pregnancies among teenagers. Failing this, the most effective strategy given the birth of one child is the prevention of subsequent births. These findings should not be interpreted to suggest that educational interventions are unimportant. It is only their impact on economic consequences, and particularly public sector costs which is low in these analyses. Other research, however, suggests that increased education is positively associated with better health, more appropriate health-seeking behavior, and better child-rearing practices, to name just a few of its benefits.

CONCLUSIONS

The economic impact of school-age childbearing is obviously enormous. The influence of pregnancy and parenthood on the education, marital status, or family size of the young parents and their eventual effect on private economic well being and public sector costs is cause for grave concern. Studies which suggest that this pattern is transmitted to children make the problem even more significant. Those who review the situation are almost unanimous in recommending more attention to the prevention of pregnancy or birth as the most effective ways to reduce the magnitude of the problem. Recently McGee (1982), in a study of services for teenage parents, urged the improvement of measures to help teenage parents delay first births including:

- Continue to investigate incentives for pregnancy prevention.
- Experiment with interventions that affect the social context in which young people make decisions.
- The time around the onset of puberty is an especially vulnerable period for young people. Consider what junior high schools, youth organizations, and parents might offer to help teenagers make career choices, make appropriate decisions about sex, and delay parenthood until they are prepared for responsibilities. Develop appealing and, where appropriate, learn-by-doing approaches. Be sure employment preparation receives appropriate stress for girls and pregnancy prevention for boys.
- Experiment with family-planning services that are accessible, low-cost, confidential, and individualized with careful client monitoring. Provide aggressive outreach where appropriate.
- Support public policies that encourage teens to postpone parenthood, for example: promote and strengthen youth employment assistance, and encourage small-scale experiments in welfare policy to determine if changes in eligibility requirements and in procedures lead to healthier patterns of service use.

Moore and Burt (1982) have a similar list:

- Increase the availability, accessibility, and privacy of subsidized contraceptive services.
- Study the impact of parental involvement and notification on contraceptive use and sexual activity. Do not mandate parental notification until research verifies that notification has positive consequences and does not entail serious negative consequences. Study how best to involve families and males in making decisions about contraceptive use and in encouraging regular, effective use.
- Develop new methods of contraception appropriate to teenagers' irregular patterns of sexual activity. Study the impact of method choice on continuation. Develop better male-oriented methods and encourage use of condoms. Encourage early and consistent use of chosen methods.

- Sponsor research on the effect of low educational and occupational opportunities on teenagers' motivation to postpone sexual activity and/ or practice effective contraception if they become sexually active.
- Use federal regulations and enforcement powers maximally to combat racial and sexual discrimination and to provide real educational and labor market opportunities for young people.
- Leave the decision of how to resolve a pregnancy up to the pregnant teenager but encourage exploratory research on the impact of each option on the teenage parents, the baby, and their families.

Both books, as well as many previous publications, perceive the provision of services to those already pregnant and carrying to term and to young parents as less effective, although obviously needed. McGee stresses improved recruitment of teenage parents in need of services, better organization of services, and experimentation with and evaluation of innovative approaches. Moore and Burt list specific recommendations in the areas of health, family planning, child care, school, work, welfare, family involvement, and child support.

The economic impact of school-age parenthood, and particularly the public sector costs, speak only to a small portion of the hardships resulting from early childbearing. The social costs to the young mother, her male partner, their child or children, and their families are probably more significant, though less quantifiable. Continued attention to the financial aspects is defensible, however, because it focuses public attention on a social problem which many believe could be markedly reduced if this society showed more concern for its youth.

REFERENCES

Alan Guttmacher Institute. *11 Million teenagers - What can be done about the epidemic of adolescent pregnancies in the United States.* New York: Planned Parenthood Federation of America, Inc., 1976.

Bacon, L. Early motherhood, accelerated role transition, and social pathologies. *Social Forces*, 1974, 52, 333–341.

Baldwin, W., and Cain, V. S. The children of teenage parents. *Family Planning Perspectives*, 1980, 12, 34–43.

Bane, M. J., and Ellwood, D. T. *The dynamics of dependence: The routes to self-sufficiency.* Cambridge, MA: Urban Systems Research and Engineering, Inc., June, 1983.

Berrueta-Clement, J. R., Schweinhart, L. J., Barnett, W. S., Epstein, A. S., and Weikart, D. P. *Changed lives. The effects of the Perry Preschool Program on youths through age 19.* Yipsilanti, MI: The High/Scope Press, 1984.

Block, A. H. *Welfare costs at the local level.* Final report, research on the societal consequences of adolescent childbearing. Washington, D.C.: Bokonon Systems, Inc., October 1981.

Burt, M. R., Kimmich, M. H., Goldmuntz, J., and Sonenstein, F. L. *Helping pregnant adolescents: Outcomes and costs of service delivery.* Final report on the evaluation of adolescent pregnancy programs. Washington, D.C.: The Urban Institute, February 1984.

Card, J. J., and Wise, L. L. Teenage mothers and teenage fathers: The impact of early childbearing on the parents' personal and professional lives. *Family Planning Perspectives,* 1978, *10,* 199–205.

Cartoof, V. G. Postpartum services for adolescent mothers: Part 2. *Child Welfare,* 1979, *18,* 673-680.

Edwards, L. F., Steinman, M. E., Arnold, K. A., and Hakanson, E. Y. Adolescent pregnancy prevention services in high school clinics. *Family Planning Perspectives,* 1980, *12,* 6–14.

Ellwood, D. T., and Bane, M. J. *The impact of AFDC on family structure and living arrangements.* Cambridge, MA: Harvard University, March, 1984.

Furstenberg, F. F., Jr. *Unplanned parenthood—The social consequences of teenage childbearing.* New York: The Free Press, 1976.

Furstenberg, F. F., and Crawford, A. G. Family support: Helping teenage mothers to cope. *Family Planning Perspectives,* 1978, *10,* 322–333.

Goldstein, N. *Unmarried teenage childbearing.* Cambridge, MA: Harvard University, April 1984. (student paper)

Hardy, J. B., and Flagle, C. D. *Results, costs and assessment of the investment opportunity.* Baltimore, MD: The Johns Hopkins Adolescent Program. (Duplicated-undated).

Hofferth, S. L., and Moore, K. A. Early childbearing and later economic well-being. *American Sociological Review,* 1979, *44,* 784–815.

Jekel, J. F., Tyler, N. C., and Klerman, L. V. Induced abortion and sterilization among women who became mothers as adolescents. *American Journal of Public Health,* 1979, *67,* 621–625.

JRB Associates, Inc. *Final report on national study of teenage pregnancy.* McLean, VA, 1981.

Kinard, E. M., and Klerman, L. V. Early parenting and child abuse: Are they related? *American Journal of Orthopsychiatry,* 1980, *50,* 481–488.

Kinard, E. M., and Klerman, L. V. Effects of early parenthood on the cognitive development of children. *In* E. R. McAnarney (Ed.), *Premature adolescent pregnancy and parenthood.* New York: Grune and Stratton, 1983.

Klerman, L. V. Adolescent mothers and their children: Another population that requires family care. *Home Health Care Services Quarterly,* 1982, *3,* 111–128.

Klerman, L. V. Evaluating service programs for school-age parents: Design problems. *Evaluation and the Health Professions,* 1979, *2,* 55–70.

Klerman, L. V. Programs for pregnant adolescents and young parents: Their development and assessment. *In* K. C. Scott, T. Field, and E. Robertson (Eds.), *Teenage parents and their offspring.* New York: Grune and Stratton, 1981.

Klerman, L. V., and Jekel, J. F. *School-age mothers. Problems, programs and policy.* Hamden, CT: Linnett Press, Inc., 1973.

Koenig, M. A., and Zelnik, M. The risk of premarital first pregnancy among metropolitan-area teenagers: 1976 and 1979. *Family Planning Perspectives,* 1982, *14,* 239–247.

Leventhal, J. M. Risk factors for child abuse: Methodologic standards in case-control studies. *Pediatrics,* 1981, *68,* 684–690.

McCarthy, J., and Radish, E. S. Education and childbearing among teenagers. *Family Planning Perspectives,* 1982, *14,* 154–155.

McGee, E. A. *Too little, too late: Service for teenage parents.* New York: Ford Foundation, 1982.

Manski, C., and Wise, D. A. *Going to college in America.* Cambridge, MA: Harvard University Press, 1983.

Millman, S., and Hendershot, G. Early fertility. *Family Planning Perspectives*, 1980, *12*, 139–149.

Moore, K. A. Teenage childbirth and welfare dependency. *Family Planning Perspectives*, 1978, *10*, 233–235.

Moore, K. A., and Burt, M. R. *Private crisis, public cost: Policy perspectives on teenage childbearing*. Washington, DC: The Urban Institute Press, 1982.

Moore, K. A., and Hofferth, S. L. *The consequences of age at first childbirth: Female-headed families and welfare recipiency*. Washington, DC: The Urban Institute, 1978.

Moore, K. A., and Waite, L. J. Early childbearing and educational attainment. *Family Planning Perspectives*, 1977, *9*, 110–114.

Moore, K. A., Waite, L. J., Hofferth, S. L., and Caldwell, S. B. *The consequences of age at first childbirth: Marriage, separation and divorce*. Washington, DC: The Urban Institute, July, 1978 (working paper).

Moore, K. A., and Wertheimer, R. Teenage childbearing and welfare: Preventive and ameliorative strategies. *Family Planning Perspectives*, 1984, *16*, 285–289.

Mott, F., and Maxwell, N. L. School-age mothers: 1968 and 1979. *Family Planning Perspectives*, 1981, *13*, 287–292.

Orr, M. T. Sex education and contraception education in U. S. public high schools. *Family Planning Perspectives*, 1982, *14*, 304–313.

Osofsky, H. J. *The pregnant teenager*. Springfield, IL: Charles C. Thomas, Publisher, 1968.

Polit, D. F., Kahn, J. R., and Stevens, D. W. *Final impacts from Project Redirection: A program for pregnant and parenting teens*. New York: Manpower Demonstration Research Corporation, 1985.

Presser, H. B. Cited in *11 Million teenagers - What can be done about the epidemic of adolescent pregnancies in the United States*. New York: Planned Parenthood Federation of America, Inc., 1976.

Presser, H. B. *Social consequences of teenage childbearing*. Revision of a paper presented at the Conference on the Consequences of Adolescent Pregnancy and Childbearing, October 29–30, 1975.

Quint, J. C., and Riccio, J. A. *The challenge of serving pregnant and parenting teens: Lessons from Project Redirection*. New York: Manpower Demonstration Research Corporation, 1985.

Sarrel, P. M. The university hospital and the teenage unwed mother. *American Journal of Public Health*, 1967, *57*, 308–13.

Scheirer, M. A., Dial, T. H., and White, A. D. *The relationships of mother's age at first birth to public assistance costs*. Final report to NICHD under Contract No. N01-HD-02837, March, 1982.

SRI International. *An analysis of government expenditures consequent on teenage childbirth*. New York: Population Resource Center, 1979.

Trussell, T. J. Economic consequences of teenage childbearing. *In* C. S. Chilman (Ed.), *Adolescent pregnancy and childbearing: Findings from research*. Washington, D.C.: U. S. Government Printing Office, 1980.

Trussell, J., and Abowd, J. *Teenage mothers, labor force participation and wage rates*. Paper presented at the Annual Meeting of the Population Association of America, Philadelphia, PA, April, 1979.

Vinovskis, M. A. An "epidemic" of adolescent pregnancy? Some historical considerations. *Journal of Family History*, 1981, 205–230.

Walentik, D. S. *Teenage pregnancy: Economic costs to the St. Louis community*. June 1983.

Wallace, H. W., Weeks, J., and Medina, A. Services for and needs of pregnant teenagers in large cities of the United States, 1979–80. *Public Health Reports*, 1982, *97*, 583–588.

Weatherley, R. A., Perlman, S. B., Levine, M., and Klerman, L. V. Patchwork programs: Comprehensive services for pregnant and parenting adolescents. Seattle, WA: Center for Social Welfare Research, School of Social Work, University of Washington, 1985.

Wertheimer, R. F., and Moore, K. A. *Teenage childbearing: Public sector costs.* Washington, D.C.: The Urban Institute, December 1982.

Wise, D. A. *The effect of government programs on youth.* Cambridge, MA: Harvard University, March 1984.

Zellman, G. L. *The response of the schools to teenage pregnancy and parenthood.* Santa Monica, CA: The Rand Corporation, 1981.

Zelnik, M., and Kim, Y. J. Sex education and its association with teenage sexual activity, pregnancy and contraceptive use. *Family Planning Perspectives*, 1982, *14*, 117–126.

19

A DEVELOPMENTAL PERSPECTIVE ON SCHOOL-AGE PARENTHOOD*

Charles M. Super

School-age pregnancy is ordinarily encountered through individuals and groups of individuals. The clinician sees a 15-year-old adolescent going into labor dangerously early; a toddler injured in a fit of anger by his 17-year-old mother; an 18-year-old mother uncooperative in the psychological evaluation of her 3-year-old child, referred by a preschool program for emotional disturbance. As Furstenberg (1980a) has noted, the researcher, too, looks at the problems of individuals. The epidemiologist finds the category "mother's age 12 to 16 years" to be an index of risk for low birth weight. The policy researcher identifies age at first birth as an important element in a causal chain that leads to poverty.

For reasons of phenomenology and epistemology, the target of inquiry has almost always been the pregnant teenager: Who is she and what risks are associated with her condition? The perspectives mentioned above are legitimate ways of knowing the world, but as strategies of scientific inquiry they risk conferring on "school-age pregnancy" a reality which it may not fully deserve. What is unique about the school-age mother, we have asked, that might cause the increased risks? By and large, scientific research aimed at identifying special characteristics of the very young mother has yielded few results commensurate with the phenomena to be explained. Instead, it is argued here, the developmental consequences of school-age pregnancy and motherhood are socially constructed. They are the result of social and

*Preparation of this chapter was supported in part by the Carnegie Corporation of New York. All statements made and opinions expressed are the sole responsibility of the author.

interpersonal forces no different in kind from those operating for more mature women, different only in their frequency and configuration. Those differences reflect, in turn, the circumstances in which school-age pregnancy occurs and in which its sequelae are played out. Therefore, there is no special, particular relationship of school-age pregnancy to the development of offspring. The relationships that exist are those constructed by the people, the community, and the society involved.

TEENAGE PREGNANCY AND THE PREGNANT TEENAGER

There appears to be two kinds of forces leading to the perception of school-age pregnancy and its consequences as features of individuals. One, referred to above, is the way it is encountered in professional institutions. The association of school-age pregnancy with a variety of poor outcomes is strong and compelling (e.g., Battaglia et al., 1963), and the clinical goal of elaborating the phenomenon as it is presented follows naturally. In addition, from the perspective of both service providers and policymakers, the most immediate locus of intervention for the purpose of reducing the incidence of this high-risk condition is the reproductive behavior of individuals. If school-age pregnancy is a bad risk, one appropriate response is to work to reduce it. The patterns of adolescent sexual behavior and contraceptive use thus gain research priority, and moral considerations raised by some observers reinforce this avenue of inquiry and intervention.

The epistemology of social and behavioral research has been a second factor in shaping a categorical, individually based approach to school-age pregnancy. In general, the social and behavioral sciences have divided their labors into two independent tasks (Super and Harkness, 1981). One, which is the basis of most clinical and psychological endeavor, takes the individual as the unit of analysis. An understanding of the workings of the individual will explain the behaviors observed. Individual patterns may be seen to derive from personality, developmental regularities, genetic variations, or other sources, but all such theories are "nativist" (Harkness, 1980) in the sense that the origin of individual characteristics is seen to reside in the person. To be sure, the environment may impinge on the individual, but it does so as a discrete force, not in interaction with the individual, or with a pattern of its own.

The second task of knowledge, realized by mainstream sociology and cultural anthropology, focuses on characteristics and structure of the humanly constructed environment. Elemental units of analysis are institutions, roles, and features of social organization. When people appear in this framework, they are the relatively passive and undifferentiated exemplars of externally defined categories: white males, socioemotional leaders, blue-collar workers, or pregnant teenagers.

There are traditions within each of the two camps that have tried to draw more clearly the connections between society and individual. In the the past half-century, however, the individual and societal approaches have developed increasingly separate networks for exchanging information, and divergent techniques for establishing facts and constructing theories. Members of the relevant disciplines also find the application of their perspectives at different places in our society, and they share important beliefs about how the world works with other professions they come in most contact with. Thus sociologists are most likely to engage the world outside academics in the realm of policy. They talk with lawyers, administrators of social institutions, and those who deal with school-age pregnancy at the level of groups and institutions. Psychologists, for their part, are more likely to be or to confer with clinicians, mental health and social service workers who see in their clinical practice individual young mothers and their children. A related division can be found in the health sciences, where epidemiologists and policy-oriented physicians work with a large-scale perspective on services to school-age mothers, while obstetricians and pediatricians focus their concern on the clinical manifestations of the risks of school-age pregnancy.

A tabulation of research published in the years 1979–1982 reflects this pair of clinical and problem-oriented policy concerns. The majority of publications (nearly 70%) focused on sexual activity and contraception, with an additional 25% being medical studies on the immediate complications and outcomes. Empirical research on long-term social, developmental, or economic outcome of school-age pregnancy constituted the small remainder (5%), and of those only a few sought clues to the developmental processes involved.

THE DEVELOPMENT OF SCHOOL-AGE PARENTS AND THEIR CHILDREN

In order to understand why school-age pregnancy is associated with the pattern of outcomes that have been found (or more precisely the *patterns* of outcome) we need to examine the developmentally relevant characteristics of the environment that is created for and by the young mother and child. The category of "school-age mother" is a social construct and the suggestion here is that to move further in our understanding of that phenomenon requires something beyond collecting more information about who falls into that category and the associated outcomes. In the next decade we should work for a functional analysis of the developmental niche for school-age mothers and their children.

Such an analysis will help us to see why the category has the correlates it does and, in turn, will suggest ways to interrupt the developmental sequences that are undesirable.

One indication of the need for breaking down the category of school-age pregnancy into its functional features —"unwrapping the package" in Whiting's (1976) phrase — can be found in the results of Broman's (1981) large-scale analysis of the long-term outcome for children of young mothers. Using the data base collected by the Collaborative Perinatal Project of the National Institute of Neurological Disorders and Stroke, she identified 23,901 births to women between the ages of 12 to 29, and was able to subdivide the sample by race and three levels of socioeconomic status (SES), as well as three age groups of the mother. A variety of measures on the children up to the age of 7 years was available, including birth weight, psychomotor performance in infancy, IQ, and physical growth. It is difficult, however, to draw from the results a sound generalization about the children of school-age mothers, for more than one-half of the effects of maternal age on child outcome were found to depend on the SES and/or race of the mother. For example, did mothers aged 12–16 years at first birth have children who, at age seven, scored below children of older mothers on a standard IQ test? For some combinations of race and SES the answer is "yes," for others "no." School-age motherhood, in short, is not by itself a straightforward influence on children.

The search for developmental processes can begin at the beginning. Indeed, some of the most provocative reports of the past few years have indicated correlates of very young motherhood in the behavior of newborns. Thompson et al. (1979), for example, administered the Brazelton Neonatal Assessment Scales to 30 newborns of mothers under 18 years of age and to a comparable group of newborns of older mothers. The infants of the adolescent mothers were significantly less responsive to social interaction, less alert, and less skillful in integrated motor behaviors. Such reports are of particular significance in light of recent advances in understanding infants as elicitors of parental behavior, and the related observation that developmental disorder is best understood as a process of continuing transaction between child and environment (Sameroff and Chandler, 1975). It seems reasonable to hypothesize, as others have done, that some of the long-term effects of school-age motherhood may derive, in part, from such initial dispositions in their babies and the kinds of interactions that follow.

Research into prenatal influences on infant behavior suggests several mechanisms through which the environment of school-age mothers might affect the process of development in their babies-to-be. Some samples of school-age mothers have been reported to show excessive rates of smoking and alcohol use. Damaging effects of the latter have been amply documented in research on Fetal Alcohol Syndrome (Majewski, 1981), a condition that is characterized by growth retardation, physical anomaly, and behavioral dysfunctions, such as, irritability and poor habituation in infancy. Intrauterine exposure to alcohol and nicotine have both been related to problems in attentional performance among preschool children (Streissguth *et al.*, 1984).

One need not look so far as specific teratogenic agents, however, to find routes for socially constructed effects on the infants of school-age mothers. Reviews of the obstetric literature (e.g., Menken, 1980; Robertson, 1981) conclude that when race, socioeconomic factors, and prenatal care are controlled, the problems most likely to occur differentially in adolescent pregnancies are hypertension and prolonged labor. Both of these are known to vary in response to social and psychological conditions.

Rosengren (1961) has demonstrated that, among mature women, physician–patient difference in attitude toward pregnancy and delivery (specifically, the perception of pregnancy as a "natural life event" vs. an illness-like condition) is associated with an increase in duration of active labor from 6 to 13 hours. Nuckolls *et al.* (1972) used a broader index of stress, derived from the work of Holmes and Rahe (1967), and found that women with low psychosocial resources who experience high life stress have a significantly higher rate of complications during delivery (including hypertension, premature rupture of membranes, and prolonged labor), as well as poorer outcome (indexed by Apgar scores and birth weight). In the presence of substantial personal and social resources, stress did not produce such effects. There are, in addition, several studies that indicate a relationship between physiological correlates of stress (especially elevated blood pressure) during pregnancy, on the one hand, and increased irritability, decreased alertness, and lower social responsiveness of the offspring, on the other (e.g., Chisholm *et al.*, 1978; Hall, 1977; Richards, 1979; Woodson *et al.*, 1979).

Pregnant adolescents, on average, undergo more psychosocial stress than their nonpregnant peers, even when pregnancy itself is excluded from the standard life events scale (Coddington, 1979). The stressors include not only difficult negotiations with parents and the father but also superficially unrelated events such as deaths in the family. The adolescent may delay prenatal care to hide the pregnancy (Bernstein and Sauber, 1960, cited in Robertson, 1981), an approach to health care that is not likely to be beneficial. In addition, many adolescents receive their reproductive care from an obstetrician who holds negative attitudes toward teenage pregnancy (Davidson, 1981).

In summary, many of the significant obstetric and neonatal risks that have been found to be excessive in school-age mothers have also been shown, in samples of mature women, to result in part from social and interpersonal factors, as well as from socially influenced habits of drinking and smoking. There is reason to suspect that many school-age mothers experience high stress, low social support, and detrimental health-related behaviors. It does not follow that such factors must account for the pattern of dysfunction in the infants of very young mothers, but it seems a plausible hypothesis.

In the months and years that follow birth, the environments of children of school-age mothers may continue to diverge from those of children of older mothers. There are a number of good reports of how this looks from the outside, from the point of view of the demographer and sociologist. In Furstenberg's (1980b) study, for example, the preschooler who was born to an adolescent mother is about twice as likely to live separated from his or her father than is a preschooler of an older mother. We also know, for several samples, the differential cumulative probability of additional pregnancy, total years of additional schooling, and other demographic facts. What we know little of is how such facts are reflected in dimensions of functional significance for the child, that is, how they join together to form the developmental niche (Harkness and Super, 1983; Super and Harkness, 1981). Are there regular differences in the physical and social setting of infancy? Are the customary methods of care and discipline the same? Do the beliefs, values, and goals of the caretakers vary systematically? Most significantly, how is the *sequence* of niches affected by differences in interbirth interval, final family size, maternal educational attainment, and so forth?

Because environments have their own structure and rules of development it is probably not the case that we are faced with an undifferentiated array of niches. The subcultural variation in parental disapproval of teenage pregnancy that Held (1981) reports, for example, is surely related to prenatal stress, the social setting for infancy, the customs of daily care, and subcultural values about family life, to list only a few relevant issues. The theoretical challenge in understanding the developmental consequences of school-age motherhood lies in identifying configurations of the environment that are related to developmental risk, and the reward of such knowledge will be a more sound basis for moderating the human damage.

CONCLUSIONS

Most research to date on the consequences of school-age pregnancy has focused on medical and economic outcomes, with the technical goal, in the best reports, of removing the influence of social class, race, and other "extraneous" factors. What are the *unique* risks, was the question, to mother and offspring of reproduction so early in the life course? The answer, by and large, has been elusive and varying from one study to another. The proposal made here is that most and possibly all developmental consequences of school-age pregnancy are socially constructed; they are the result of social and interpersonal forces no different in kind from those operating for more mature women.

It follows from this argument that when the package of school-age pregnancy is unwrapped, there will be little, if anything, inside. What is unique about school-age motherhood in modern America is, in fact, the wrapping we provide. There are probably several different types of wrapping, as Hamburg (Chapter 7, this volume) also suggests, that is, several different configurations of the developmental niche. A fruitful next step in understanding and ameliorating the consequences of school-age pregnancy may be to reverse the strategy of isolating it from extraneous influences, and to examine instead in detail what the configurations of those influences are and how they form a sequence of environments for the developing mother and child.

REFERENCES

Battaglia, F. C., Frazier, T. M., and Hellegers, A. E. Obstetric and pediatric complications of juvenile pregnancy. *Pediatrics*, 1962, *32*, 902–910.

Broman, S. H. (1981). Longterm development of children born to teenagers. In K. G. Scott, T. Field, and E. Robertson (Eds.), *Teenage parents and their offspring*. New York: Grune and Stratton, 1981, pp. 195–224.

Chisholm, J. S., Woodson, R. H., and da Costa, E. Maternal blood pressure in pregnancy and newborn irritability. *Early Human Development*, 1978, *2(2)*, 171–178.

Coddington, R. D. Life events associated with adolescent pregnancies. *Journal of Clinical Psychiatry*, 1979, *40*, 180–185.

Davidson, E. C. An analysis of adolescent health care and the role of the obstetrician-gynecologist. *American Journal of Obstetrics and Gynecology*, 1981, *139(7)*, 845–854.

Furstenberg, F. Burdens and benefits: The impact of early childbearing on the family. *Journal of Social Issues*, 1980, *36(1)*, 64–86. (a)

Furstenberg, F. The social consequences of teenage parenthood. In C. S. Chilman (Ed.), *Adolescent pregnancy and childbearing: Findings from research*. NIH Publication No. 81-2077, 1980, pp. 267–308.

Hall, F. Prenatal events and later infant behavior. *Journal of Psychosomatic Research*, 1977, *21*, 253–257.

Harkness, S. The cultural context of child development. In C. M. Super and S. Harkness (Eds.), Anthropological perspectives on child development, *New Directions for Child Development*, 1980, *8*, 7–14.

Harkness, S., and Super, C. M. The cultural construction of child development: A framework for the socialization of affect. *Ethos*, 1983, *11*, 221–232.

Held, L. Self-esteem and social networks of the young pregnant teenager. *Adolescence*, 1981, *16(64)*, 905–912.

Holmes, T. M., and Rahe, R. M. The social readjustment rating scale. *Journal of Psychosomatic Research*, 1967, *11*, 213–218.

Majewski, F. Alcohol embryopathy: Some facts and speculations about pathogenesis. *Neurobehavioral Toxicology and Teratology*, 1981, *3*, 129–144.

Menken, J. The health and demographic consequences of adolescent pregnancy and childbearing. In C. S. Chilman (Ed.), Adolescent pregnancy and
childbearing: Findings from research. NIH Publication No. 81-2077, 1980, pp.
177–206.
Nuckolls, K. B., Cassel, J., and Kaplan, B. Psychosocial assets, life crisis and
the prognosis of pregnancy. American Journal of Epidemiology, 1972, 95,
431–441.
Richards, M. P. M. Conception, pregnancy and birth—a perspective from developmental psychology. In L. Carenza and L. Zichella (Eds.), Emotion and
reproduction: Proceedings of the Serono conference (Vol. 20). New York: Academic Press, 1979.
Robertson, E. G. (1981). Adolescence, physiological maturity, and obstetric
outcome. In K. G. Scott, T. Field, and E. Robertson (Eds.), Teenage parents
and their offspring. New York: Grune and Stratton, pp. 91–101.
Rosengren, W. R. Some social psychological aspects of delivery room difficulties. Journal of Nervous and Mental Disease, 1961, 132, 515–521.
Sameroff, A. J., and Chandler, M. Reproductive risk and the continuum of
caretaking casualty. In F. A. Horowitz, M. Hetherington, S. Scarr-Salapatek,
and G. Siegal (Eds.), Review of child development research (Vol. 4). Chicago:
University of Chicago Press, 1975, pp. 187–244.
Streissguth, A. P., Martin, D. C., Barr, H. M., Sandman, B. M., Kirchner, G.
L. and Darby, B. L. Intrauterine alcohol and nicotine exposure: Attention
and reaction time in 4-year-old children. Developmental Psychology, 1984,
20(4), 533–541.
Super, C. M., and Harkness, S. Figure, ground, and gestalt: The cultural context
of the active individual. In R. M. Lerner and N. A. Busch-Rossnagel (Eds.),
Individuals as producers of their development: A life-span perspective. New
York: Academic Press, 1981, pp. 69–86.
Thompson, R. J., Cappleman, M. W., and Zeitschel, K. A. Neonatal behavior
of infants of adolescent mothers. Developmental Medicine and Child Neu-
rology, 1979, 21, 474–482.
Whiting, B. B. The problem of the packaged variable. In K. F. Riegel and J.
A. Meacham (Eds.), The developing individual in a changing world (Vol.
1). The Hague: Mouton, 1976.
Woodson, R. H., Blurton Jones, N. G., da Costa Woodson E., Pollack, S., and
Evans, M. Fetal mediators of the relationship between increased pregnancy
and labour blood pressure and newborn irritability. Early Human Development, 1979. 3, 127–139.

INDEX

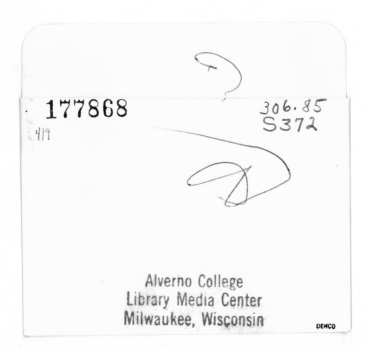